Bionanotechnology

Connecting theory with real-life applications, this is the first textbook to equip students with a comprehensive knowledge of all the key concepts in bionanotechnology. By bridging the interdisciplinary gap from which bionanotechnology emerged, it provides a systematic introduction to the subject, accessible to students from a wide variety of backgrounds. Topics range from nanomaterial preparation, properties and biofunctionalisation, and analytical methods used in bionanotechnology, to bioinspired and DNA nanotechnology, and applications in biosensing, medicine and tissue engineering. Throughout the book, features such as 'Back to Basics' and 'Research Report' boxes enable students to build a strong theoretical knowledge and to link this to practical applications and up-to-date research. With over 200 detailed, full-colour illustrations and more than 100 end-of-chapter problems, this is an essential guide to bionanotechnology for any student or researcher exploring this exciting, fast-developing and interdisciplinary field.

LJILJANA FRUK is a reader in BioNano Engineering in the Department of Chemical Engineering and Biotechnology, University of Cambridge. She has taught bionanotechnology in Germany and the UK, both at undergraduate and postgraduate level. Her group works on the design of enzyme-like catalysts, hybrid biopolymers for applications in sensing and optoelectronics, as well as drug nanocarriers for senescent cells and hard-to-treat cancers. A fellow of the Royal Society of Chemistry and council member of the Cambridge Philosophical Society, Dr Fruk is also a science populariser and co-editor of the book *Molecular Aesthetics* (with Peter Weibel, 2013).

ANTONINA KERBS is a scientific team coordinator at Miltenyi Biotec, Germany. Before joining Miltenyi in 2019, she was a postdoctoral researcher in Dr Fruk's group in the Department of Chemical Engineering and Biotechnology, University of Cambridge, where she worked on the preparation and biofunctionalisation of nanoparticles, and the designing of biosensing devices.

Bionanotechnology

Concepts and Applications

Ljiljana Fruk
University of Cambridge

Antonina Kerbs
Miltenyi Biotec, Germany

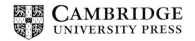

CAMBRIDGE
UNIVERSITY PRESS

CAMBRIDGE
UNIVERSITY PRESS

University Printing House, Cambridge CB2 8BS, United Kingdom

One Liberty Plaza, 20th Floor, New York, NY 10006, USA

477 Williamstown Road, Port Melbourne, VIC 3207, Australia

314–321, 3rd Floor, Plot 3, Splendor Forum, Jasola District Centre, New Delhi – 110025, India

79 Anson Road, #06–04/06, Singapore 079906

Cambridge University Press is part of the University of Cambridge.

It furthers the University's mission by disseminating knowledge in the pursuit of education, learning and research at the highest international levels of excellence.

www.cambridge.org
Information on this title: www.cambridge.org/9781108429054
DOI: 10.1017/9781108690102

First published 2021

Printed in Singapore by Markono Print Media Pte Ltd

A catalogue record for this publication is available from the British Library.

ISBN 978-1-108-42905-4 Hardback
ISBN 978-1-108-45290-8 Paperback

Additional resources for this publication at www.cambridge.org/bionanotechnology

Contents

Preface

Bionanotechnology is a field at the intersection of nanotechnology and biology. It employs *nanomaterials* and *biomolecules* (and increasingly also whole organisms) to design new functional materials and devices. At the same time, it also learns from biological systems and turns what evolution has perfected over the past millennia into solutions we can apply to resolve some of the challenges we are facing now.

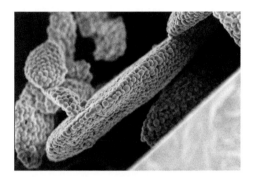

Figure P.1

Transmission electron microscopy image of spheric polydopamine nanoparticles. Images obtained by Leander Crocker and Maxime Crabe (Fruk group), University of Cambridge.

In simple terms, bionanotechnology is a bit of everything: there is lots of *chemistry* (synthesis and modification of nanomaterials), *physics* (rules of the nanoworld and principles of analytical methods), *biology* (all those proteins and microorganisms), *medicine* (drug delivery, diagnostics) and *engineering* (device and material design). However, bionanotechnology is not just a mix-and-match collection of concepts, but it has, over the past decades, continuously grown into a field with a clear identity and goals.

This textbook aims to combine the concepts and bridge the gaps between different disciplines from which bionanotechnology emerged, and give a more systematic view of the basics and application across the field. Knowing that there will be students and researchers from a wide range of disciplines reading the book, we often give broad description of a particular principle, and provide literature sources for those who want to learn more. The book begins with the an overview of basic physics and chemistry behind nanomaterial engineering, then moves onto the composition of the cell and scales of biomolecules, and continues with chapters on topics such as DNA nanotechnology, nanomaterial biofunctionalisation, bioinspired nanotechnology and nanomedicine. Throughout the book, we summarise basic concepts from different scientific fields in the form of **Back to Basics** boxes and highlight the latest scientific developments in

Research Reports. Important terms are highlighted in bold throughout and certain **Key Concepts** are gathered at the end of each chapter as a revision aid before the **Problem** sections. We hope that our book will be used as a reference book not only by lecturers and undergraduate students, but also postgraduates and researchers working in the field and trying to refresh their knowledge or learn basic concepts to help them in their projects. We wanted to make sure that concepts are clearly presented, and of huge help was our collaboration with an engineer and talented graphic designer Dr Nan Li from the University of Cambridge. She helped design many of the figures and provided valuable input that eased our creative process.

In the past decades, interdisciplinarity has been embraced as a more natural way to enable technological and scientific advances in various research fields. Students, however, still start by studying traditional scientific disciplines and move into more interdisciplinary areas in their final undergraduate year and postgraduate research. While working in German and UK universities, we have witnessed an increased number of undergraduates and graduates venturing into the fields only remotely related to their first degree. The bionanotechnology and chemical product design classes in Cambridge are often attended by engineers working on their biomedical devices and trying to learn some chemistry and biology, and biologists working with nanoparticles but struggling to understand how to modify the surface to prevent their aggregation. That means that a good part of the lecture is spent introducing basic terminology and concepts before moving onto the developments in bionanotechnology and recent applications and challenges. Students with physics and engineering background often struggle with the basic bionano principles, since they have not been taught organic synthesis, protein structure or genetics. The other way around, those with a background in medicine or chemistry might be challenged by instrumental design or physics behind the nanophenomena. Students are also often encouraged to consult a particular chapter written by a group of experts in an edited collection, which can be too advanced for their background or simply too difficult for them to grasp. We believe that one of the ways to resolve these challenges is to provide them with a textbook that would ease their journey through various disciplines, and combine the basic concepts with the most recent applications in the fields of drug design, biomimetics, biosensing, optoelectronics, just to name a few.

We hope that *Bionanotechnology* will manage to bridge some gaps between the basic scientific concepts and advanced applications, and inspire a new generation of researchers to embrace interdisciplinarity as the natural way of finding the most sustainable innovative solutions to ongoing challenges.

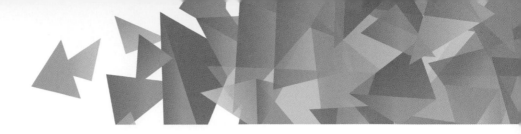

1 Nanomaterials

Principles and Properties

1.1 Bionanotechnology: Concept and History

Bionanotechnology is an interdisciplinary field at the intersection of nanotechnology and biology. Whereas nanotechnology provides tools and platforms for exploration and transformation of biological systems, biology is a source of inspiration and building blocks, all with the aim to design new materials and devices.

Historically, it is believed that the emergence of nanotechnology was hinted in the lecture of Richard Feynman (1918–1988) at Caltech in 1959 and in an article published in 1960 entitled 'There's plenty of room at the bottom' (Feynman, 1960; 25 years later he gave an updated talk 'Tiny machines' available online at https://youtu.be/4eRCygdW--c). Although his lecture and article give a vivid description of science that can enable manipulation of matter at the atomic and molecular level, the word **nano** (from Greek for dwarf) is not mentioned nor is there any description of the technology that will enable this manipulation. Nanotechnology was touched upon more in Feynman's lecture 'Infinitesimal machinery' given in 1983 and published as an article in 1993, in which he discusses design of silicon micromotors and touches upon many topics including potential application of such tiny machines in computing (Feynman, 1993). The term **nanotechnology** was independently coined by Norio Taniguchi (1912–1999) in 1974, and then again by Eric Dexler in the late 1970s. Dexler's paper published in 1981 entitled 'Molecular engineering' talks about design of protein machines by precise positioning of reactive groups on atomic level, and use of such technology for computing and manipulation of biological materials (Drexler, 1981). This sounds much like the bionanotechnology of today.

There were several discoveries in the 1980s to mid 1990s, which marked the beginning of **bionanotechnology** as a separate field. One was the exploitation of DNA as a structural element for a design of programmed nanostructures predicted in 1981 and then demonstrated in 1983 by Ned Seeman, a pioneer of DNA nanotechnology (Seeman, 1981; Kallenbach et al., 1983; see also Chapter 6). A few years later, in the mid 1990s, a method was patented that demonstrated DNA sequencing with the help of protein nanopore (Dreamer, 2016), and Chad Mirkin and his coworkers described DNA biosensors based on DNA-modified gold nanoparticles (Mirkin et al., 1996; Chapter 6). Around the same time Doxil, a liposomal formulation of powerful chemotherapeutic doxorubicin was approved by the US Food and Drug Administration (FDA), making it a first nanoformulated drug in use and on the market. This ultimately led to development of nanomedicine, which is closely linked to bionanotechnology and will be explored in Chapters 8 and 9.

1.2   Nanomaterials in Bionanotechnology

It is important to remember that rules are different down at the bottom. Properties of materials change as the size and the scale decrease and as we approach the molecular and atomic world. Surfaces become larger, surface energy bigger, electrons get confined in small spaces. In the past decades, the number of different nanomaterials has grown, but they can be grouped into a few main classes, all of which have found use in bionanotechnology (Table 1.1). These are **metallic nanomaterials**, mainly nanoparticles (NPs) and nanorods made of noble metals (Au, Ag, Pt, Cu), **metal oxides** such as magnetic nanomaterials based on iron oxide (Fe_3O_4), or titanium oxide (TiO_2), semiconducting nanomaterials such as **quantum dots** (note that the definition of quantum dots in physics will differ from the one we use in nanotechnology), **carbon nanomaterials** (graphene, carbon nanotubes and nanodiamonds) and **(bio)polymeric/organic nanoparticles** made either from man-made or natural polymers such as polysaccharides and organic molecules such as lipids or peptides.

Table 1.1 Most widely used nanomaterials in bionanotechnology and their characteristic properties

Nanomaterials	Typical representatives	Characteristic property
Noble metal nanoparticles	Au, Ag, Cu, Pt	Surface plasmon
Metal oxides	SiO_2, TiO_2, Fe_3O_4	Superparamagnetism, photocatalysis
Quantum dots	CdS, CdSe, CdSe–ZnS,	Fluorescence, photocatalysis
Carbon nanomaterials	Nanotubes, graphene, nanodiamonds	Biocompatibility conductivity
(Bio)polymer-based nanoparticles	Polysaccharides (chitosan, cellulose), man-made polymers	Adaptability, soft materials, biocompatibility
Others i.e. supramolecular structures, porous materials	Metal organic frameworks, mesoporous silica	Porosity, loading capacity, large surface area

In this chapter we will explore characteristic properties of these materials such as their high surface area and surface energy, their interaction with light and size-dependent fluorescence, and have a look at why they differ from their bulk counterparts.

1.3   Nanosized vs Bulk Materials

As a result of their small size, materials at the nanoscale behave more like molecules than a bulk material. Surface effects and quantum confinement determine physical and chemical properties, including increased catalytic activity, tunable fluorescence, surface plasmons and change in magnetic properties and conductivity.

Atoms at the surfaces of nanomaterials have fewer neighbours than their bulk counterparts and their unsatisfied, dangling bonds make the system more unstable. The smaller the particle, the larger the number of atoms on its surface and the larger the binding energy per atom. Such a system will have a high affinity to bind other species or to engage in various interactions that can minimise the surface energy, making nanosized systems excellent catalysts (materials that speed up chemical reactions).

As we approach the world of atoms, quantum size effects start to play an important role. In metals and semiconductors the electronic wave functions of conduction electrons are delocalised over the entire system; these electrons can be described as 'particles in a box'. The density of state (DOS) and the energies of the particles depend on the size of this box. As the box becomes smaller, properties such as light absorption, light emission, ionisation potential, and the number of electrons available for bond formation change.

What happens at the small scales and within small spaces? If we consider a reaction between two molecules in a dilute solution, we know that the reaction will be governed by the concentration of these molecules and the reaction rate constant. But when reacting species are confined within a small space, electrostatic or hydrophobic interactions become more intense easing the intramolecular interactions and product formation. Chemists often say that the effective molarity of the system increases. This effect is particularly important in biological systems; molecules concentrated in a particular cell compartment will react much faster than when they are dispersed throughout the entire cell interior. In fact, we know that the reactions that rarely occur in bulk may be driven by an increased effective molarity when they are packed within structures such as nanowells or nanopores. Design of nanoreactors and artificial compartments has already made an impact in the field of catalysis. Confining reagents within nanostructures often leads to an increase of reaction rates and yields. A perfect example of such a system are proteins, in particular catalytic proteins (enzymes), which accelerate a myriad of reactions within the cell by confining reagents within the small volume of their reactive pocket.

What about the quantum effects at the nanoscale? How do they affect the properties of the materials? We will try to illustrate this without getting into the complexity of the quantum mechanics (see Further Reading at the end of this chapter for more details). Let us consider a spherical metal nanoparticle with a radius of 2 nm. Depending on the material, this nanoparticle might contain tens or thousands of atoms (see In Numbers 1.1 for a calculation).

In Numbers 1.1   How Many Atoms Are There in a Nanoparticle?

Taking 166 pm as the atomic radius of gold, calculate the number of gold atoms in a spherical 2 nm gold nanoparticle.

Solution
Assuming that both nanoparticle and atom are spheres, we can calculate the volumes (keeping in mind that 2 nm refers to the diameter of the nanoparticle):

$$V = \frac{4}{3}\pi r^3$$

$$V_{\text{nanoparticle}} = 4.19 \times 10^{-27} \text{m}^3$$

$$V_{\text{gold atom}} = 1.92 \times 10^{-29} \text{m}^3$$

The number of gold atoms is therefore:

$$N_{\text{atoms}} = V_{\text{nanoparticle}} / V_{\text{gold atom}} = 2194.$$

This is an approximation, as atoms will be packed within the nanoparticle following the rules of crystal packing, which means there will be some empty space between them.

Interacting atoms result in distribution of a large number of energy levels that form energy bands. In a single atom, two energy levels will be separated by a significant energy gap. Two interacting atoms produce two new energy levels (four all together), four atoms eight (Figure 1.1). With each new atom added, levels become closer in energy, resulting in densely packed bands and energy gaps which are easier to cross. After a certain number of atoms is packed together, the bands will overlap and the electrons will be able to move freely among the atoms.

Figure 1.1

Energy levels and the
band gap for single and
multiple metal atoms.

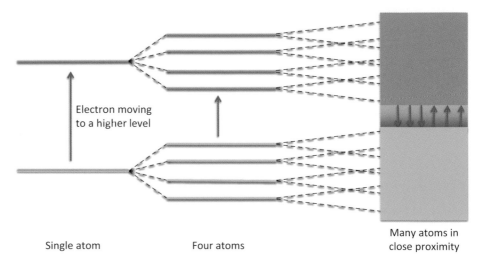

Single atom   Four atoms   Many atoms in
close proximity

The overlap and the gap between energy bands will differ for metals, semiconductors and insulators (Figure 1.2). An important concept to introduce at this point is the Fermi level, which describes the top filled electron energy level in a given material at absolute zero. It is a hypothetical concept also used to describe work needed to be done to add one electron to a given system.

Figure 1.2

Energy bands and band
gap for different classes
of materials. The dashed
line represents the
Fermi level.

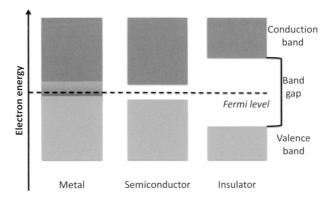

Insulators are characterised by a Fermi level, which lies between two bands of different energy, in a large band gap that prevents electrons from transitioning from one band to another. In metals, the Fermi level lies within the highest occupied band, which means there is no energy gap to overcome and the electrons can move freely between the bands. Note that only those electrons very close to the Fermi energy are excited above it.

The average spacing between the energy states ΔE is given by

$$\Delta E = \frac{4E_F}{3N}, \tag{1.1}$$

where E_F is the Fermi energy and N is the total number of valence electrons.

We can see that for a bulk metal with a large number of valence electrons, the spacing is small, and ultimately a continuous band is formed. As dimensions decrease and fewer atoms are present within a given volume, there are fewer valence electrons and the spacing between energy states increases. In short, energy levels become discrete and a small volume of materials starts to resemble the electronic structure of an atom. This is known as **quantum confinement**.

To achieve quantum confinement, at least one of the dimensions needs to be less than 100 nm. As the volume decreases, the density of state function D_s – a mathematical model that explains how the number of available electron energy states vary with unit volume and energy – becomes more discrete (see Back to Basics 1.1).

For metals in which the Fermi level lies within the bands, discrete density of states exist further away from the Fermi level (Figure 1.3) and as a result, quantum confinement can be achieved only when the size is significantly decreased (to a few nm) and there is a small number of atoms within the given volume (see In Numbers 1.2).

Figure 1.3

Energy bands of nanosized metal and a semiconductor. Changes in density states and relative position of the bands to the Fermi level will determine the extent of the quantum confinement.

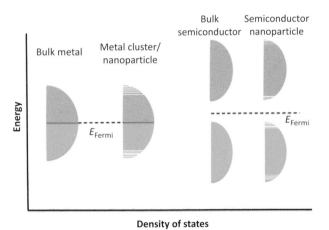

Back to Basics 1.1   Density of States of a Solid

Electrons organise themselves into a number of electron energy states within many energy sublevels. If there are many electrons as in a bulk material, energy levels will be very close and ultimately blend into a band.

The total number of energy states N_s with energy up to E (material will have a certain amount of energy, which is distributed among free electrons) is:

$$N_s = \left(\frac{8\pi}{3}\right)(2m_e E)^{\frac{3}{2}} \frac{D^3}{h^3},$$

where m_e is the mass of the electron, D^3 is volume and h is Planck's constant.

The number of energy states per unit volume n_s is then:

$$n_s = \frac{N_s}{D^3} = \left(\frac{8\pi}{3}\right)\frac{(2m_e E)^{\frac{3}{2}}}{h^3}.$$

The density of state function D_s, the derivative of the above equation with respect to energy, refers to the number of available electron energy states per unit volume, per unit energy:

$$D_s = \frac{8\sqrt{2}\pi m_e^{\frac{3}{2}}}{h^3}\sqrt{E}.$$

It is important to remember that D_s is only a mathematical model, and unlike the model, the real density of states function becomes more discrete as the volume changes and dimensions move towards the nanometre scale. In bulk materials, the energy levels are continuous, for 2D materials in which one dimension is on the nanoscale (thin films for example) the energy levels can change stepwise. As we go towards 1D materials (two dimensions on the nanoscale, for example nanowires), the separation is more discrete and finally in 0D materials (three dimensions on the nanometre scale), they will be clearly separated.

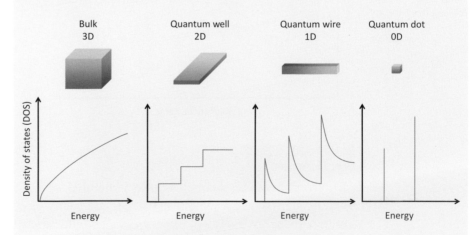

In Numbers 1.2	At What Diameter Does a Gold Nanoparticle Achieve Quantum Confinement at 25 °C?

Some electrons can be excited above the Fermi energy and need to have energy larger than $k_B T$. For quantum confinement, the following must be true:

$$\Delta E = \frac{4E_F}{3n_v} > k_B T,$$

where n_v is a number of valence electrons, k_B is Boltzmann's constant and E_F for gold is 5.53 eV. By rearranging the above equation we get:

$$n_v < \frac{4E_F}{3k_{BT}}$$

$$n_v < \frac{4(8.86 \times 10^{-19}\ \mathrm{J})}{3(1.38 \times 10^{-23}\ \mathrm{J\ K^{-1}})(298\ \mathrm{K})} = 288.$$

This means that particle needs to have fewer than 288 valence electrons. Gold has a density of $19\,320\ \mathrm{kg\,m^{-3}}$ and atomic mass is $79\ \mathrm{g\,mol^{-1}}$. Density of atoms is:

$$\frac{19\,320\ \mathrm{kg\,m^{-3}} \times N_A}{0.079\ \mathrm{kg\,mol^{-1}}} = \frac{(19\,320\ \mathrm{kg\,m^{-3}})(6.02 \times 10^{23}\ \mathrm{atoms\,m^{-3}})}{0.079\ \mathrm{kg\,mol^{-1}}}$$

$$= 1.5 \times 10^{29}\ \mathrm{atoms\,m^{-3}}.$$

The volume of the particle is given by

$$V_P = \frac{288\ \mathrm{atoms}}{1.5 \times 10^{29}\ \mathrm{atoms\,m^{-3}}} = 1.92 \times 10^{-27}\ \mathrm{m^3}.$$

If we assume that the nanoparticle is spheric, volume will be defined as

$$V = \frac{4}{3}r^3\pi$$

and

$$r = \left(\frac{3V}{4\pi}\right)^{1/3} = \left(\frac{3(1.92 \times 10^{-27}\ \mathrm{m^3})}{4\pi}\right)^{1/3} = 7.7 \times 10^{-10}\ \mathrm{m}.$$

Taking this into account the gold particle will achieve quantum confinement and behave as non-metal when its diameter is less than 1.4 nm.

However, as the size gets smaller, a significant role in metal nanoparticles is played by the large number of surface atoms and electrons, which results in formation of an electron cloud known as a **surface plasmon**. Surface plasmon describes the collective excitation of free electrons in metals, which can oscillate when stimulated by an energy source (Back to Basics 1.2). Surface plasmon has been extensively exploited in bionanotechnology, in particular for design of biosensors.

Back to Basics 1.2 Surface Plasmon

The early work on surface plasmon (SP) was done by Rufus H. Ritchie (1924–2017) in the 1950s – the impact of his 1957 paper becoming clearer only decades later with the development of nanotechnology (Ritchie, 1957). Understanding surface plasmons opened up the fields of nanoplasmonics and nanophotonics, and resulted in a number of applications in optoelectronics, solar energy conversion and medicine.

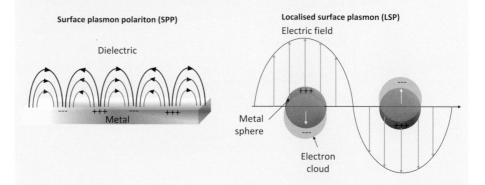

A plasmon is a quantum of the collective excitation of free electrons in solids. A surface plasmon is an electromagnetic wave that propagates on the metallic–dielectric interface of metallic thin films. Essentially, surface plasmons are the light waves that are trapped on the metal surface because of their interaction with the free electrons, which respond collectively by oscillating in resonance with the wave of light. A combined excitation consisting of a surface plasmon and the electromagnetic field of light is called a surface plasmon polariton (SPP) at a planar interface, or a localised surface plasmon (LSP) for the closed surface of a metal nanosphere.

By interaction of the incident electromagnetic field of light with the metal nanoparticle, the conduction electrons at the nanoparticle surface oscillate with respect to the nanoparticle lattice due to the Coulomb attraction between electrons and metallic nuclei. This resonant oscillation, known as a **localised surface plasmon resonance** (LSPR), produces large, wavelength-selective increases in absorption, scattering and electromagnetic field at the nanoparticle surface.

Using a set of equations postulated by Gustav Mie (1868–1957) (Mie, 1908), which will not be discussed here, it could be shown that the size, shape and chemical composition, which determine their dielectric constant, as well as the refractive index of the surrounding media and the wavelength of incident light affect the LSPR of a metal nanoparticle (Fong and Yung, 2013). As a result, the nanoparticle shape or size can be affected in such a way to obtain a desired response at the particular wavelength. For example, addition of a biomolecule to a surface of a plasmonic nanoparticle changes the refractive index at the nanoparticle surface, which results in a shift of the LSPR peak frequency utilised for LSPR-based biosensing (see Chapters 5 and 9).

The situation is different in the case of nanosized semiconductors in which the Fermi level is positioned between the conduction and valence bands, and discrete energy levels are present at the edges of these bands on each side of the Fermi level (Figure 1.3). As a result, the quantum effects do not depend so much on the number of atoms (and electrons N) as in metals, but rather on the band gap and the position of the Fermi level. In semiconductors, even large structures with up to 10 000 atoms can be much more different than their bulk counterparts. For example, in the case of semiconducting quantum dots, absorption and emission of light strongly depend on the nanoparticle size. This is due to the fact that the boundaries of the band gaps can be readjusted by addition or removal of several atoms. As the photon with the right amount of energy hits the quantum dot nanoparticle, the electron is excited from valence into a conductive band. When this electron relaxes back to the valence band, energy matching the energy of the band gap is emitted, and as a consequence, semiconducting quantum dots are fluorescent. The emitted wavelength will depend on the band gap energy, which, in turn, depends on the size of the nanoparticle. Simply put, smaller quantum dots will emit light of higher energy, since the energy levels are more discrete and band gaps larger for smaller (and more confined) volumes. Ultimately, the fluorescence emission of the quantum dots can be tuned by controlling their size (Figure 1.4), which played an important role in development of new classes of fluorescent materials for labelling (more in Chapter 5).

(a) Band gap and (b) emission wavelengths for quantum dots of different sizes. As the size of the nanoparticle increases, the band gap becomes smaller, resulting in high wavelength emissions (red shift).

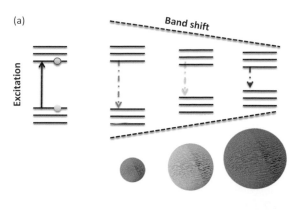

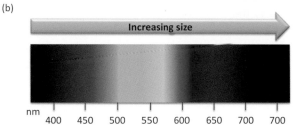

Semiconducting materials are also characterised by formation of exciton, an electron–hole pair created when a valence electron is excited into the conduction band and becomes mobile. There is a characteristic dimension for each semiconductor in which the exciton is strongly confined and its mobility severely constricted. Formation of excitons plays an important role in design of oxidative materials for medical applications (see Research Report 2.1) and enzyme-like catalysts.

Until now, we have mainly discussed metals and semiconductors. What about carbon nanomaterials? These materials, such as graphene, a thin layer of graphitic carbons, and carbon nanotubes (CNT), have remarkable thermal and electronic conductivities. In fact, carbon nanotubes have been shown to behave both as metals and semiconductors and can even switch between the two states. Electron transport through carbon nanotubes occurs in the pair of sub-bands within the electron states closest to the Fermi level. When these bands overlap, the electron flow is not hindered, which results in carbon nanotubes with a distinct metallic character (Matsuda et al., 2010). The distance between the bands depends on the wrapping, chirality and the diameter of the carbon nanotubes. For example, all armchair-type carbon nanotubes are metallic, whereas zigzag and chiral can be both metals and semiconductors depending on the wrapping parameters (more on this in Chapter 2). The band gap of semiconducting nanotubes can even be tuned by addition of dopants. Continuous development of new strategies for nanotube preparation has already resulted in enhanced quality and more control over their properties, which will be discussed in Chapter 2.

Different nanomaterials are often referred to as *0D, 1D and 2D materials*, which can sometimes be confusing. It is important to remember that numbers 0, 1 and 2 describe how many dimensions are *not* nanosized. This means that 0D materials will have all three dimensions on a nanoscale, such as nanoparticles of different shapes (Figure 1.5a), 1D materials such as nanorods have one dimension (usually length), which is not at nanoscale (Figure 1.5b), whereas 2D materials, such as thin films, have two non-nanoscale dimensions (Figure 1.5c). For example, graphene usually has a thickness of one to three atom layers, but could be produced in larger sheets and it is considered a 2D material. In bionanotechnology, there is an additional term which is often used and it refers to **nanocomposite materials**. They can be considered **3D nanomaterials** as they are not confined to nanoscale, but can be considered as dispersions of nanomaterials or bundles of nanowires, and nanoscale layers. Such are multi-phase solids with one or more dimensions at the nanometre scale, which can be prepared by addition of nanomaterials to a bulk material such as polymer (nanocomposite hydrogels, Chapter 9) or cement, or by introduction of regular nanometre spacings to bulk material such as found in butterfly wings or abalone shells (Chapter 7).

Figure 1.5

Nanomaterials are grouped into 0D, 1D and 2D based on their dimensions: (a) 0D refers to zero dimensions which are not on a nanoscale; (b) 1D, one dimension (usually length) not at nanometre scale; (c) 2D, two dimensions not on a nanometre scale, such as in graphene and nanoplates.

(a)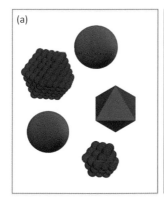

(b)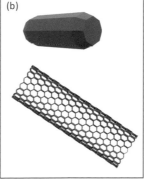

(c)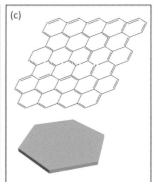

1.4 The Ratio of Surface Atoms to Volume

Nanosized materials have a large ratio of the number of surface atoms to nanoparticle volume. This is best visualised by looking at the idealised example of a cuboctahedral gold nanoparticle shown in Figure 1.6, and calculation of the surface atom numbers. The resulting values indicate that this percentage decreases with the increase in particle size.

Atoms in a cuboctahedral gold nanoparticle. Percentages indicate the number of surface gold atoms.

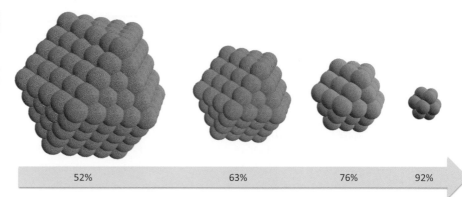

52%   63%   76%   92%

In an ideal case of a regular cuboctahedral particle made of a single metal, the percentage can be easily calculated. However, determining the percentage of surface atoms in real samples is not straightforward, as these systems do not fit into idealised geometric forms. For example, complex hydrogen-binding experiments and use of X-ray diffraction analysis were required to determine the number of palladium atoms in nanoparticles of different sizes (Figure 1.7). The plot of experimental data clearly shows that the percentage of surface atoms decreases rapidly as the size of the particles increases from 10 nm to several µm.

Experimental data showing the change of surface atom percentage with the diameter of palladium nanoparticle (d_{NP}). Adapted by permission from Springer Nature: Nützenadel (2000).

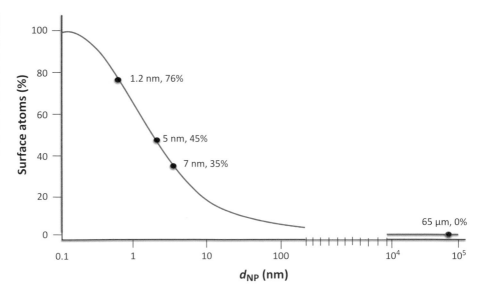

A large number of surface atoms results in a large surface energy, which means that nanosized materials are often unstable or metastable. In order to minimise the energy, nanostructures have a tendency to grow into bigger structures, and even aggregate. Consequently, nanoparticle preparation methods need to be optimised to account for this thermodynamic aspect. As we will see in Chapter 2, various strategies have been employed to increase the stability of inherently metastable nanostructures.

1.5 Surface Energy

It is not easy to measure **surface energy at the nanoscale**. In recent years this has been improved by use of supercomputers to quantify the properties of small nanostructures called clusters, which are composed of tens or hundreds of atoms. Earlier studies on crystalline structures, such as cubic sodium chloride (NaCl) crystals, provided some insight into the scales of the surface energy of a specific surface area. Taking into account the surface energy and edge energy of 1 g NaCl cube (2×10^{-5} J cm^{-2} and 3×10^{13} J cm^{-1}, respectively), surface energy can be calculated for each smaller cube obtained by successive division of a large starting structure. As seen in Table 1.2, surface energy increases dramatically with decrease in crystal dimensions from macro to nanoscale.

Table 1.2 Cube dimensions, surface area and surface energy of sodium chloride (NaCl) crystal

Side (cm)	Surface area (cm^2)	Surface energy (J g^{-1})
0.77	3.6	7.2×10^{-5}
0.1	28	5.6×10^{-4}
0.01	280	5.6×10^{-3}
0.001	2.8×10^3	5.6×10^{-2}
10^{-4} (1 μm)	2.8×10^4	0.56
10^{-7} (1 nm)	2.8×10^7	560

How can we explain these results? Imagine atoms on the surface of a cube. Being on the surface, they are exposed to the environment and possess fewer atomic neighbours than the atoms in the interior of a crystal. As a result, their coordination number is lower and they have a number of dangling or unsatisfied bonds. Due to the presence of these unsatisfied bonds, the inwardly directed force that pulls atoms closer is stronger, and as a consequence the bond lengths between the atoms on the surface and those in the interior decrease.

When solid particles are very small, such a decrease in bond length becomes significant and the lattice dimensions of the entire solid particle become smaller (for more on lattice types see the Appendix). Ultimately, there is extra energy possessed by the surface atoms: surface energy γ (Equation 1.2). As atoms on the surface are being pulled inwards, energy required to keep them in their original position is equal to:

$$\gamma = \frac{1}{2} N_b \varepsilon \rho, \tag{1.2}$$

in which N_b represents the number of broken bonds, ε the bond strength, and ρ the surface atom density (number of atoms per area in a new surface).

What does this mean for a metal nanoparticle? One of the most common lattices encountered in metals is a **face-centred crystal** (FCC) lattice (Figure 1.8 and see the Appendix).

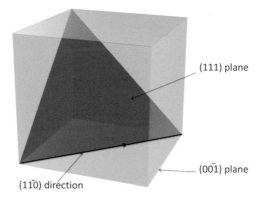

Figure 1.8

Face-centred crystal (FCC) lattice. Planes of this lattice are represented by three digit numbers, Miller indices (001) corresponding to their orientation in three dimensions.

(111) plane

(00$\bar{1}$) plane

(1$\bar{1}$0) direction

If we now consider different planes (facets) within this lattice and calculate the surface energy taking into account Equation 1.2, we see that there is a difference for atoms positioned along (100) or (110) planes (see Back to Basics 1.3 for more details on crystal facets and the calculation).

From the calculations of FCC crystal facet surface energy, it can be seen that low index facets such as (100), (110) and (111) have lower surface energy that decreases from (100) to (111). High index facets (those with larger sum of Miller indices) are characterised by much higher energy.

This plays an important role in synthesis of differently shaped nanoparticles, as the facets have a different affinity for binding of chemical species depending on their surface energy. Generally, the systems aim to minimise the energy, resulting in high index facets being more susceptible to interactions.

Back to Basics 1.3	Crystal Facets and Their Surface Energy

If we put crystal within the coordinate system, we can label different facets according to their position in 3D space describing the crystal symmetries. For example cube has 6 (100) facets, but it can evolve into more complex shapes ultimately leading to octahedron with 8 (111) facets.

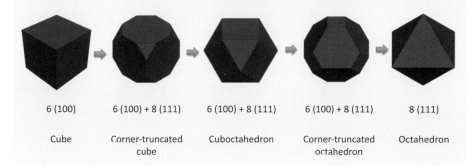

6 (100)	6 (100) + 8 (111)	6 (100) + 8 (111)	6 (100) + 8 (111)	8 (111)
Cube	Corner-truncated cube	Cuboctahedron	Corner-truncated octahedron	Octahedron

One of the most common lattices encountered in metals is a face-centred crystal (FCC) lattice. If we consider two different facets with length a within this lattice we can calculate their surface energy.

Four bonds will be broken for an atom within (100) facet ($N_b = 4$), the number of atoms per unit area (a^2) will be 2 and according to Equation 1.2, the surface energy amounts to:

$$\gamma = \left(\frac{1}{2}\right) 4\varepsilon \frac{2}{a^2} = 4\frac{\varepsilon}{a^2}.$$

Along the same line, the surface energy of (110) facet is $\gamma = 3.5\frac{\varepsilon}{a^2}$.

1.6 Strategies to Reduce Surface Energy

The laws of thermodynamics tell us that any material or system is stable only when it is in the state of the lowest Gibbs energy (Back to Basics 1.4). Therefore, there is a strong tendency for a solid (or liquid) to minimise its total surface energy.

Back to Basics 1.4 Laws of Thermodynamics and the Gibbs Energy

The thermodynamic universe contains two parts, the system (cell, reaction vessel, engine etc.) and its surroundings (the region outside the system where the measurements are done). The system can be *open* (matter can be transferred through the boundary between the system and its surroundings), *closed* (matter cannot pass through the boundary) and *isolated* (the system has no mechanical or thermal contact with its surroundings).

In a molecular world, the internal energy U is the total kinetic and potential energy of the molecules in the system. ΔU represents internal energy when a system changes from an initial state i with internal energy U_i to a final state f of internal energy U_f: $\Delta U = U_f - U_i$. It is experimentally shown that for the isolated system no change in internal energy takes place. This observation was summarised in the **first law of thermodynamics**, which states that *the internal energy of an isolated system is constant*:

$$\Delta U = q + w,$$

where q is the heat added to the system and w work done on the system.

The first law uses the internal energy to identify the permissible changes. The spontaneous changes (process that occurs without the addition of external energy) within these permissible changes can be identified by the entropy.

The **second law of thermodynamics** states that *the entropy of an isolated system increases in the course of a spontaneous change*:

$$\Delta S_{universe} = \Delta S_{system} + \Delta S_{surroundings} > 0.$$

When the process occurs at constant temperature and pressure the second law of thermodynamics can be rearranged and written as:

$$\Delta G = \Delta H - T\Delta S,$$

where ΔG is the change in Gibbs free energy ($[G] = J$), ΔH and ΔS are changes in enthalpy and entropy of the system.

If $\Delta G < 0$, the process occurs spontaneously and is referred to as exergonic.

If $\Delta G = 0$, the system is at equilibrium.

If $\Delta G > 0$, the process is not spontaneous as written, but occurs spontaneously in the reverse direction.

Finally, the **third law of thermodynamics** states that *the entropy of all perfect crystalline substances is zero at $T = 0$.*

There are a few routes that can lead to the reduction of surface energy. **Surface relaxation** occurs more readily in the liquid phase than in the solid and it is characterised by inward shifting of surface atoms and ions. When dangling bonds engage in formation of new chemical bonds we talk about the **surface restructuring**. Surface energy can be decreased by adsorption of various chemical species onto the surface through electrostatic or van der Waals forces through the process of **surface adsorption**. In solids, surfaces can be enriched through solid–solid diffusion such as **impurity enrichment**.

In nanostructures, there are two general pathways that lead to surface energy reduction. One involves controllable formation of larger structures (hence a lower surface energy) from individual components or by **random aggregation**, and the other the adsorption of the molecules onto the nanostructured surface (more on this in Chapter 4). Controlled growth of larger structures is usually achieved through **sintering** (Figure 1.9a) or **Ostwald ripening** (Figure 1.9b).

Sintering can be considered as a process in which a solid–vapour interface is replaced by a solid–solid interaction. This is achieved through reshaping of the structures and a sealing of the gaps. Such a process is not desirable in preparation of nanostructures as it can have dramatic impact on the properties of obtained nanomaterials. Fortunately, sintering usually requires high temperatures. In Ostwald ripening, two individual nanostructures become a single one through growth of the larger one at the expense of the smaller until the latter completely disappears. This process is very important for nanomaterial formation and will be discussed in more detail in Chapter 2.

Random aggregation leads to formation of agglomerates (Figure 1.9c) within which many nanostructures are associated with one another through chemical bonds or/and physical attraction at interfaces. Agglomerates are difficult to destroy and difficult to separate into their individual components. Their formation also alters the surface accessibility and material properties, and it should be avoided during nanomaterial preparation.

Figure 1.9

Surface energy can be
reduced by formation of
larger structures. During
synthesis of crystalline
materials this can be
achieved through (a)
sintering or (b) Ostwald
ripening. (c) Random
aggregation leads to
formation of large
irregular structures.

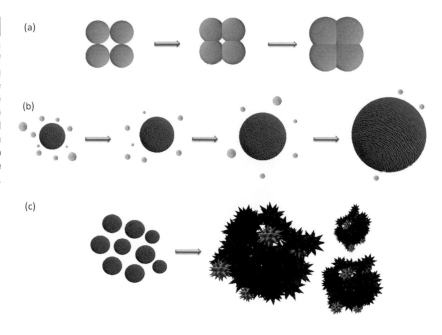

Understanding the underlying principles behind nanomaterial properties
can help us to come up with the set of guidelines to ease their preparation and
tune them to suit various applications. We will take a closer look at some
aspects of nanomaterial synthesis, before we cover various strategies in
Chapter 2.

1.7 Principles of Nanomaterial Synthesis

Preparation protocols vary across nanomaterial classes and depend on their
application. However, there are some general guidelines that help us to
develop and fine-tune synthetic protocols. Ideally, nanomaterials should be
uniform in size (monosized) and **well-dispersed**, without the presence of
agglomerates. This is particularly important for subsequent modification
and (bio)applications. The size not only determines the optical and electronic
properties, but also guides the choice of the molecules and procedures used for
subsequent functionalisation. Although we often aim to achieve uniform size
distribution, aggregates are desirable for some applications. For example,
surface-enhanced resonance Raman scattering (SERS, Chapter 5), benefits
from the presence of random aggregates of noble metals, which enhance the
surface plasmon and consequently the read-out signal. Even when the narrow

distribution of sizes cannot be achieved, the preparation protocol should lead to nanomaterials that have **identical shape**, **chemical composition** and **crystal structure** (in the case of crystalline materials). Shape, composition and crystallinity play an important role in defining the surface energy and binding of surface ligands, as well as inherent electronic and optical properties.

The chemistry behind the synthesis of nanomaterials, in particular in the case of widely used metal nanoparticles and metal oxides, is often simple and based on already established protocols of chemical reduction or sol–gel synthesis adapted from inorganic, organic or organometallic chemistry. However, the processes of **crystal nucleation** and **size and shape control** are far from straightforward and in many cases, still not fully understood. A small change in the ratio or reagents or reducing agents can result in dramatically different nanoshapes despite the starting material being the same as it is the case with nanoparticles shown in Figure 1.10.

Figure 1.10

Transmission electron micrographs of differently shaped gold nanoparticles. Tetrachloroauric acid (HAuCl$_4$) is used as a starting material, whereas temperature and reducing agents were changed.

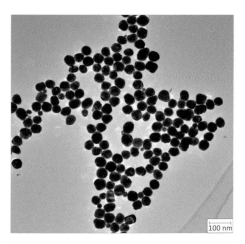
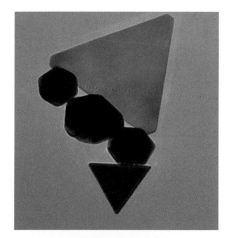
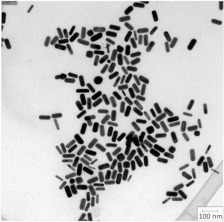
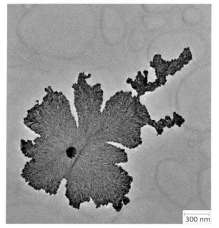

Gold nanoparticles are not only one of the most widely used nanoparticle classes in bionanotechnology, but, historically, they were among the first ones to be prepared. Red gold colloids (for more on colloids check Back to Basics 1.5) were used for glass staining in ancient Rome, although, as far as we know, Roman glassblowers were not aware of the nanospecies they had produced.

One of the most common methods to obtain metallic nanostructures such as spherical particles, is in-solution reduction (Back to Basics 1.6) of the metal salt precursors in the presence of various stabilisers.

Back to Basics 1.5   Colloids

Colloids are mixtures of insoluble, dispersed particles of different sizes but small enough to be evenly distributed throughout another substance. A colloid is composed of colloid particles and the dispersing medium and examples can be found all around us. For example, milk is the colloidal mixture of fatty acid and proteins (very complex) in water, other examples include different creams and even paper. Colloids, unlike solutions, show strong Tyndall effect, or Tyndall scattering; scattering of light as it passes through the mixture of small particles.

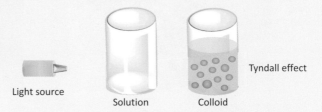

Thomas Graham (1805–1869), the Scottish physical chemist, postulated Graham's law of diffusion in 1848. The law describes the relative permeation laws of two gases and was instrumental for understanding colloids. He explained that low diffusivity exhibited by colloidal solutions results from the larger size of colloids in relation to ordinary molecules. Graham is considered to be the 'father of colloid chemistry'. He also introduced sol–gel terms, extensively used in nanomaterial synthesis.

Gold nanoparticles are prepared using $HAuCl_4$ precursor and various reducing agents to afford elemental gold Au(0):

$$AuCl_4^- (aq) \rightarrow Au(s) + 4\,Cl^-.$$

The most frequently used method for preparation of gold nanoparticles, the Turkevich method, employs hot citrate solution to reduced HAuCl$_4$ precursor. The method was published in 1951 (Turkevich et al., 1951), and since then a number of studies have been performed to decipher the mechanism and growth of gold nanoparticles. The overall equation can be written as:

citrate   acetone dicarboxylate

Acetone dicarboxylate is an intermediate product that degrades to acetone at high temperature (100 °C) in the presence of water:

acetone dicarboxylate   acetone

Acetone can further act as a reducing agent for AuCl$_4^-$ ions:

acetone   formaldehyde

This double-act reduction in which both the citrate and the intermediate product act as reducing agent ensures that there is a substantial amount of small gold nuclei formed. The danger at this stage is that the presence of too many nuclei can lead to uncontrollable agglomeration. Small nuclei are characterised by large surface energy, which makes them prone to formation of large random aggregates in order to minimise the overall energy of the system. However, aggregation can be avoided if the solution of precursor and a reducing agent is diluted and as we will see later in the chapter, there is a thermodynamic reason behind this dilution.

Back to Basics 1.6 Oxidation and Reduction Reactions

Oxidation is the loss of electrons by a substance during a chemical reaction. The substance, which accepts these electrons is called the **oxidising agent**.

Reduction is the gain of electrons and the substance which donates these electrons is called the **reducing agent**.

The substances being oxidised and reduced, and the oxidising and reducing agents, can be identified in ionic equations.

For example in preparation of $FeCl_3$:

$$Cl_2(g) + 2Fe^{2+}(aq) \rightarrow 2Cl^-(aq) + 2Fe^{3+}(aq)$$

Cl_2 is an oxidising and Fe^{2+} is a reducing agent.

Additional control over the growth of nanoparticles is aided by the presence of carboxylate (C=O) groups in both the citrate and the oxidation product acetone dicarboxylate. Carboxylates coordinate gold nuclei and enable further interaction between Au(0) nuclei and Au (III) ions in the solution, easing the subsequent growth.

Initially, Turkevich and his colleagues observed remarkable differences in the shapes of nanoparticles as they replaced citric acid with sodium citrate (Figure 1.11).

Figure 1.11

Slightly different reducing agents can lead to dramatically different nanoparticle solutions. Transmission electron micrographs of gold nanoparticles prepared using (a) citric acid and (b) sodium citrate with $HAuCl_4$ as a precursor.

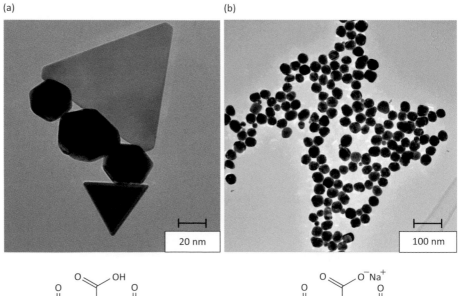

The reason for these dramatic variations in shape is the pH of the solution. Unlike citric acid, sodium citrate acts both as a reducing agent and a buffer, stabilising the pH, which leads to more control over the nucleation and first stages of nanoparticle formation. Ultimately, this control results in slower growth, which produces smaller, monodispersed and spherical nanoparticles. The underlying mechanism of this strategy was fully described as late as 2014 and it involves several stages (Thahn, 2014). At low pH (3.7–6.5), an intermediate complex species is first formed, which undergoes fast nucleation within 10 s, followed by fast random attachment and particle ripening, ultimately leading to larger particles (Figure 1.12). At higher pH values (6.5–7.7), another pathway with a much longer nucleation time followed by a slow growth produces more defined, monodispersed and smaller nanoparticles.

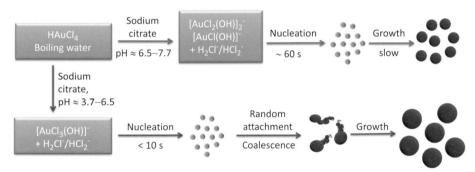

Figure 1.12

Detailed mechanism of gold nanoparticle growth in the presence of sodium citrate.

The mechanisms of nanoparticle growth are often rather complex, but it is important to understand them to establish a set of rules to aid their synthesis and ultimate scale up. The example of gold nanoparticle preparation highlights how important it is to control different stages of particle growth, which can be sensitive to a range of variables such as temperature, concentration, pH and even the rate and sequence of reagent addition.

1.8   (Nano)crystal Growth

The development of X-ray crystallography enabled extensive studies of crystal formation. In 1952, Pound and La Mer published the theory which described three distinct stages of crystal formation; generation of atoms, nucleation and growth, and summarised it in a diagram known as the **La Mer diagram** of crystal growth (Pound and La Mer, 1952; Figure 1.13).

Figure 1.13

La Mer diagram of crystal growth. Notice the three distinct areas in the diagram that correspond to different stages of crystal growth and the changes in the monomer concentration over time.

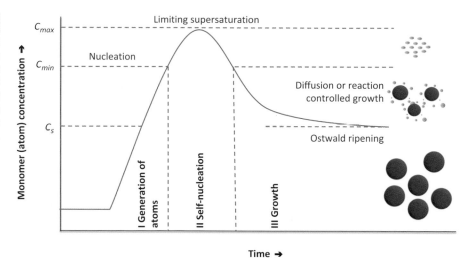

Figure 1.13 La Mer diagram of crystal growth. Notice the three distinct areas in the diagram that correspond to different stages of crystal growth and the changes in the monomer concentration over time.

The three stages of crystal formation are:

Stage I This is characterised by rapid increase in concentration of atoms or nucleating species, which are sometimes referred to as monomers. For example, these can be formed by chemical reduction of a starting reagent such as $HAuCl_4$ and assembly of initial species into small atomic assemblies or clusters.

Stage II After some time, monomers start forming nuclei or seeds (C_{min}), which undergo rapid nucleation when the concentration maximum C_{max} is reached. Such nucleation significantly reduces their concentration in the solution. As long as the concentration of reactants is kept below the critical level, further nucleation is suppressed.

Stage III With the continuous supply of monomers produced by reduction, growth of nanocrystals occurs under the control of monomer diffusion through the solution. An important process within the growth stage is Ostwald ripening, which is discussed in more detail later in the chapter.

If a solution of monodispersed and uniformly sized nanocrystals is required, nucleation must occur in a very short timeframe in order to generate a large number of uniform nuclei. This can be achieved by ensuring a rapid increase in the amount of nuclei (reaching supersaturation) either by increasing temperature or by lowering the concentration of the precursors followed by quick addition of the reducing agent.

When the concentration of monomers is less than C_{min}, nucleation ceases but the growth continues. This growth depends on several distinct processes, all of which work in synergy: diffusion of monomers to the surface of the growing nuclei, adsorption of the monomers and irreversible incorporation of the surface species into the nanocrystal. Diffusion of the monomers from solution to the surface of nuclei is the one that is probably the easiest to control and can be used to engineer particular sizes and shapes.

Let us have a closer look at the underlaying principles of diffusion-controlled growth, and start by quickly reviewing the work of the German physician and physiologist Adolf Fick (1829–1901). Adolf Fick studied diffusion of fluids through membranes and explained how the diffusion flux (J) depends on the concentration gradient (Tyrrell, 1964). The law he proposed, named **Fick's law** in his honour, established the relationship between the radius of a growing nuclei, time and concentration:

$$J = 4\pi x^2 D \frac{dC}{dx},\tag{1.3}$$

in which J is the diffusion flux, D is a diffusion constant, and C is the concentration at distance x from the surface of the nanocrystal (Figure 1.14).

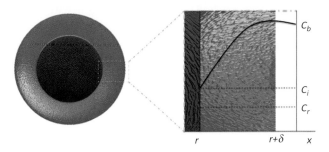

Figure 1.14

Growing crystalline nanoparticle in the solution of monomers. C_b is the concentration of monomer in bulk solution and C_r at the surface of a growing nanocrystal, r is the radius of a nanocrystal and x, distance of the monomers from the surface.

Due to the steady state of solute diffusion, J is a constant irrespective of x and the integration of $C(x)$ from $(r + \delta)$ to r results in:

$$J = 4\pi Dr (C_b - C_i).\tag{1.4}$$

When the concentration of the growth species (C_b represents concentration of the monomer in the bulk solution) is kept low and the diffusion distance very large, the limiting factor of growth will be diffusion of the monomers to the surface. Thus, the particle size will change with time as shown below:

$$\frac{dr}{dt} = \frac{Dv}{r} (C_b + C_r),\tag{1.5}$$

where D is the diffusion coefficient, C_b and C_r are the concentrations of the monomer in the solution and at the surface, respectively, r is the radius of the crystal, and v is the molar volume of the nuclei.

As can be seen from Equation 1.5, there is a particular radius above which particles will start growing (critical radius) and the larger the particle, the slower will be the growth.

Fick's law indicates that in order to control growth, the concentration of the monomers should be kept low and the diffusion distance large. This can be achieved by changing the viscosity and concentration of the solution, or by introducing the surface barriers.

However, when diffusion is rapid, the limiting factor will be the **kinetics of the surface reactions**, addition and possible reduction of the monomers on the surface:

$$\frac{dr}{dt} = kv(C_b + C_r), \tag{1.6}$$

in which k is the rate of the surface reaction.

In a kinetically or reaction-controlled growth of a nanoparticle, the rate will largely depend on the surface properties. Species attached to the surface such as various ions that either promote or block the reactions and the chemical reactions catalysed or quenched by the nanocrystal will all affect crystal growth. For example, some types of silver and gold nanoparticles engage in self-catalysis of various reactions, which determine the outcome of the growth stage.

The famous physicist Wolfgang Pauli (1900–1958) once said that when God made the bulk, he left the surfaces to the Devil. Indeed, surfaces are very complex systems and it is not easy to describe the kinetics of surface reactions, not to mention trying to control them.

But let us consider what the above equations can tell us about the growth of gold nanoparticles – our model system chosen to illustrate the principles of nanocrystal formation. In short, to achieve a monodispersed solution of uniformly sized and shaped gold nanoparticles, the concentration of the precursor ($HAuCl_4$) should be kept low to increase the diffusion path, but the reducing agent added rapidly. To slow down diffusion of gold monomers to the particle surface the viscosity of the bulk solution can be increased, or the access to the surface hindered. This can often be achieved by the addition of various polymers to the solution, or by introduction of surface-binding molecules, which can slow down or completely arrest the growth.

1.9 Ostwald Ripening and Coalescence

After the particles of particular radius are grown, two processes, Ostwald ripening and coalescence/oriented attachment, are responsible for further growth into larger, more regular nanocrystals. Both processes can be explained by taking into account the surface energy of the nanoparticle. High surface energy of smaller nanoparticles is responsible for their high instability and dispersibility. If we have a dispersion of smaller and larger nanoparticles, smaller nanoparticles will tend to dissolve into monomers, which can then be used for further growth of the larger nanoparticles. This is the principle behind Ostwald ripening. A mathematically elegant theory of Ostwald ripening was postulated by Wilhelm Ostwald (1853–1932) in 1896, and fully explored by Evgeny Lifshitz, Vitaly V. Slyozov (1915–1985) and Carl Wagner (1901–1977), whose work on kinetics of ripening in dilute systems resulted in LSW (Lifshitz–Slyozov–Wagner) theory (Baldan, 2002).

Depending on the process, Ostwald ripening can either widen or narrow the crystal size distribution. Ostwald ripening is often not desirable in preparation of bulk materials as it results in abnormal grain growth, which significantly changes the mechanical properties. However, in the case of nanomaterials it can be used to control the size distribution and afford monodispersed solutions of large crystalline particles. While Ostwald ripening is characterised by growth of large particles at the expense of the smaller ones present in the solution, coalescence and oriented attachment refer to the fusion of crystalline particles. **Coalescence** and **oriented attachment** are very similar, and differ only in the orientation of the crystal lattice at the grain boundary. For orientated attachment a crystallographic alignment occurs so that continuous crystallographic planes appear on either side of grain boundaries, whereas for coalescence there is no particular preference of crystal orientation (Figure 1.15).

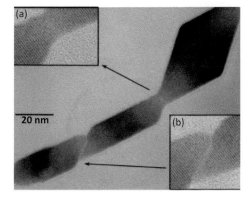

Figure 1.15

Scanning electron micrograph of titanium dioxide (TiO_2) nanocrystal. Crystal growth can occur by oriented attachment (a) or coalescence, which is characterised by dislocated planes (b). Adapted from Penn and Banfield (1999), with permission from Elsevier.

One can imagine coalescence as a conjoining of the crystal facets. Studies have shown that in order to coalesce, nanocrystals can sometimes 'jump' a distance of as much as 1 nm and move closer to one another. Once they are in proximity, the space between the facets is filled within 10–100 seconds under the influence of Coulombic attraction forces and weak van der Waals inter-actions (Back to Basics 1.7).

It is important to note that coalescence can also precede the growth of nanoparticles and can aid the formation of seeds from very small nuclei (1–2 nm). In fact, it has been shown to occur throughout different stages of gold nanoparticle preparation (Figure 1.16), and confirmed by transmission electron microscopy studies of seeds (Thahn et al., 2014).

Back to Basics 1.7 Van der Waals and Coulomb Interactions

Van der Waal interactions, named after Dutch physicist Johannes Diderik van der Waals (1837–1923), are weak distance-dependent interactions between neutral atoms or molecules. It can be described by a potential energy that is inversely proportional to the sixth power of the distance between the interacting molecules $\sim 1/r^6$. Being weak compared to another chemical forces, van der Waals interactions still have significant effect on the properties of substances and materials. The prominent example of the van der Waals power is the ability of gecko lizards to climb on glass surfaces. This was attributed to the van der Waals interactions between the β-keratin lamellae structures on a gecko's toe pads and the surface (Chapter 8).

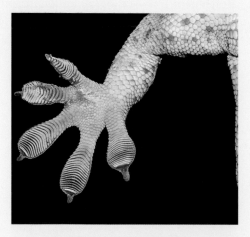

Source: ePhotocorp/iStock/Getty Images Plus.

Frequently, van der Waals force is used as a synonym for all weak intermolecular interactions, such as dispersion forces (London forces or instantaneously induced dipole interaction), dipole-induced dipole inter-action (Debye forces) and dipole–dipole interactions (Keesom forces).

Coulomb's law, first described in 1784 by French physicist Charles-Augustin de Coulomb (1736–1806), explores a force interacting between distinct point charges, which are stationary with respect to each other. **Coulomb force** is directly proportional to the magnitude of charges and inversely proportional to the square of the distance between them:

$$|F| = k_e \frac{|q_1 q_2|}{r^2},$$

where k_e is Coulomb's constant ($k_e = 8.987\,551\,787\,368\,1764 \times 10^9\,\mathrm{N\,m^2\,C^{-2}}$), q_1 and q_2 are the magnitudes of the charges, and the r is the distance between them. The force is attractive if the interacting charges have opposite signs and repulsive if charge signs are same.

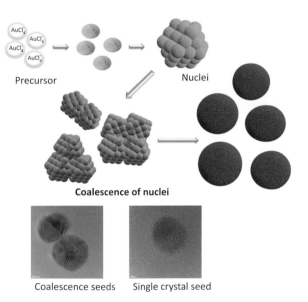

Figure 1.16

Coalescence of small nuclei is responsible for growth of multi-facet seeds.

We have explored the formation of nanoparticles, and looked at the crystal growth stages, but how much do we know about the formation of the first, small nuclei which ultimately lead to the formation of larger nanoparticles?

1.10 Nuclei Formation and the Control of the Nanoparticle Shape

Formation of nuclei or seeds is not only important for initiation of the crystal growth, but it also plays an important role in determining the shape of the nanoparticle. Particularly useful systems to shed more light on the initial stages of growth and the fate of the seeds are **clusters**. Clusters contain fewer atoms than a regular nanoparticle and enable more precise calculation of physiochemical changes over different stages of the crystal growth. They are also the first atom assemblies formed in the monomer solution, and due to the large number of surface atoms, have been shown to be powerful catalysts. For example, gold clusters loaded onto an active solid support were shown to be excellent oxidants of carbon monoxide at low temperature (Hasmi and Hutchings, 2006), and copper nanoclusters containing from 2 to 20 atoms were used for reduction of some common dye pollutants (Vilar-Vidal et al., 2012).

One of the most widely studied systems are gold clusters, and with the help of imaging techniques and computational chemistry, the detailed mechanism of what happens to the chloroauric ions, $AuCl_4^-$, in solution after addition of a reducing agents could be described. First, the ions form dimers and trimers bridged by chloride ions (Figure 1.17), which subsequently coalesce into clusters, but still contain chloroauric complexes coordinated to the surface. These complexes facilitate surface binding and coalescence of other species present in the solution until and after the nuclei are formed.

Figure 1.17

Initial stages of gold nanoparticle formation are characterised by cluster formation.

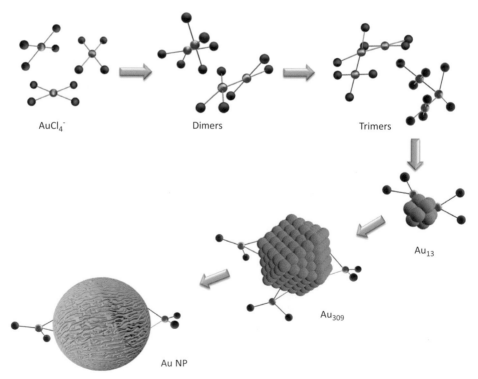

AuCl$_4^-$ Dimers   Trimers

Au$_{13}$

Au$_{309}$

Au NP

Clusters of noble metals form closed shell packing lattices following the **magic number** rule. The existence of the magic numbers can be explained by the noble gas analogy. Noble gases such as helium, argon and others found in the eighteenth group of the periodic table, are characterised by their inertness, which stems from their saturated electron shells and unavailability of electrons to engage in bonding with other elements. Unlike in noble gases, in the case of clusters, magic numbers refer to the saturation of the crystal shells (more on magic numbers in Back to Basics 1.8) not the electron shells.

Back to Basics 1.8   Clusters and Magic Numbers: Case of Noble Metals

Nuclei of noble metals have cubic crystal lattices. From a geometrical/mathematical point of view this means that atoms can be packed in a regular manner to achieve a stable atomic structure and form shells (imagine an onion and different layers and the atoms packed within these layers). Each shell can contain only a certain number of atoms and this can be represented by $N = 10\,n^2 + 2$ where N is the number of atoms and n is the number of the shell.

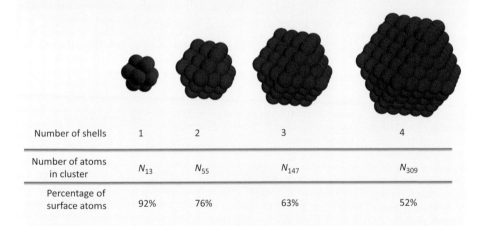

Number of shells	1	2	3	4
Number of atoms in cluster	N_{13}	N_{55}	N_{147}	N_{309}
Percentage of surface atoms	92%	76%	63%	52%

In such a way, if we consider gold nanoparticle, the core will have $N = 10 \times 1^2 + 2 = 12$ atoms in addition to the one which is at the centre of the cluster. The addition of the second shell of atoms would mean that to the existing 13 atoms, additional $N = 10 \times 2^2 + 2 = 42$ atoms are added, resulting in 55 atoms and so on (check the figure).

The noble metal magic numbers are 13, 55, 147 and so on. These will differ for other cluster classes. More on clusters and the significance of the magic numbers can be found in Wilcoxon and Abrams (2006).

The introduction of magic numbers eased the understanding of cluster formation and led to the development of reproducible methods for seed design and growth of nanoparticles of various shapes. As mentioned earlier, the shape, not only the size, of nanoparticles determines their physiochemical properties. For example, at the nanoscale, interaction with incoming light, and consequently optical properties are controlled not only by type and size of the nanomaterial, but also by its symmetry and shape. To achieve the desired properties, we need to understand the various factors responsible for the size and shape control. We also need to keep in mind that the bigger the nanoparticle, the slower it grows. As a consequence, it is difficult to manipulate the shape of the larger nanostructures. However, smaller monomers and seeds are coalescing and dissolving, and the geometry of these dynamic structures can be controlled by the addition of different chemical additives and solvents, or by changing the temperature.

Experimental studies have shown that the number of defects, such as those introduced by coalescence of differently oriented crystal facets (see Figure 1.15), within crystal seeds can have a remarkable effect on the final shape of the nanoparticles. Such defects which are a result of a fusion between different crystal domains are often referred to as **twin defects**. The appearance and frequency of twin defects will strongly depend on the reaction conditions. We will not go into the detailed mechanisms of twin defect formation, as these will depend on the nanomaterial type. However, it is important to remember that in the case of metal and metal oxides, the shape of the seeds and the number of twin defects will determine the final shape of the nanostructures (Figure 1.18).

Figure 1.18

The quality of seeds determines the shape of noble metal nanoparticles. The defects in seeds (shown in orange) determine the growth direction and the shape of the nanoparticles. Adapted from Lu et al. (2009).

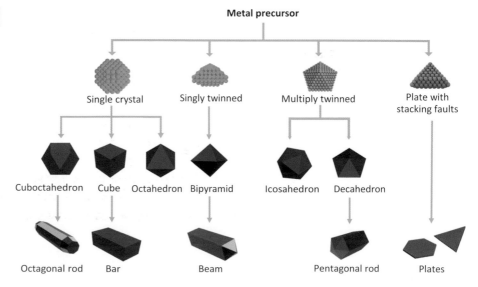

For example, a single crystal seed without defects could result in octahedral, cuboctahedral, or cubic nanoparticles, whereas multiply **twinned seeds** will grow into rods. Initial defects can sometimes be removed to improve the quality of the seeds. This is usually achieved by oxidative etching, a process in which oxidising species such as oxygen or chloride ions are introduced to the solution to smooth the defects and afford a large number of single-crystal seeds. In fact, halide ions such as chloride or bromide, can have a dramatic impact on the final shape of noble metal nanoparticles due to their ability to act as surface passivation agents. By attaching to the surface they can control the growth kinetics and formation of defects. Preparation protocols of nanoparticles are reported which involve the exclusion of oxygen by addition of oxygen scavengers such as iron (III) complexes, or use of inert atmosphere. Such conditions often result in formation of multiply twinned seeds useful for the growth of rod-shaped nanoparticles.

More often than not, before a protocol to prepare a monodispersed solution of single-shaped nanostructures can be established, a mix of shapes and sizes is obtained (Figure 1.19) and careful optimisation of the synthesis is needed. If this cannot be achieved, polydispersed solutions of nanoparticles need to be treated by different purification steps such as selective precipitation.

Figure 1.19

Transmission electron microscopy image of triangular silver plates and spherical silver nanoparticles prepared from a mixture of different seeds.

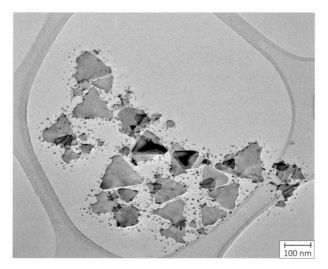

Key Concepts

Band gap: a minimum energy that is required to excite an electron up to the conduction band from the valence band. It is large for insulators and small for semiconductors, whereas in metals there is no energy gap to overcome and electrons can move freely between the bands.

Bionanotechnology: an interdisciplinary field at the intersection of nanotechnology and biology, and closely linked to nanomedicine.

Clusters: assemblies of small number of atoms formed in initial stages of metal nanoparticle formation with excellent catalytic properties.

La Mer diagram: a diagram that describes three distinct stages of crystal growth from the production of monomers, through nucleation and crystal formation.

Nanoparticle growth: is diffusion- and kinetics-controlled. Different phenomena that guide the growth of nanoparticles in solution and can be controlled by the composition of the solution and the properties of monomers and growing interfaces.

Nanotechnology: study of properties, preparation and application of man-made nanosized structures.

Ostwald ripening: a process of growth of larger (nano)crystals through dissolution of smaller crystals and structures present in the solid or in the solution.

Quantum confinement: change of electronic and optical properties as materials approach few nm in size. The spacing between the energy levels becomes more discrete, the band gap increases and the electronic structure of materials starts to resemble the electronic structure of an atom, as they reach sub-10 nm sizes.

Quantum dots: in nanotechnology quantum dots is a term that describes semiconductor nanoparticles with distinct optical and electronic properties that stem from their small size.

Random aggregation: a process by which large agglomerates of small nanoparticles are formed through chemical bonds or more often, through physical attraction at interfaces.

Surface energy at the nanoscale: is larger than its bulk counterpart and it can be reduced by surface relaxation, surface restructuring or surface modification.

Surface plasmon: collective oscillation of free electrons at the interface between conductors and dielectrics. Most used surface plasmon phenomena in biotechnology are localised surface plasmons on noble metal nanoparticles, and the surface plasmon resonance on thin gold films.

Twinned seeds: small crystal seeds with defects that can be used to control the growth of metal and metal oxide nanoparticles of different shapes.

Problems

1.1 Silicon has a density of $2330\ kg\,m^{-3}$ and an atomic weight of 28.05. Use these data to estimate the volume occupied by a silicon atom.

1.2 A typical silicon chip embedded in a computer ranges in size from a few to $600\ mm^2$. How many transistors can be fitted onto a chip if each could be made from 100 atoms of silicon in a monolayer?

1.3 Electrons in the highest occupied energy level of an atom are called valence electrons. How many valence electrons are present in (a) gold, (b) copper, (c) sodium and (d) carbon atom?

1.4 Calculate the wavelength of an electron ($m = 9.11 \times 10^{-31}$ kg) moving at $100\ 000\ m\,s^{-1}$ (hint: use the de Broglie equation found in Chapter 5).

1.5 Using the particle in the box model, estimate how much energy is emitted when an electron in an atom jumps from the fourth to the fifth energy level. Assume that the atom has a radius of 100 pm. What is the wavelength of the emitted photon? The energy of the particle in the box can be calculated using the following equation

$$E = \left(\frac{h^2}{8mL^2}\right)n^2,$$

where h is the Planck constant (6.626×10^{-34} J s), L is the distance between the opposite walls of the box corresponding to the diameter of the particle, m is the mass of the particle and n is the energy level.

1.6 Compare the surface energy of a (111) and (110) facet within FCC lattice and discuss which facet would probably be coated more quickly with a ligand X present in the solution.

1.7 A quantum dot emits a photon with a frequency of 600 THz as it drops to the valence band. Determine the band gap energy.

1.8 The properties of particles are largely dependent on their surface-to-volume ratio. Derive the equation for surface-to-volume ratio as a function of a particle radius (treating the particle as a sphere).

1.9 Explain Ostwald ripening process. How does Ostwald ripening kinetics change with particle size?

1.10 Explain the diffusion-controlled synthesis of nanoparticles using Fick's law. How do the surface properties influence the growth of nanoparticles?

1.11 Name two factors that play an important role in determining the shape of nanocrystals.

Further Reading

Lindsay, S. M. (2010). *Introduction to Nanoscience*, Oxford University Press.

Natelson, D. (2015). *Nanostructures and Nanotechnology*, Cambridge University Press.

Raether, H. (1988). *Surface Plasmons on Smooth and Rough Surfaces and on Gratings*, Springer Tracts in Modern Physics, vol. 111, Springer-Verlag.

Rogers, B. Adams, J. and Pennathur, S. (2015). *Nanotechnology: Understanding Small Systems*, CRC Press.

Simpson, M. L. and Cummings, P. T. (2011). Fluctuations and correlations in physical and biological nanosystems: the tale is in the tails. *ACS Nano*, **5**(4), 2425–2432.

Toumey, C. (2005). Apostolic succession. *Engineering and Science*, **1–2**, 16–23.

Zayats, A. V. and Smolyaninov, I. I. (2003). Near-field photonics: surface plasmon polaritons and localised surface plasmons. *Journal of Optics A: Pure and Applied Optics*, **5**, 16–50.

References

Baldan, A. (2002). Progress in Ostwald ripening theories and their applications to nickel-base superalloys, *Journal of Materials Science*, **37**, 2171–2202.

Deamer, D., Akeson, M. and Branton, D. (2016). Three decades of nanopore sequencing. *Nature Biotechnology*, **34**(5), 518–524.

Drexler, E. K. (1981). Molecular engineering: an approach to the development of general capabilities for molecular manipulation. *Proceedings of the National Academy of Sciences of the USA*, **78**(9), 5275–5278.

Feynman, R. (1960). There's plenty of room at the bottom. *Engineering and Science*, **23**(5), 22–36.

Feynman, R. (1993). Infinitesimal machinery. *Journal of Microelectromechanical Systems*, **2**(1), 4–14.

Fong, K. E. and Yung, L.-Y. L. (2013). Localised surface plasmon resonance: a unique property of plasmonic nanoparticles for nucleic acid detection. *Nanoscale*, **5**(24), 12043–12071.

Hasmi, A. S. K. and Hutchings, G. J. (2006). Gold catalysis. *Angewandte Chemie International Edition*, **45**, 7896–7936.

Kallenbach N. R., Ma R.-I. and Seeman N. C. (1983). An immobile nucleic acid junction constructed from oligonucleotides. *Nature*, **305**, 829–831.

Lu, X., Rycenga, M., Skrabalak, S. E., Wiley, B. and Xia, Y. (2009). Chemical synthesis of novel plasmonic nanoparticles. *Annual Reviews in Physical Chemistry*, **60**, 167–192.

Matsuda, Y., Thahir-Kheli, J. and Goddard, W. A. (2010). Definitive band gaps for single walled carbon nanotubes. *Journal of Physical Chemistry*, **1**, 2946–2950.

Mie, G. (1908). Beiträge zur Optik trüber Medien, speziell kolloider Metallösungen. *Annalen der Physik*, **25**, 377–445.

Mirkin, C. A., Letsinger, R. L., Mucic, R. C. and Storhoff, J. J. (1996). A DNA based method for rationally assembling nanoparticles into macroscopic materials. *Nature*, **382**, 607–609.

Nützenadel, C., Züttel, A., Chartouni, D., Schmid, G. and Schlapbach, L. (2000). Critical size and surface effect of the hydrogen interaction of palladim clusters. *The European Physical Journal D*, **8**, 245–250.

Penn, R. L. and Banfield, J. F. (1999). Morphology development and crystal growth in nanocrystalline aggregates under hydrothermal conditions: insight from titania. *Geochimica et cosmochimica acta*, **63**(10), 1549–1557.

Pound, G. M. and La Mer, V. K. (1952). Kinetics of crystalline nucleus formation in supercooled liquid tin. *Journal of the American Chemical Society*, **74**(9), 2323–2332.

Ritchie, R. H. (1957). Plasma losses by fast electrons in thin films. *Physical Review*, **106**, 874–881.

Seeman, N. C. (1981). Nucleic acid junctions: building blocks for genetic engineering in three dimensions. In R. H. Sarma (ed.), *Biomolecular Stereodynamics*, Adenine Press, pp. 269–277.

Thahn, N. T. K., Maclean, K. and Macchidine, S. (2014). Mechanism and growth of nanoparticles in solution. *Chemical Reviews*, **114**, 7610–7630.

Turkevich, J., Stevenson, P. C. and Hiller, J. (1951). A study of the nucleation and growth processes in the synthesis of colloidal gold. *Discussions of the Faraday Society*, **11**, 55–75.

Tyrrell, H. J. V. (1964). The origin and present status of Fick's diffusion law. *Journal of Chemical Education*, **41**(7), 397–400.

Vilar-Vidal, N., Rivas, J. and Lopez-Quintela, M. A. (2012). Size dependent catalytic activity of reusable subnanometer copper (0) clusters. *ACS Catalysis*, **2**(8), 1693–1697.

Wilcoxon, J. P. and Abrams, B. L. (2006). Synthesis, structure and properties of metal nanoclusters. *Chemical Society Reviews*, **35**, 1162–1194.

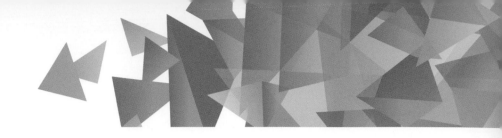

2 Nanomaterials

Preparation Strategies

Despite the relative youth of the term nanotechnology, as far as we know nanomaterials have been around for centuries. Hundreds of years ago, dispersions of **gold and silver nanoparticles** were used by master glassblowers to produce coloured decorative glass for church windows (Figure 2.1a) or luxury glassware such as the Lycurgus Cup from fourth century CE Rome (Figure 2.1b). In the late nineteenth and early twentieth centuries, industrialists used **carbon black** to reinforce rubber and thus improve its strength, tensile

Figure 2.1

(a)

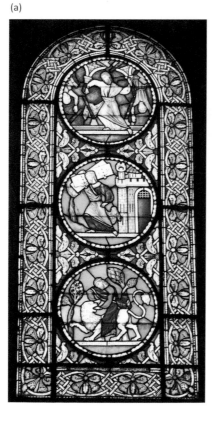

(b)

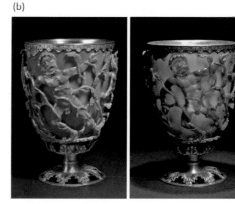

(c)

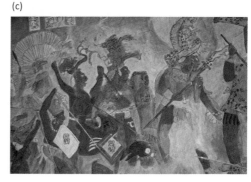

Examples of early use of nanoparticles. (a) Stained church windows were usually made using glass doped with silver and gold colloids (stained window in Ely Cathedral, UK). This work is licensed under a CC BY-SA 3.0 licence. (b) Lycurgus Cup from the fourth century appears green under daylight and red under transmitted light due to the presence of silver and gold nanoparticles. © The Trustees of the British Museum. (c) Mayan blue pigment is made by mixing indigo dye with nanoporous clay to improve the stability of the colour and prevent the photodegradation. mofles/iStock/Getty Images Plus.

properties and tear. We know now that carbon black is made of carbon particles that can vary in size, and some of them are nanosized spheres. But practical uses of early nanotechnology were not constrained only to Europe. A corrosion resistant **azure pigment** known as Mayan blue, first produced in 800 CE, was discovered in the pre-Columbian Mayan city of Chichen Itza (Figure 2.1c). It is a complex material made of nanoporous clay used to stablise the blue indigo dye. **Damascus steel swords** made in the Middle East between 300 CE and 1700 CE were known for their impressive strength and exceptionally sharp cutting edge, and studies have shown that the steel contains nanotubes and nanowire structures (Reibold, 2008). Swords were produced in a process of forging and forming that employs coal, iron powder, high temperatures and high pressures applied during hammering, a protocol that is in many ways similar to how the nanotubes are made today (see Section 2.4.2).

With the development of modern science, and in particular in the nineteenth century, colloidal solutions of nanoparticles were prepared using the more scientific methods of chemical synthesis, although the products were not always what were expected. For example, the red colloidal gold solution made by Michael Faraday (1791–1867) in 1857, still on display in Faraday Museum at the Royal Institution in London, was made accidentally by washing thin gold metal leaf with a mix of chemicals that included a reducing agent – white phosphorus. Michael Faraday studied and described the colloidal solutions he prepared, paving the way to colloid science and later nanotechnology. But it was not until powerful microscopes were designed during the latter half of the twentieth century that nanomaterials could be properly characterised and new synthetic methods developed.

Although there are numerous protocols available for preparation of a wide range of nanostructures, old strategies are continuously improved and new ones introduced with the aim of minimising the energy input, removing the use of toxic and expensive reagents, and enabling scale up. Production of large amounts of nanomaterials is particularly challenging. There are several reasons for that, one being the sensitivity of many bottom-up processes to concentration, temperature, diffusion rate, all of which need to be transferred from micro to macro scale without compromising the quality of the product. Considering that the range of applications is increasing, the next decade could see the development of affordable processes capable of achieving controllable shape and sizes of nanostructures on a larger scale.

2.1   Bottom-Up and Top-Down Strategies

To illustrate how different types of nanostructures can be prepared and modified, in this chapter we will focus mainly on bottom-up in-solution strategies. **Bottom-up processes** employ synthesis and self-assembly (more on self-assembly in Chapter 4) of smaller elements (molecules or atoms) to obtain larger structures (Figure 2.1) in solution. The most important aspect of the bottom-up approaches is the use of physical and chemical forces that act on a nanoscale to achieve larger assemblies. Biomolecules are made by bottom-up approach, and it is not surprising that this strategy is particularly well-suited for preparation of hybrid bio–nano structures. In-solution prepared nanomaterials and hybrids are often easier to stabilise and modify with hydrophilic biomolecules. The processing and extraction of desired materials from solution can be done using readily available strategies such as size-dependent precipitation or size exclusion chromatography, and the whole process can be scaled up and optimised using process engineering and microfluidics, although such strategies are not without their challenges.

Contrary to the bottom-up, **top-down approaches**, as the name states, encompass such processes like carving out the bulk material, or printing or patterning the surfaces to contain defined nanopatterns (Figure 2.2). Such are different lithographic methods (Back to Basics 2.1), which can be used to design patterns of molecules down to 100 nm resolution, although the processes involved in lithography tend to be slow, expensive and require significant expertise.

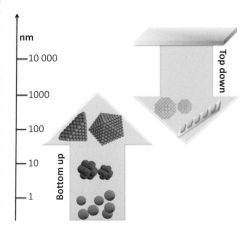

Figure 2.2

Nanomaterials and bio–nano hybrids can be prepared using bottom-up or top-down strategies. Whereas bottom-up starts with smaller elements (molecules and atoms) to build larger structures through assembly, top-down usually starts with much larger structures and bulk materials from which nanostructures can be carved out, etched or patterned through lithography or printing.

Top-down strategies have been extensively employed in nanoelectronics for design of integrated circuits, and in the field of biosensing to prepare sensor components. The fabrication of top-down structures is generally more expensive and slower than the bottom-up structures. Whereas top-down methods might require more physics and engineering, and are limited by instrumentation (which can be really expensive) and not easily scaled up, bottom-up involve wet chemistry and can be easily adapted by any lab. Ultimately, the nanosized hybrid materials prepared using both approaches make use of the same biofunctionalisation strategies (Chapter 4). In reality, devices and intelligent, adaptable materials for medical use and beyond require a combination of top-down and bottom-up strategy. For example, tissue engineering of a bone (Chapter 9) often requires design of a nanopatterned scaffolds obtained by carving of a bulk metal, and bottom-up assembly of nanoparticles and biomolecules to create a structure that resembles natural bone tissue.

Details on top-down strategies can be found in recommended reading material, and in the following sections we will focus on various bottom-up strategies to synthesise different types of nanostructures.

| Back to Basics 2.1 | Top-Down Method: Lithography |

Photolithography refers to design of nanostructured surfaces with the help of light. A substrate (i.e. glass) is covered with the layer of photoresist (light-sensitive polymer, such as PMMA: polymethylmethacrylate). A mask, which can be made of anything that blocks the light, is prepared separately and physically attached to the surface of the photoresist. Irradiation (usually UV) leads to the scission of carbon–carbon bonds in polymer at the sites exposed to light. Smaller polymer fragments, which are produced can easily be removed by washing. This strategy is known as **positive photoresist**. Light exposure can also cause hardening of the photoresist, and in that case we talk about **negative photoresist**, which remains insoluble upon irradiation and removal of the mask. Although the role of the mask is to block the light, the light will be diffusing around the edges of the mask pattern, and therefore maximum resolution set by the original mask is seldom achieved. Rather, there is a resolution limit, determined by the Rayleigh equation in which the minimum resolvable feature, r, is:

$$r = \frac{k\lambda}{NA},$$

where NA is a numerical aperture depending on a refractive index and the angle (called collection angle) between the light source and the obstacle, and k is a material determined factor with values usually between 0.5 and 1.0. As can be seen from the equation, smaller features can be achieved with decrease in the wavelength λ of the incoming light; for nanometre features one should use laser light with wavelengths smaller than 200 nm, which is not readily available.

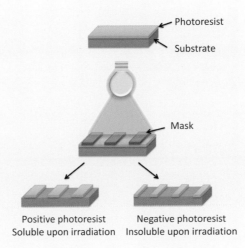

Other than UV light, the photoresist can be etched using electron beam (**e-beam lithography**) or X-ray (**X-ray lithography**), both of which require expensive equipment and handling expertise.

Soft lithography methods use printing, stamping and moulding of polymers and the principle of self-assembly instead of light and electrons to create patterns. An example of such lithography is microcontact printing, in which a polymer stamp is designed (usually employing a mould prepared by photolithography). The stamp is then immersed into 'ink', a solution of molecules that can form self-assembly layers on the printed surface. These might be thiol molecules on gold surface, for example (Chapter 4). Resolution down to 100 nm has been achieved by printing biomolecules for biosensor design.

2.2 Preparation of Metallic Nanostructures

In the previous chapter, we mentioned that bottom-up, in-solution procedures involve reduction of salt precursors to zero valent metal M(0) with the help of various **reducing agents**. To allow for the control of nucleation and growth of nanomaterials, different additives such as polymers or ions may be added. Most common precursors are metal salts or complexes, although some nanoparticles can also be made electrochemically using metal anodes (Table 2.1).

Table 2.1 Some precursors and reducing agents for the preparation of metal nanoparticles

Common precursors	Chemical formula	Reducing agents	Chemical formula
Tetrachloroauric (III) acid	$HAuCl_4$	Sodium borohydride	$NaBH_4$
Silver nitrate	$AgNO_3$	Citric acid	$C_6H_8O_7$
Silver perchlorate	$AgClO_4$	Hydrogen peroxide	H_2O_2
Hexachloroplatinic (VI) acid	H_2PtCl_6	Hydrogen	H_2
Palladium (II) chloride	$PdCl_2$	Methanol	CH_3OH
Copper (II) acetylacetonate	$Cu(C_5H_7O_2)_2$	Formaldehyde	$HCHO$
Rhodium (III) chloride	$RhCl_3$	Ketyl radical	$(CH_3)_2\dot{C}O$

The choice of reducing agents will depend on the type of reaction, the desired rate of the seed formation and compatibility with other chemicals present in the solution. If the reducing agent is too strong, it might engage in reaction with other components in the solution and lead to unwanted side products. One such strong reducing agent is the widely used sodium borohydride $NaBH_4$. When milder conditions are required, reducing agents such as citric or ascorbic acid (vitamin C) can be used. There are also a number of reducing agents that play a double role and can both reduce the metal precursor and coordinate the surface of the grown seeds and small nanoparticles making them more stable – such as some acids, for example, citric acid or alcohols such as ethylene glycol. There are also a number of biomolecules, in particular different enzymes and sugars that have been used to prepare a variety of metal nanoparticles although with limited success in terms of monodispersity.

2.2.1 Use of Strong Reducing Agents: A Case of Gold Nanoparticles

A significant advance in preparation of small, stable and well-dispersed metal nanoparticles (2–10 nm) was made by Mathias Brust and David J. Schiffrin and colleagues in 1994. Making such small and monodispersed structures was not an easy task, and to overcome the issues of aggregation, Brust et al. introduced a two-phase synthesis of gold nanoparticles. They employed **sodium borohydride, NaBH$_4$**, to afford fast reduction at the water–organic solvent interface followed by immediate capping with thiol-containing compounds for particle stabilisation (Figure 2.3).

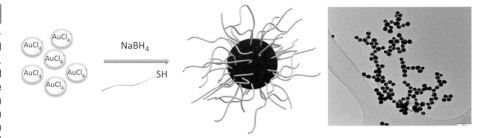

Figure 2.3

Preparation of thiol-capped gold nanoparticles (red). AuCl$_4^-$ ions are reduced using NaBH$_4$ in the presence of thiol (−SH) ligands. Transmission electron micrograph shows regular spherical nanoparticles.

It is worth looking into this strategy in more detail as it marked the beginning of controllable synthesis of monodispersed solutions of various metal nanoparticles. The first step of the procedure is dissolving a gold precursor, tetrachloroauric acid HAuCl$_4$ followed by addition of tetraoctylammonium bromide (TOAB) in toluene. Tetraoctylammonium bromide acts both as a stabilising agent and a phase-transfer catalyst, which means that it can facilitate the transfer of AuCl$_4^-$ ions from the aqueous solution to toluene to be reduced at the water–organic interface with NaBH$_4$ dissolved in water. As soon as the reducing agent is added, the colour of the solution changes from yellow to red due to the growth of gold nanoparticles (Figure 2.4). They are immediately stabilised by thiol ligand capping and can be extracted from the mixture.

The Brust–Schiffrin method is characterised by ease of reduction and production of small, but stable, nanoparticles, which are obtained as a monodispersed solution of spherical gold. Important innovation was also the use of thiol molecules as surface capping agents; different thiol-containing compounds could be used depending on the requirements of the subsequent application. The choice of the thiol could make nanoparticles more hydrophilic or hydrophobic, therefore changing their behaviour in various solvent mixtures. Although this particular strategy has been replaced with other

Figure 2.4

Gold nanoparticle preparation by the Brust–Schiffrin method. Gold nanoparticles (red) are formed from HAuCl₄ precursor (yellow). The procedure involves use of a reducing agent at the organic solvent–water interface and capping with thiol ligands.

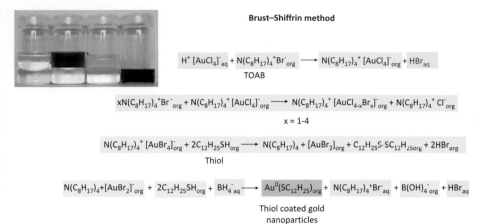

strategies, both $NaBH_4$ and thiols are used as common reagents not only for preparation of gold but also other metallic nanomaterials.

2.2.2   Use of Mild Reducing Agents: A Case of Platinum Nanoparticles

Being a strong reducing agent, $NaBH_4$ cannot always be used for reduction of precursor salts as it is very reactive and could react with other chemicals present in the solution. When this is the case, milder reducing reagents need to be employed. One such reagent is methanol, which was successfully used for the preparation of platinum nanoparticles from H_2PtCl_6 precursor in the presence of polyvinylpyrrolidone (PVP) as a stabilising ligand. Ligands such as PVP form a protective layer around nanoparticles to prevent further growth and aggregation (check Chapter 1 for details and diffusion and surface-controlled growth). A two-step reduction of the precursor can be represented by chemical equations shown below (Duff, 1995):

$$PtCl_6{}^{2-} + CH_3OH \rightleftharpoons PtCl_4{}^{2-} + HCHO + 2\,H^+ + 2\,Cl^-$$

$$PtCl_4{}^{2-} + CH_3OH \rightleftharpoons Pt^0{}_{sol} + HCHO + 2\,H^+ + 4\,Cl^-.$$

Understanding the steps involved in the reduction can help us to predict the effect of various additives on the growth of nanoparticles. This can be done utilising the **Le Chatelier's principle**, which states that the position of chemical equilibrium changes to counteract any disturbance caused by the change of conditions. In the case of the above reactions, the principle implies that an increase of the Cl^- ion concentration will move the equilibrium towards the left-hand side, and slow down the nucleation. Namely, the supply of Pt(0) monomers will be limited due to the decrease in the amount of the PtCl$_4^{2-}$ intermediate, subsequently slowing down the formation of nuclei. Low concentration of monomers will favour a diffusion-controlled growth of platinum nanoparticles, resulting in monodispersed solution of nearly spherical particles. If, on the other hand, pH is increased or Cl$^-$ is removed, for example by precipitation, this will push the equilibrium towards Pt(0) production. Consequently, a large number of nuclei will be generated, resulting in faster burst nucleation, and ultimately seed defects and growth of larger particles of varied shapes. The PVP polymer added as a stabiliser to this reaction mixture increases the amount of regular, spherical nanoparticles. By acting as a growth barrier, it forms a protecting layer around the surface and increases the viscosity of the surrounding solution, therefore promoting the diffusion-controlled growth of spherical particles.

2.2.3   Micelle-Guided Reduction

Micelles are supramolecular aggregates with liquid cores formed in thermodynamically stable liquid mixtures usually composed of a minimum of three but more often four components: oil, water, and one or more surfactants. Droplet size used for metal nanoparticle synthesis is usually around 100 nm and the ratio of water to surfactant (w/s ratio) to achieve these sizes needs to be larger than 15. The simplest micelles are spherical clusters of a surfactant in water, which results in formation of hydrophobic core, and they are known as direct micelles. Reverse micelles, on the other hand, are formed when the water to surfactant ratio is smaller than 15, and they are smaller droplets (size 1–10 nm) with hydrophilic, usually water, core. Reverse micelles are kinetically unstable and can exchange the content when they collide. The size and shape of micelles can be controlled by a careful combination of all components, which can have obvious advantages for the synthesis of nanoparticles. Besides metallic nanoparticles, many different types have been prepared using **micelle-guided strategies**.

Typical synthesis of metallic nanoparticles using micelles involves preparation of two (or more) types of micelles, each loaded with a different component necessary for nanoparticle formation. For example, for preparation of platinum nanoparticles, a reducing agent such as NaBH$_4$ is loaded in one, and H$_2$PtCl$_6$ precursor in another batch of micelles. The content of two different droplets can be exchanged through fast particle fusion–fission process, with both reagents combining and reacting at the interface to form nanoparticles (Figure 2.5).

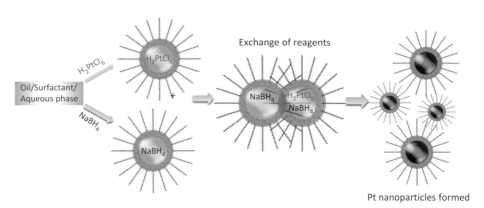

Figure 2.5

Microemulsion strategy for preparation of Pt nanoparticles. Precursor and the reducing agent are packed within nanodroplets which fuse and enable formation of monosized nanoparticles.

The size of nanoparticles is generally related to the initial size of the droplets and obtained nanomaterials are monodispersed. Additional control over size and kinetics of droplet fusion can be achieved by use of various surfactants such as sodium dioctyl-sulfosuccinate (AOT), which minimise the tension between two immiscible liquid phases (oil and water).

Micelle-guided synthetic approaches are desirable strategies when control over the shape and size of nanoparticles is needed; precursor and reducing agents can be entrapped within the droplet core and either allowed to merge or to exchange the content to ensure the nucleation and growth. Such synthesis also does not involve the use of high temperature or toxic compounds making it environmentally desirable. In addition, in the case of reverse micelles, the tail of the interface surfactants can be modified to contain specific molecules suitable for binding onto the growing nanoparticles, easing the surface stabilisation and addition of functional groups suitable for further modifications.

Finally, once prepared, nanoparticles are usually extracted by the destruction of micelles, which can be achieved by pH change or temperature increase.

2.2.4   Polyols and Surface Capping Agents for Shape Control

Polyols are organic compounds containing multiple OH groups and their most prominent member is ethylene glycol, $HOCH_2CH_2OH$. They can act both as efficient solvents and reducing agents ensuring continuous production of uniformly shaped seeds. The addition of a well-chosen surface capping agent, which selectively binds to a particular crystal facet of initially formed seeds, can then guide the growth into various geometrical shapes. For example, when silver nitrate (AgNO₃) is heated in ethylene glycol, small silver nanoparticles are obtained, which can grow further into regular cuboctahedra upon controlled addition of polyvinylpyrrolidone (PVP), a non-toxic polymer that contains a hydrophilic component and hydrophobic carbon chain. The PVP binds onto (100) facets of small silver seeds, stabilising them and allowing deposition of further Ag seeds (Figure 2.6).

Figure 2.6

PVP-aided synthesis of silver nanoparticles. Monodispersed silver nanocrystals with regular polyhedral shapes are synthesised by reduction of silver nitrate using polyvinylpyrrolidone (PVP) as a capping polymer. (a) During the nucleation and growth silver deposits continuously onto the (100) facet of the fcc crystal lattice, resulting in formation of octahedron with completely bound (111) facets. (b)–(f) SEM images of cubes, truncated cubes, cuboctahedra, truncated octahedra and octahedra (scale bar: 100 nm). Adapted from Tao et al. (2006), by permission of John Wiley and Sons.

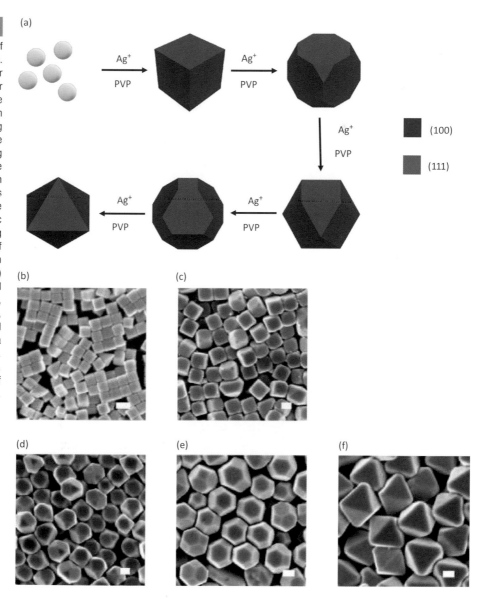

Overall, reduction of Ag$^+$ ions to Ag nanoparticles can be written as:

$$2HOCH_2CH_2OH \xrightarrow{\Delta} 2CH_3CHO + H_2$$

$$2CH_3CHO + 2Ag^+ \xrightarrow{\Delta} 2Ag^0 + 2H^+ + CH_3COCOCH_3.$$

The PVP acts as an excellent capping agent, and has been also used to passivate the surface and ease the preparation of porous and cage-like metal nanostructures. A range of porous metallic structures can be made using a principle of **galvanic replacement**, a redox process in which one metal gets oxidised by ions of another with higher reduction potential. Hollow cubes or cages can be prepared using cubic silver seeds, which are selectively etched/replaced by gold ions (Figure 2.7). The reaction starts locally at the cube facets and as it proceeds Ag is oxidised, further releasing electrons. Those are captured by AuCl$_4^-$ resulting in the production of Au(0) which grows onto the cube. As the gold layer is generated, the initially formed hole within the Ag cube (Figure 2.7b) serves as the site for Ag dissolution (Figure 2.7c) and, ultimately, the cube turns into a porous nanobox (Figure 2.7d).

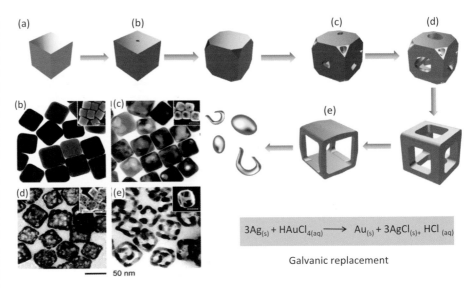

Figure 2.7

Preparation of porous gold structures by galvanic replacement. In the presence of chloroauric acid (HAuCl$_4$) silver atoms from a template nanocube (a) are continuously replaced by gold atoms (b→c→d), resulting in a caged structure (e). Transmission electron micrographs show these different stages of galvanic replacement. Adapted with permission from Skrabalak et al. (2008). © 2008 American Chemical Society.

$$3Ag_{(s)} + HAuCl_{4(aq)} \longrightarrow Au_{(s)} + 3AgCl_{(s)} + HCl_{(aq)}$$

Galvanic replacement

Further reaction leads to the production of cages (Figure 2.7e) and finally, complete dissolution. To control the wall thickness and porosity as well as to obtain pure Au frames, wet etchants such as Fe(NO$_3$)$_3$ can be employed, which speed up complete dissolution of the remaining Ag template.

Gold hollow nanostructures prepared by galvanic replacement of silver nanoparticles have already found an application in sensor design. They are excellent substrates for enhancement of Raman signal in surface plasmon resonance scattering (SERS, see Chapter 5). Such cage/hollow structures also absorb near-infrared light and can be used to induce hyperthermia useful for heating up and eliminating cancer cells (Chapter 9).

2.2.5 Metallic Nanoparticles: A Brief Overview of Other Methods

The **light-induced reduction** is an excellent strategy to afford spatial and temporal control over the growth of nanoparticles. In light-induced reduction, reducing agents are **radical species** produced upon irradiation of an otherwise inert precursor. The activation energy for such processes is usually high and requires the use of UV/visible light. Light-induced reduction is particularly suitable for in situ growth of nanomaterials and conductive layers within different non-conductive materials such as polymers or hydrogels (see Back to Basics 2.5). For example, to prepare silver nanoparticles, silver nitrate ($AgNO_3$) precursor can be reduced using UV illumination of acetone in 2-propanol, resulting in the production of ketyl radical, which acts as a reducing agent:

Ketyl radical

Although irradiation without the presence of coordinating ligand often results in a polydispersed solution of nanoparticles, its advantage is the external control over reduction by control of the irradiation (ON–OFF switching). Such control was used to design switchable electronic devices in which the conductivity is switched on by the growth of conducting silver nanoparticles of different sizes within an inert matrix under UV irradiation (Hung et al., 2015).

Electrochemical reduction of the metal anode to produce nanoparticles has several advantages. High purity of the particles can be achieved, the set-up is cheap and easy, and the current density can be used to control the nucleation and growth of nanoparticles. On the other hand, the method is limited by the availability of the electrode material and deposition of reduced metal on the cathode, which causes the system deactivation and arrest of the particle production. In order to prepare stable nanoparticles and prevent their aggregation, stabilising ligands should be added to the electrolyte (Figure 2.8).

Figure 2.8

Electrochemical
production of Ag
nanoparticles. Silver
anode is used as a
source of silver ions and
current density can be
used to control the
nucleation and growth of
nanoparticles.

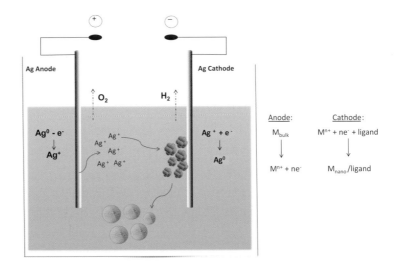

Decomposition of metallo-organic complexes has often been used in prep-aration of platinum and copper nanoparticles and it is based on the use of metal complexes containing organic ligands such as dibenzylideneacetone (DBA).

DBA

Decomposition can be achieved by control over the solvent combinations, temperatures, and pressures and depending on conditions different shapes such as nanowires and rods can selectively be prepared (Ramirez et al., 2007).

Laser-induced size reduction is a relatively new method based on the use of powerful lasers to ablate the surface of larger nanoparticles into various sizes. It works best for plasmonic materials such as noble metals as the wavelength of the laser can be adjusted to their plasmon resonance. In such a way, more control over shape and size can be achieved. To make sure that nanoparticles are not simply fried and destroyed, a pulsed laser is commonly used, which makes the whole strategy pretty expensive (Werner and Hashi-moto, 2013).

There are numerous variations of all of the mentioned strategies to prepare different shapes and sizes of metal nanoparticles. The choice will largely depend on the final product requirements: size, shape, surface charge and ligand and, ultimately, the application.

2.3   Preparation of Metal Oxide Nanomaterials

General principles of nanoparticle growth discussed in Chapter 1 such as burst nucleation, diffusion-controlled growth apply to metal oxide nanomaterials, although they are much less understood than in the case of metallic nanoparticles. Metal oxides are more thermally and chemically stable than metals, so the nanoparticle growth is not as easily manipulated. For example, Ostwald ripening, which plays an important role in determining the size and homogeneity of shapes by directing the growth of the larger particles at the expense of the smaller, has been shown to be less effective and to require prolonged heating after nucleation.

The most common method for preparation of metal oxide nanomaterials is **sol–gel processing** (Back to Basics 2.2). Depending on the class of precursors and conditions used, the sol–gel strategy for oxide nanomaterials preparation can be divided into the hydrolysis of alkoxide precursors and the hydrolysis of metal salts.

Back to Basics 2.2   Sol–Gel Processing

Sol–gel processing refers to a wet chemical route for the synthesis of colloidal dispersions of inorganic and organic–inorganic hybrids, particularly oxides and oxide–base hybrids. It usually consists of hydrolysis and condensation of precursors, which can be either metal alkoxides or inorganic/organic salts. Catalysts are often added to promote hydrolysis and condensation reactions. Alkoxides are strong bases with a formula RO^-, where R is the organic substituent. An example of sol–gel processing is the preparation of Si dioxide nanoparticles from tetramethyl orthosilicate, $Si(OCH_3)_4$, as a precursor.

Step 1 is the hydrolysis of the precursor to achieve replacement of alkoxide groups:

$$Si(OR)_4 + x\,H_2O \rightarrow Si(OR)_{4-x}(OH)_x + x\,ROH.$$

Step 2 is condensation and there are two different routes by which it can be achieved:

(a) condensation with formation of water:

or

(b) condensation with formation of alcohol:

Both hydrolysis and condensation consist of several additional steps, which are not further discussed here.

Other common methods for preparation of metal oxide nanoparticles are high-temperature non-hydrolitic and the reverse micelle strategy described earlier. For example, titanium dioxide (TiO_2) nanoparticles have been made using micelles made of Triton surfactant which were packed with titanium (IV) tetrachloride ($TiCl_4$) precursor. In the presence of water, titanium salt hydrolyses, affording nanoparticles with sizes which correspond to the initial size of the micelles. To obtain pure nanoparticles, micelles are usually destroyed by heating or a change of pH, and isolated nanoparticles can either be used as prepared or employed as seeds for further growth through Ostwald ripening.

2.3.1   Hydrolysis of Alkoxide Precursors

There are a few classes of oxide nanomaterials that are of particular interest for bionanotechnology. Such as iron oxide (Fe_2O_3 or Fe_3O_4) nanomaterials, characterised by their exceptional magnetic properties, and silica nanomaterials, in particular, porous silica (SiO_2) nanoparticles, shown to be effective vehicles for encapsulation and delivery of drugs (see Chapter 9). Both classes have made it all the way to clinical trials with iron oxide nanomaterials making it all the way into clinical use, and silica-based systems being approved as imaging tools.

Hydrolysis of alkoxide precursors is used to prepare the majority of silica and titanium dioxide (TiO_2) nanomaterials. The reactivity of alkoxide compounds is inversely proportional to their size, and generally, tetrapropyl silicate $Si(OC_2H_5)_4$ with a larger organic unit is less reactive than smaller tetramethyl silicate $Si(OCH_3)_4$. Consequently, the choice of the precursor determines the rate of nuclei production and subsequent nanoparticle growth. But there are also other factors that impact the nanoparticle shape and size such as the temperature and pH, as well as the presence of organic compounds, which can be used to control the hydrolysis. In the case of SiO_2 nanoparticles, reaction rate and size of the particles are strongly dependent on solvents, precursors, amount of added water, and the presence of bases such as ammonia. Ammonia is critical for the condensation step and it has been shown to aid the formation of the well-defined geometric shapes.

The method in which the hydrolysis and condensation are facilitated by the addition of the base in ethanol/water mixture is known as the Stöber method after Werner Stöber and his coworkers who described sol–gel synthesis of silica nanoparticles ranging in size from 50 nm to 2 μm in 1968 (Stöber et al., 1968; Figure 2.9).

Contrary to the use of the base, preparation of silica under acidic conditions results in linear polymer-like chains, which ultimately lead to large amorphous structures.

Figure 2.9

Stöber method for preparation of silica nanoparticles. (a) Hydrolysis and condensation reactions and (b) the original electron macrograph. Adapted from Stöber et al. (1968) with permission from Elsevier.

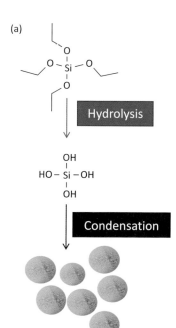

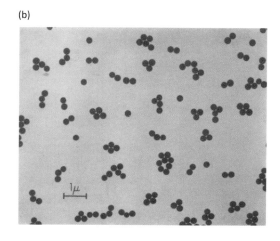

2.3.2 Hydrolysis of Inorganic or Organic Metal Salts

In the 1970s, Egon Matijević (1922–2016) and his coworkers extensively studied magnetic colloids (the term nanoparticle had not yet been coined), particularly formation of different shapes and sizes of iron oxide forms such as haematite (α-Fe$_2$O$_3$) and akagancite (β-FeOOH) through hydrolysis of iron (III) chloride, FeCl$_3$:

$$FeCl_3 + 3H_2O \rightarrow \alpha\text{-}Fe_2O_3/\beta\text{-}FeOOH + HCl.$$

Depending on the conditions, iron oxide nanoparticles of different morphology can be obtained, and akageneite is often just an intermediate compound that results in magnetic iron oxide nanoparticles. Commonly, the strategy to prepare magnetic nanoparticles involves the use of diluted precursor solutions to afford diffusion control and an addition of hydrochloric acid to control the kinetics of particle formation by shifting equilibrium to the left. To obtain different shapes, ageing of the solution at high temperature (100 °C) is important as it affects the Ostwald ripening process (Figure 2.10).

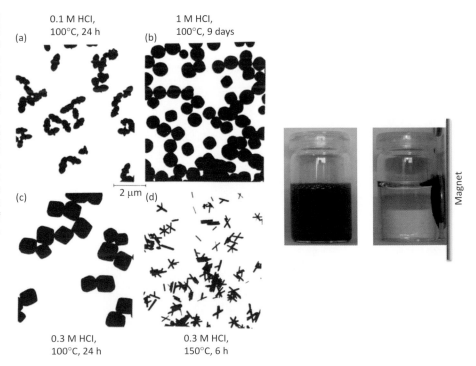

Figure 2.10

Iron oxide nanoparticles prepared from FeCl$_3$ precursor. Different sizes and shapes of nanoparticles can be achieved by varying the concentration of HCl, temperature and time of reaction (left) (adapted from Matijević, 1977, with permission from Elsevier), and magnetic nanoparticles in the absence and presence of an external magnet.

While studying magnetic nanoparticles, Matijević realised that it is crucial to report the exact information on the synthetic procedure, and noted that the solutions of the identical chemical composition can result in entirely different morphology and size of the nanoparticles. He stressed the importance of a treatment after the initial colloids are formed, correctly predicting the value of the controlled Ostwald ripening (Matijević, 1977).

Thus far, there are eight different crystal forms of iron oxide. Three lattice structures of these eight – *magnetite* (Fe_3O_4), *haematite* (α-Fe_2O_3) and *maghemite* (γ-Fe_2O_3) – have been used profusely due to their distinct magnetic and catalytic properties. Magnetite and maghemite nanoparticles have been particularly useful for bionanotechnology as they are the most magnetic of the forms. They have also been among the first nanoparticles to make it from the lab to the clinic and have been used as contrast agents for magnetic resonance imaging (MRI) and magnetically controlled delivery of drug cargo to different tumour sites (see Chapter 9).

In general, magnetic properties of iron oxide nanoparticles differ significantly from the properties of the bulk material and are characterised by superparamagnetism, magnetism which can be switched on by the applied magnetic field but disappears when the field is removed (Back to Basics 2.3).

| Back to Basics 2.3 | Types of Magnetism |

Diamagnetism, often referred to as 'negative' magnetism, was named and studied by Michael Faraday. All substances are diamagnetic: the strong external magnetic field speeds up or slows down the electrons orbiting the atoms in such a way to oppose the action of the external field. For diamagnetic materials the value of the susceptibility (a measure of the relative amount of induced magnetism) is always negative and typically near negative one-millionth.

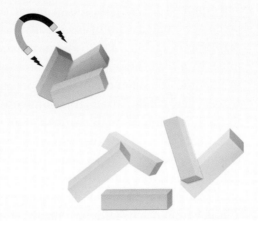

Ferromagnetism is characterised by net magnetisation independent of the external magnetic field. Ferromagnets are strong magnets and the typical examples are ferrite, α-iron and magnetite, iron oxide Fe_3O_4.

Paramagnetism does not show net magnetisation, but rather a magnetic moment is induced by a magnetic field and not retained after the field is removed. A large number of elements and compounds are paramagnetic as this is the consequence of the unpaired electrons in the atomic or molecular orbitals. This type of magnetism is often exhibited by compounds containing iron, platinum or rare-earth elements, but there are a few other groups of materials that might show weaker or stronger paramagnetism.

Superparamagnetism is a paramagnetism characterised by a much larger magnetic susceptibility. This type occurs in small ferri- and ferro-magnetic nanoparticles. Superparamagnetism makes nanoparticles very attractive for nanomedicine, in particular to be used as probes for magnetic resonance imaging (MRI) or for design of magnetically guided drug delivery.

The magnetisation of the particles depends strongly on their size, shape, crystallinity, and the presence of doping metals and defects. Since the 1970s, various hybrid magnetic nanoparticles have been synthesised using variations of principles established by Matijević and his coworkers. Some of them have also been successfully scaled up and today we can make iron oxide-based nanoparticles on a kilogram scale.

2.3.3   High-Temperature Non-Hydrolytic Methods

This method for preparation of metal oxide nanoparticles uses various salt precursors, but reactions are usually performed in organic solvents at temperatures as high as 300 °C and in the presence of surfactants such as oleylamine to afford nanoparticle stabilisation. High temperature ensures rapid production of monomers and the supersaturation needed for burst nucleation. Under these conditions, a large number of small nuclei is formed, which leads to the formation of small particles. The ratio of surfactant oleylamine to the precursors can additionally be used to control the shape and size of nanoparticles. For example, when bimetallic oxides are produced using iron and manganese acetylacetonate ($Fe(acac)_3$ and $Mn(acac)_2$), cubic nanoparticles are obtained if the ratio of oleylamine to the iron salt is less than 3:1, whereas a larger ratio results in cuboctahedra (Figure 2.11).

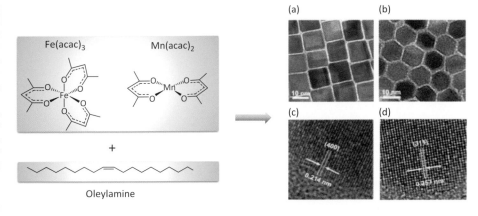

Cuboctahedral nanoparticles are the result of formation of smaller, unstable nuclei prone to coalescence, which results in seed defects and seed-guided nanoparticle growth as described in Chapter 1.

2.4 Synthesis of Quantum Dots

Tunable fluorescence (Chapter 1) makes semiconducting quantum dots particularly interesting for use in biological imaging and development of novel cancer diagnostics. Unlike organic dyes, quantum dots (QDs) often have a broad excitation range and narrow emission. Broad absorption allows multiple readouts from differently sized quantum dots after irradiation with a single light source. Quantum dots also have large molar absorption coefficients (1×10^5–25×10^5 $M^{-1} cm^{-1}$) compared to organic dyes (0.25×10^5–2.5×10^5 $M^{-1} cm^{-1}$) and exhibit longer fluorescence lifetimes (larger than 10 ns) compared to organic fluorophores (1–5 ns). This behaviour results in significant improvement of signal-to-noise ratio and ease of detection when materials with intrinsic fluorescence such as biological tissues are imaged.

Since the properties of QDs depend on their size, it is crucial to control their synthesis to afford the narrow size distribution. This is often achieved under high temperatures (150–370 °C) to afford rapid production of large amounts of nuclei and formation of smaller nanoparticles, and in the presence of surfactants such as trioctylphosphine (TOP) or trioctylphosphine oxide (TOPO) to arrest further growth (Murray et al., 1993).

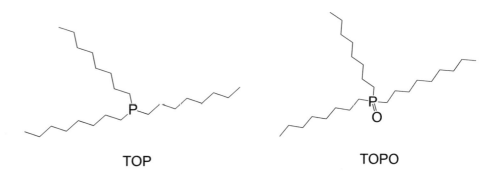

TOP   TOPO

Precursors for synthesis of the first generation of quantum dots were metal alkyls such as dimethyl cadmium, $Cd(CH_3)_2$, to which various metal powders such as selenium, Se (to afford CdSe nanoparticles) or sulphur, S (for CdS nanoparticles) are added. First prepared by Louis E. Brus, quantum dots were extensively explored in the 1990s and the high-temperature synthesis has since been adapted to afford various compositions and different levels of fluorescence efficiency. However, high-temperature synthesis is not economically viable and does not allow for the use of heat-sensitive organic surfactants and solvents. These drawbacks prompted the development of low-temperature synthesis. In one such example, a precursor is first heated in oleylamine surface ligand at 90 °C, after which the addition of elemental sulphur and further heating to 140 °C affords CdS nanoparticles of various sizes depending on the heating time.

Optical properties of quantum dots depend not only on the size of the nanoparticles but also on the presence of surface defects. Often, a crystalline layer (a shell) is added on top of the core nanoparticle, to remove the detrimental defect, resulting in **core–shell nanoparticles** (Figure 2.12).

The addition of a shell increases the overall size of the quantum dot, and since the fluorescence depends on the size, only certain fluorescence emissions

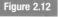

Figure 2.12

Core–shell ZnS–CdSe quantum dot. It consists of inner core of cadmium selenide (CdSe) coated with the stabilising shell of zinc sulphide (ZnS).

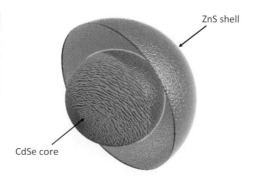

ZnS shell

CdSe core

can be achieved with core–shell systems. However, shells such as zinc-sulphide (ZnS) are useful to prevent the leakage of toxic core elements such as cadmium (Cd) and selenium (Se). The majority of the quantum dots used in biology and medicine are based on Cd-systems, composed of cadmium and elements such as sulphur and selenium. Others involve a combination of groups III and V (InP, InAs) or IV and VI (PbSe, PbTe) of the periodic system of elements. Many of the elements used for preparation of quantum dots are toxic, and although the addition of a stabilising shell prevents their leakage, they are often not suitable for use in biological systems, with the exception of applications requiring cell death such as photodynamic therapy of pathogens (see Research Report 2.1). The issues with biocompatibility motivated the development of quantum dots free of toxic components by using elements from group I, II and VI ($CuInS_2$, $AgInS_2$) (Xu et al., 2016).

Research Report 2.1 | Quantum Dots for Improved Antibiotic Activity

Tunable fluorescent properties of quantum dots, in particular those made of non-toxic elements such as CuI–ZnS, are useful probes for labelling of different cell compartments. However, quantum dots are also semiconductors and when illuminated with light they can generate excited electrons and holes called **excitons** across their nominal energy band gap. Once produced, such excitons are available for reduction and oxidation reactions.

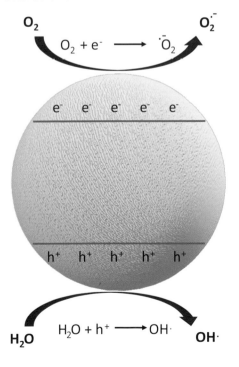

$$O_2 \qquad\qquad O_2^{\cdot-}$$
$$O_2 + e^- \longrightarrow \cdot O_2^-$$
$$e^- \quad e^- \quad e^- \quad e^- \quad e^-$$
$$h^+ \quad h^+ \quad h^+ \quad h^+ \quad h^+$$
$$H_2O \qquad H_2O + h^+ \longrightarrow OH^\cdot \qquad OH^\cdot$$

In the presence of water and oxygen excited electrons and holes can be used to generate radical species such as hydroxyl (OH$^{\bullet}$) and superoxide (O$_2$$^{\bullet-}$) radicals, which in turn can activate various proteins or induce damage of the cancer cells (photodynamic therapy).

Light activated quantum dots can also be used to remove pathogens. Researchers from the University of Colorado, Boulder, designed small CdTe QDs, which penetrated the cell membrane of multi-drug resistant bacteria and produced large amount of intracellular superoxide radical. These radical species enhanced the effects of antibiotics in such a way that more bacteria could be killed with less antibiotic. The drawback of this approach was the use of 520 nm light to induce the production of super-oxide radical; light of such wavelength does not have large penetration depth (only 1 2 cm) making this approach suitable only for treating skin infections and wounds, or contaminated surfaces (Courtney et al., 2017).

2.5 Preparation of Carbon Nanomaterials

Being one of the essential building blocks of the life on Earth, carbon atoms form a vast number of molecules. In nature, elemental carbon can be found in three crystalline (allotropic) forms (Figure 2.13). In **graphite**, each carbon is covalently bound to three other carbons, the carbon atom is sp^2 hybrid-ised, resulting in basic trigonal geometry, with trigonal units further joining into hexagons. Formation of three bonds leaves one electron free to move within the graphite layer making it very conductive. In fact, graphite is often used to make electrodes. Due to the layered structure, it is also soft and greasy. Contrary to graphite, each carbon within the **diamond** structure engages in four bonds with neighbouring carbon atoms and it is sp^3 hybrid-ised. Trigonal geometry we see in graphite is replaced by tetragonal in diamond, and carbons form a perfect tetrahedral unit within the cubic cell. All electrons are localised and diamonds are bad conductors of electricity. They are also the hardest naturally occurring material (the wurtzite structure of boron nitride is harder than diamond but it can only be made synthetic-ally), have a high melting point and a high refractive index. The third form of carbon, **fullerene**, was first described in 1985, and it has a large symmet-rical structure composed of 60 atoms arranged into 20 hexagons and 12 pentagons (Kroto et al., 1985).

Figure 2.13

Allotropic forms of
carbon. Graphite is
characterised by a
layered arrangement of
hexagonal carbons,
carbon atoms in diamond
engage in four bonds
with neighbouring
carbons, and fullerene is
composed of pentagons
and hexagons of carbon
atoms arranged in a ball-
like shape.

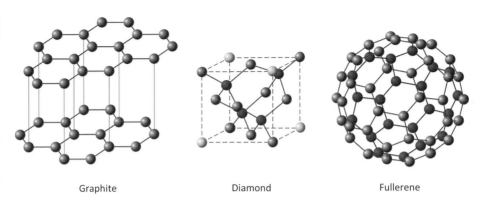

Graphite   Diamond   Fullerene

2.5.1   Synthesis of Fullerene

Initially, fullerene was synthesised using a cluster beam apparatus in the lab of
Richard Smalley (1943–2005) at Rice University in Texas, USA (Kroto et al.,
1985). He was interested in studying the formation of small clusters, which he
prepared using a focused laser beam that could achieve temperatures 1000 °C
or more and produce hot atomic vapor. Such vaporised atoms assemble into
clusters when cooled, which are then analysed by mass spectrometry. When
graphite was used as a target, a large amount of soot was produced that
contained a number of yet unknown carbon structures such as 'carbon snakes'
and ball-like fullerene. After the existence of fullerene was confirmed, controlled synthesis of fullerene in larger amounts was demonstrated by Wolfgang Krätschmer and his coworkers in 1990 with the help of arc discharge of
graphite electrodes in helium atmosphere.

   In the following years, vaporisation of graphite was also achieved by
pyrolysis and the use of radio-frequency plasma, but such procedures usually
involve several steps and make large-scale synthesis expensive. To reduce the
costs, chemical synthesis emerged as an alternative to vaporisation techniques, and although many strategies have been proposed, only a few were
successful. Synthetic approaches usually involve preparation of individual
molecular units, which are then joined together into curved structures until
the fullerene is fully assembled (Mojica et al., 2013). However, such
approaches require extensive use of catalysts, excellent understanding of
organic synthesis, and control over complex cyclisation processes. Due to
the difficult and low yielding synthesis, fullerenes are an expensive material,
and the cost has limited their use in bionanotechnology.

2.5.2   Carbon Nanotubes and Graphene

When pure graphite electrodes are used for **arc discharge** during which a direct-current arc voltage is applied in an inert atmosphere, fullerenes are usually found deposited as soot inside the chamber (15% of total product) and **multi-walled carbon nanotubes (MWCNTs,** Figure 2.14b) on the cathode. When a graphite anode contains metal catalysts such as iron or cobalt, **single-walled carbon nanotubes (SWCNTs,** Figure 2.14a) are generated in high yields, usually larger than 75%.

Figure 2.14

Carbon nanotubes. (a) Single-walled carbon nanotubes (SWCNT) are made of a single and (b) multi-walled carbon nanotubes (MWCNT) of multiple curved layers of graphitic carbon atom.

(a) SWCNT   (b) MWCNT

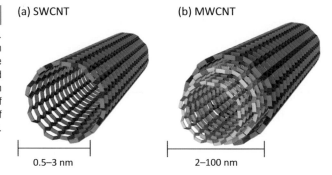

0.5–3 nm   2–100 nm

Arc discharge was the method used for preparation of the first single-walled carbon nanotubes in 1993 by Sumo Iijima and his team (Iijima and Ichihashi, 1993), and it is often used for preparation of both the high purity single and multi-walled carbon nanotubes. The synthesis of SWCNT is significantly improved by the addition of various metal powders such as nickel, cobalt, iron, tungsten and others, which act as catalysts. For example, it was shown that use of nickel–yttrium–graphite as a starting material results in high yield (larger than 90%) of pure SWCNTs. Metal atoms form alloy clusters, which can anneal all initially produced carbon structures into hexagons, and in such a way promote the lengthening and orientation of the tube. Single-walled nanotubes of controllable length, diameter and chirality can be obtained using various catalytic clusters (Figure 2.15). In the final stages of tube formation, metal clusters at the edge of the tube aggregate and become less reactive and less mobile. When they reach a particular size, the adsorption energy decreases and the large cluster peels of the edge. In the absence of the clusters, defects cannot be annealed effectively, resulting in closing of the tube edges and formation of multi-walled carbon nanotubes. Besides arc discharge, carbon nanotubes can be produced by laser ablation and chemical vapour deposition (CPD). **Laser ablation** is very similar to arc discharge in that it is using high-power pulsed laser to heat up graphite inside a quartz tube in inert atmosphere at temperatures around 1200 °C. Although this method is not economically viable as it uses plenty of energy, it results in high yields and excellent control over physical parameters. For example, it has been shown that by changing the laser power, the diameter of tubes can be changed, and the use of high-power laser pulses resulted in thinner tubes.

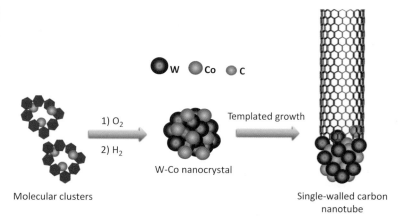

Figure 2.15

Tungsten (W) and cobalt (Co) clusters used in directed synthesis of carbon nanotube using chemical vapour deposition. Clusters are used as templates to direct the growth of single-walled carbon nanotubes (SWCNT). Adapted from Yang et al. (2014).

The most common method for tube preparation today is **chemical vapour deposition**, which employs chemical breakdown of hydrocarbons within a tubular silica substrate containing metal nanocrystal catalysts. In the first stage of the process, hydrocarbon gas such as acetylene and a process gas such as hydrogen are introduced to the system. Acetylene is decomposed at the surface of the catalysts, and carbon atoms accumulate on its edges and grow into the tube. In many cases, initially used high-temperature CVD has been replaced with a low-temperature method, which employs temperatures lower than 800 °C.

All of the methods currently in use can produce both single- and multi-walled carbon nanotubes, although the latter are usually made in the absence of metal catalyst. Multi-layer assembly found in MWCNT can be achieved through one of two routes, the Russian doll or the parchment route. As the names suggest, Russian doll MWCNTs contain smaller nanotubes inserted within the larger ones, and the parchment type MWCNTs are made by multiple folding of the graphene sheet, a process similar to the rolling up of a scroll of paper. Although single-walled and multi-walled CNT generally have similar properties, there are some differences (Table 2.2). For example, inner nanotubes in multi-walled structures are shielded from chemical reactions and provide a higher tensile strength, whereas single-walled tubes are easily twisted and more pliable.

Table 2.2 Comparison between single-walled and multi-walled carbon nanotubes

Single-walled carbon nanotubes (SWCNT)	Multi-walled carbon nanotubes (MWCNT)
Single graphene layer	Multiple graphene layers
Diameter range: 0.5 to 3 nm	Diameter range: 2 to 100 nm
Length: several micrometres	Length: up to a few centimetres
Synthesis requires catalysts	Synthesis can be achieved in the absence of catalysts
Bulk synthesis is difficult; stringent control over growth and conditions required	Bulk synthesis is less complex
Low purity	High purity
More defects introduced during functionalisation	Less defects during functionalisation
Easily twisted and more pliable	High tensile strength; more rigid
Low accumulation in body	Accumulate in body more readily

Note: Adapted from Eatemadi (2014). https://doi.org/10.1186/1556-276X-9-393. This work is licensed under the Creative Commons Attribution 4.0 International License.

Due to the nature of the strong covalent carbon–carbon bond, carbon nanotubes are as stiff as diamond, and their Young's modulus, a measure of stiffness, is as high as 900 GPa. As a comparison, the Young modulus of steel is 200 GPa, rubber 0.01 GPa, and DNA 0.3 GPa. Their tensile strength can be 10 times that of steel and thermal conductivity nearly 15 times that of copper ($6000\,\mathrm{W\,m^{-1}K^{-1}}$ vs $385\,\mathrm{W\,m^{-1}\,K^{-1}}$). But one of the most interesting properties of carbon nanotubes is that they can behave either like metal (they can be 1000 times better conductor than silver) or semiconductor depending on external conditions (Motta et al., 2007; Ando, 2009).

Such electronic properties stem from their parent material graphene, an atom-thick sheet of hexagonally distributed carbon atoms, and the way it wraps into nanotubes. If we imagine this wrapping to be similar to the wrapping of the flat sheet of paper into a tube, this can be described by a wrapping vector C_h that points across the sheet to connect atoms that coincide in the tube. A **graphene wrapping vector** is a combination of basis vectors a_1

and a_2 of the graphene sheet (Figure 2.16) and it determines if the carbon nanotube will be metallic or semiconducting.

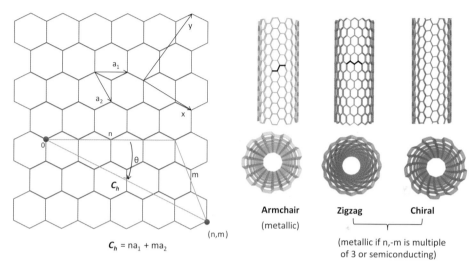

Figure 2.16

Graphene wrapping and different orientations of carbon nanotubes. Electronic properties of nanotubes depend on graphene folding and and C_h wrapping vector. Armchair and zigzag wrapping is illustrated by black lines within the carbon nanotubes.

$C_h = na_1 + ma_2$

Armchair (metallic)   Zigzag   Chiral

(metallic if n,-m is multiple of 3 or semiconducting)

We will not go deeper into the theory behind this phenomenon, which takes into account the distribution of electrons between s and p orbitals and the changeable energy gap between the π and π^* valence and conduction bands. More details can be found in the recommended further reading at the end of the chapter.

Carbon nanotubes are one of the most widely used nanomaterials, although there are some concerns about their toxicity, particularly if they are inhaled (see Chapter 9). One of the most promising applications of carbon nanotubes in biomedicine is neuron wiring, in which disconnected neurons can communicate again through the carbon tube bridge (see Research Report 2.2). They have also been used in tissue engineering as components of implantable hydrogels or in design of biosensors (Chapter 9).

Research Report 2.2   Activity of Neurons Restored by Carbon Nanotubes

Carbon nanotubes are characterised by high electric conductivity. Taking this into consideration, researchers from the University of Trieste, Italy, set out to check whether electrical stimulation delivered via carbon tubes can induce signalling between neuronal cells. They have grown neuronal cells on a layer of carbon nanotubes, applied a voltage and then monitored them for any communication between tubes and cells. They found that indeed carbon nanotubes can stimulate neuronal activity, making them suitable for design of interfaces between man-made materials and brain tissue (Mazzatenta et al., 2007). The same group showed in 2016 that neurons can regrow and reconnect when added to 3D mesh of carbon nanotubes. Such 3D mesh was also implanted in the brain of the adult rat, showing complete regeneration of the healthy tissue around the carbon nanotube implant (Usmani et al., 2016). The arrow shown here in (f) points at the contact point of the carbon nanotube bundle and the neuronal cell.

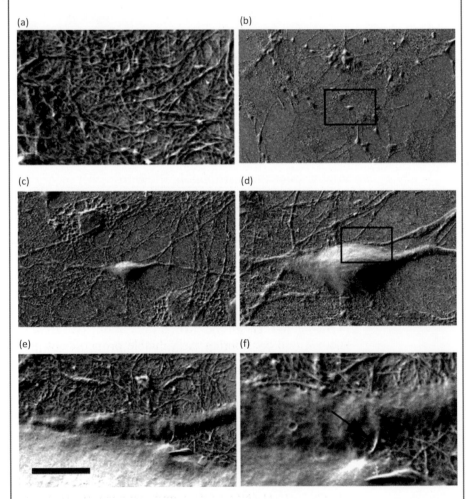

Source: Mazzatenta et al. (2007), https://doi.org/10.1523/JNEUROSCI.1051-07.2007. © 2007 Society for Neuroscience.

The carbon nanotube parent material, **graphene**, is also finding applications in medicine, mainly as a biosensor component. This atom-thick layer of hexagonal carbon atoms resembling atomic chicken wire is characterised by high conductivity and tensile strength. Although the application potential of graphene is big, the obstacle to its wider use is the deterioration of properties as the size of the sheets increases, increasing the number of defects. This makes the preparation of graphene on a large scale challenging. Graphene is usually prepared by exfoliation of graphite. To achieve graphite peeling, alkali ions such as Li^+, whose sizes match the graphite interlayer distance, are inserted between graphite layers. Recent developments in preparation of graphene are moving in the direction of 'green' peeling strategies, which do not involve use of chemicals such as electrochemical exfoliation (Achee et al., 2018). Besides graphite exfoliation, purely chemical strategies such as oxidation of graphite in the presence of strong acids have also been developed. The oxidation results in graphite carboxylic acids from which graphene is obtained by reduction with hydrazine (Figure 2.17).

Figure 2.17

Preparation of graphene by hydrazine reduction of graphite carboxylic acid.

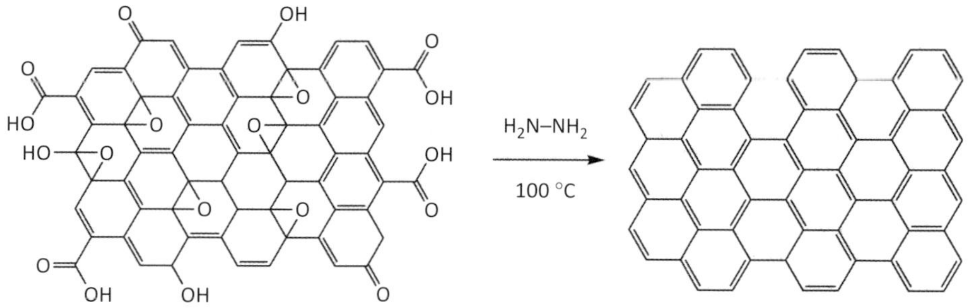

Over the years various physiochemical techniques for large-scale synthesis of defect-free graphene sheets have been employed with varying levels of success, and considering the valuable properties of graphene, this remains a very active field of research.

2.5.3   Preparation of Carbon Nanodiamonds

Nanodiamonds were discovered during an attempt to synthesise artificial diamonds, which involves the use of powerful explosives. One of the strategies for nanodiamond preparation is based on a **controlled explosion** of a mixture of TNT ($C_6H_2(NO_2)_3CH_3$) and hexogen ($C_3H_6N_6O_6$) explosives (60 wt% TNT and 40 wt% hexogen) under a negative oxygen atmosphere. This method, which has been known since the 1960s, yields mainly 4–5 nm carbon nanodiamonds (CND) although sometimes larger (up to 10 nm) nanodiamonds can be obtained. Overall yield usually does not exceed 4–10% per weight of explosives used, which prompted the development of other methods such as the electrochemical treatment of lithium carbonate (Li_2CO_3) doped with graphite (Kamali and Fray, 2015). Although yields can be improved by other methods, the largest amounts of nanodiamonds are produced within large explosion chambers. Spherical nanodiamonds prepared by high-energy explosions are coated by layers of graphite and also contain hydrocarbon chains and oxygen-rich functional groups such as carboxylic acid (COOH) and hydroxyl (OH) groups (see Figure 2.18). Hydrocarbon and graphite impurities can be removed by oxidation with oxygen plasma or strong acids to afford highly ordered nanodiamond core with a large number of OH or COOH groups. Such a nanodiamond surface is particularly well-suited for further modification and attachment of various functional groups, which will be discussed in Chapter 4. Carbon nanodiamonds are particularly interesting for applications in bionanotechnology and nanomedicine due to their biocompatibility and chemical stability. They can also be made fluorescent by the presence of **nitrogen-vacancy centres (NV)**, which can be created by either irradiation of nanodiamonds with high-energy particles (electrons, protons, helium atoms) followed by vacuum annealing at 600–800 °C, or by microsecond laser irradiation of carbon powders in organic solvents. Vacancies formed by high-energy irradiation can migrate through the structure during annealing and get trapped by nitrogen, the common diamond impurity. Unlike carbon, which engages in four bonds, nitrogen can only form three, easing the vacancy trapping. Once nitrogen-vacancy centres are formed, electrons can cross between the ground and excited state with the

Figure 2.18

Carbon nanodiamonds usually contain oxygen (red) and nitrogen-rich groups (blue) on the surface. Each nanoparticle is made of a highly ordered diamond core. Reprinted by permission from Springer Nature: Mochalin et al. (2011).

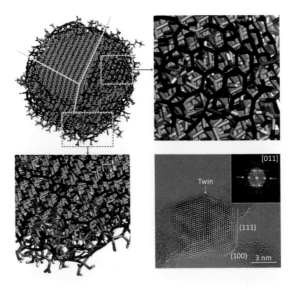

input of energy and emit a photon when they relax back to the ground state. This generates fluorescence that can be utilised for imaging of cells and tissues. Nitrogen-vacancy containing nanodiamonds can also be used as pressure and temperature probes (Research Report 2.3) as the transition frequency of electrons is temperature and pressure dependent. Detected fluorescence can therefore be directly correlated to quantitative change in temperature since nanodiamonds are excellent thermal conductors and the recorded temperature is the same as that in their immediate surroundings.

Research Report 2.3	Carbon Nanodiamonds As Cell Thermometers

Measuring temperature variations on a nanometre scale is challenging. It is difficult to design a thermometer that can measure small temperature changes across the cell. But such temperature information would tell us more about the heat dissipation through cell compartments, tumour metabolism or the effects of the drug treatment.

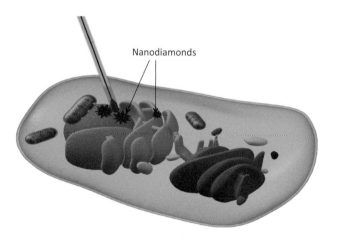

Nanodiamonds

In order to enable sensitive, nanoscale temperature measurements, researchers from Harvard University injected a single nanodiamond 100 nm in size into a human cell. Using nitrogen-vacancy centres, the temperature in the proximity of the nanodiamond could be determined by measuring the wavelength of emitted light after excitation with the laser light. By using a second nanodiamond, it was also possible to measure the temperature difference between two locations within the same cell. The length scales of the measurements were as short as 200 nm, which is smaller than some organelles, and temperature fluctuations as small as 0.05 K could be recorded (Kucsko et al., 2013).

2.6   Preparation of Polymeric Nanoparticles

Natural and man-made polymers can be made on nanoscale using either the pre-formed polymers or direct synthesis from monomer elements (Back to Basics 2.4).

Back to Basics 2.4	Polymer Synthesis

Polymers, from Greek *poly*, 'many' and *mer*, 'part', are large natural (DNA, proteins, cellulose) or synthetic (polyethylene, polystyrene, polyethylene glycol) molecules composed of repeating units known as monomers. Depending on the type of monomers, polymers can be classified as **homo** (single type of repeat units) and **co** (two or more types of repeat units) polymers.

Synthetic polymers are usually prepared by linking monomers through a polymerisation reaction, which can proceed through two mechanisms: **chain-growth polymerisation** and **step-growth polymerisation** (growth by reaction between bi-functional or multi-functional monomers).

The **chain-growth polymerisation** mechanism is based on growth of the polymer by reaction between monomers and active sites on the growing chain. The active site is regenerated after each growth stage. Monomers are present throughout the reaction, and their concentration decreases steadily over time. The reaction speed depends on the presence of an initiator, and in most cases there is also a termination phase. Depending on the nature of the initiator, chain-growth polymerisation reactions can be classified as radical, cationic, anionic or coordination polymerisation.

Most commonly used polymers such as polyethylene (PE), polypropylene (PP) or polyvinyl chloride (PVC) are prepared using chain-growth polymerisation.

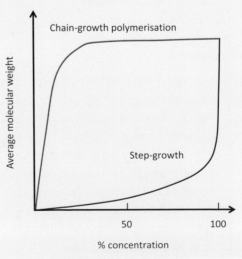

Step-growth polymerisation mechanism describes the growth of polymers through reaction between bi-functional or multi-functional monomers catalysed by the presence of acids, bases, metal catalysts or by heat. When a monomer has three or more reactive functional groups, branched polymers are formed. Long reaction times are needed for preparation of long polymers, and there is no termination step and polymers remain active throughout the reaction. Polyesters such as polyethylene terephthalate (PET), polyamides (PA) such as nylon and polyurethanes (PUR) are all prepared using step-growth polymerisation.

Polymer nanoparticles can be prepared using methods such as precipitation and dialysis to turn synthesised polymers into nanoparticles or sheets, or by radical-induced polymerisation and emulsion processes to make nanoparticles directly from monomers (Figure 2.19). The processes employed for preparation will depend on the applications, and those nanoparticles used in medical applications need to be prepared using strategies that are devoid of toxic reagents and additives.

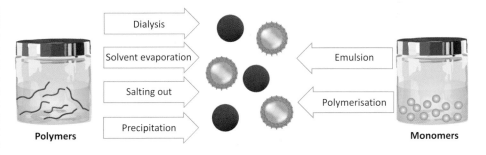

Figure 2.19

Preparation of polymer nanoparticles (nanospheres and nanocapsules). Nanoparticles can be prepared using two routes: either from polymers using such processes such as precipitation or salting out, or from monomers by controlled polymerisation or various emulsion strategies.

Polymer nanoparticles can generally be grouped into **polymer nanospheres**, which are entirely made of rigid polymer, and **polymer nanocapsules**, that contain a cavity consisting of a liquid core surrounded by a polymer shell (Figure 2.19). As nanomaterial building blocks, polymers have a number of advantages such as tunable mechanical and thermal properties, and availability of various functional groups within their backbone, which are suitable for further modification. This makes polymer nanoparticles particularly interesting for applications in drug delivery (Research Report 2.4).

Research Report 2.4   Biocompatible Polymer for Drug Formulation

Poly-lactic-co-glycolic acid (PLGA) is a co-polymer of polylactic (PLA) and polyglycolic acid (PGA), and in terms of design and performance is the best defined biomaterial available for drug delivery. Its popularity stems from several properties, which are desirable for biomedical applications. PLGA hydrolyses into lactic and glycolic acid, which are easily metabolised and therefore biocompatible. The polymer can also be processed into almost any shape and size, and as such be used for encapsulation of molecules of virtually any size. The most common method to prepare PLGA nanocapsules for drug encapsulation is the **emulsification–solvent evaporation** technique. Initially, a polymer is dissolved in solvent, which is immiscible with water. Then a drug is added and a polymer–drug mixture is subsequently introduced to a large volume of water in the presence of emulsifier under constant stirring and controlled temperature. Finally, the organic solvent is allowed to evaporate to harden the droplets.

Another strategy involves precipitation of a polymer and a drug in the presence of a surfactant. There are numerous variations of these strategies, the choice of which will largely depend on the properties of the drug and the application requirements. PLGA formulations have been approved by the FDA and European Medicine Agency (EMA) for use in various drug delivery systems including anti-cancer therapies. Such are, for example, Lypron Depot® (containing leuprolide) and Trelstar® (containing triptorelin) PLGA microspheres used in the treatment of breast and advanced prostate cancers. PLGA nanoparticles have still not made it onto the list of approved formulations but there are several in ongoing clinical trials (Rezvantalab et al., 2018).

PLGA

Lactic acid   Glycolic acid

There is a particular interest in using biocompatible nanostructures made of natural polymers such as chitosan, bacterial cellulose and hyaluronic acid (Figure 2.20). For example, chitosan nanoparticles are extensively explored as drug delivery platforms suitable for oral and nasal delivery.

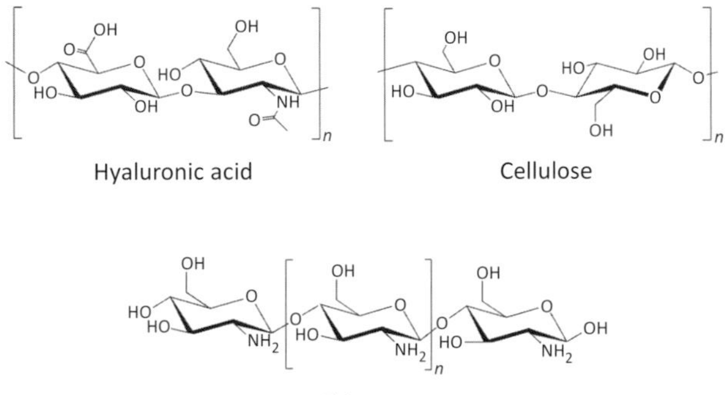

Figure 2.20

Biocompatible polymers used as nanomaterial precursors. n denotes the number of monomer units and can range from few to several thousands.

Hyaluronic acid

Cellulose

Chitosan

2.7 Preparation of Porous Nanomaterials

Porous nanomaterials are characterised by the presence of nanosized pores. There are many different materials within this class, all of which can be made using a wide range of strategies, which can be found in dedicated textbooks and will not be discussed here in great detail. Instead we will give a short overview of various types of porous nanomaterials and their uses in bionanotechnology.

Traditionally, porous materials can be divided into **microporous** (pores are smaller than 2 nm), **mesoporous** (pore size between 2 and 50 nm) and **macroporous** (pore size larger than 50 nm). The best-known **microporous materials** are zeolites, which are characterised by rigid crystal frameworks of pores, which form tunnels within the core. Naturally occurring zeolites are aluminosilicates with the basic SiO_2 tetrahedral units in which some Si atoms are substituted with aluminium (Al) (Figure 2.21a).

There are also a number of synthetic zeolites containing other elements and featuring larger pores. Similar to zeolites are recently discovered **metal-organic frameworks (MOFs)**, man-made porous structures made of organometallic building blocks composed of metal nodes (clusters or small metal units) and organic linkers (Figure 2.21b). There are around 70 000 MOFs known to date, which have been either theoretically predicted or synthesised, and the number is growing. Both zeolites and MOFs are characterised by a large surface area which makes them excellent catalysts, while their pores and

Figure 2.21

Natural and synthetic zeolite structures. (a) Typical unit of natural aluminosilicate zeolites and structures of zeolite A and Y. (b) Assembly of organic linkers and metal nodes results in metal-organic frameworks (MOFs) such as MOF-5. Yellow sphere illustrates the volume of the pore. Courtesy of Dr David Fairen-Jimenez, University of Cambridge.

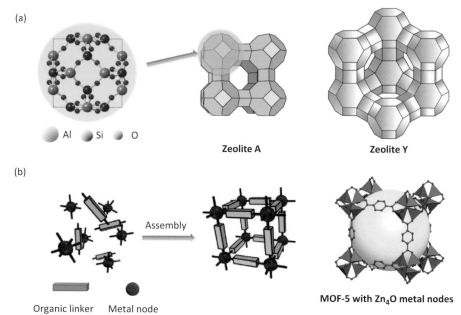

cavities are suitable for encapsulation of 'guest' molecules, such as small organic drugs or biological therapeutic cargos, such as nucleic acids or peptides. For this reason, they are interesting as drug delivery systems and extensively explored for targeted delivery strategies in cancer treatment. The main challenges still to be addressed concern their thermal and long-term stability within complex biological liquids.

Mesoporous materials have larger pores (up to 50 nm). One of the most widely used classes of mesoporous nanomaterials in bionanotechnology is **mesoporous silica**, extensively used in imaging and drug delivery (Kresge et al., 1992). With the adjustable pore size, a surface that can be easily functionalised and biocompatibility, mesoporous silica nanoparticles have numerous advantages over other materials. Due to their structural features and surface properties, they have been successfully used for engineering of hard tissues such as bone (Research Report 2.5), and in the design of biosensors.

Research Report 2.5   Mesoporous Silica for Bone Regeneration

Mesoporous silica nanoparticles have a few advantages over some other porous nanomaterials. Besides high surface area, the chemistry for surface modification is well understood, and the pore size can be tuned.

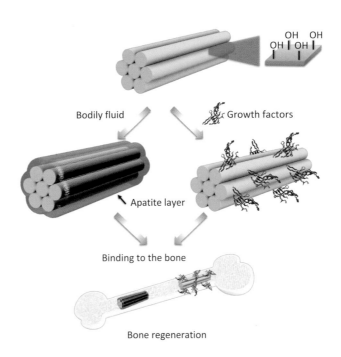

Besides being used for drug delivery, mesoporous silica has proved an excellent material to promote bone regeneration. Silanol groups on the surface of nanostructured silica react with body fluids to produce a layer of apatite, the basic mineral component of human hard tissue, which can bind to the bone promoting its regeneration (Izquierdo-Barba et al., 2005). In addition, the mesoporous silica nanostructures can be modified with different biomolecules such as growth factor proteins and peptides to aid the bone healing and tissue strengthening.

Mesoporous silica is prepared by a templating method using cationic surfactants. In the first step, silicate–surfactant clusters are formed which then undergo self-assembly under different pH to afford porous structures. Different templates have been successfully used, ranging from soft ones such as micelles to the hard ones such as polymer beads or other nanoparticles (gold has been often used) (Wu et al., 2013). Some successful procedures also involve a modified Stöber method used for the synthesis of silica nanoparticles and treatments of pre-synthesised silica particles with harsh reagents such as $NaBH_4$. Many methods of porous silica synthesis rely on careful control of pH and dilution of reacting mixture so that the final yields are usually low and scale-up challenging.

Besides silica (SiO_2), other mesoporous materials such as alumina (Al_2O_3) or mesoporous bioactive glasses (SiO_2–CaO–P_2O_5) have been prepared and successfully used in bone replacement and dentistry (Zhang et al., 2016).

Macroporous materials with pores larger than 50 nm are composed of a variety of mainly polymeric materials obtained by cross-linking strategies. Macroporous materials such as hydrogels, hydrophilic polymer networks, can absorb a high percentage of water – sometimes 1000 times their dry weight. Hydrogels can be made by non-covalent or covalent cross-linking of synthetic, natural or hybrid building blocks (Back to Basics 2.5). The choice of cross-linking strategy will define their physiochemical properties. Covalent cross-linking often results in chemically and mechanically stable gels, whereas electrostatic cross-linking based on formation of cation bridges produces reversible hydrogels that can disintegrate easily. In general, if the cross-linking strategy involves formation of hydrogen bonds, or use of ionic or hydrophobic forces, such gels can be easily disrupted and reconstructed using various additives. This together with their moulding capability and high absorption of water-soluble molecules makes them particularly suitable for medical applications such as tissue engineering (Chapter 9). Recent years have seen revived interest in responsive hydrogels that alter their mechanical properties when irradiated, heated or are exposed to magnetic force which can be applied in biosensing (De France et al., 2018).

Back to Basics 2.5 | Hydrogels

Hydrogels are three-dimensional, physically or chemically bonded polymeric networks capable of adsorbing water in the intermolecular space. The water content of hydrogels can reach to over 90% of their total mass. The ability to absorb water arises from hydrophilic functional groups such as –OH, –COOH, –CONH, –$CONH_2$, –SO_3H attached to the polymeric backbone, while their insolubility in water results from chemical and/or physical cross-links between network chains. The term hydrogel, first introduced in 1894 (van Bemmelen, 1894), implies that the material is already swollen in water, while the dried hydrogel is usually referred to as **xerogel**. If the hydrogel is dried under supercritical conditions so that the network is not affected and remains highly porous the hydrogel is called an **aerogel**.

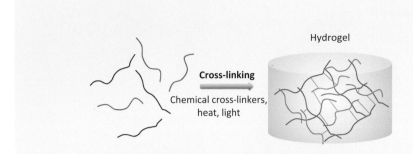

Hydrogels can be prepared using either natural polymers such as collagen and chitosan, or synthetic polymers such as polyacrylic acid (PAA) and polyvinyl alcohol (PVA), or a combination of both. Hydrogels can be classified based on the nature of the cross-linked junction into **physically bonded networks** formed due to ionic interactions, hydrogen bonds or hydrophobic interactions as well as polymeric chain entanglements, and **chemically cross-linked networks** formed through strong covalent bonds.

Physical gels are often 'reversible', as they can be decomposed into monomers by changing environmental conditions such as pH, ionic strength of the solution or temperature. Chemical gels are considered more 'permanent' and can be prepared using different chemical reactions.

2.8 Biosynthesis of Nanomaterials

As we have seen in previous sections, there are various physiochemical strategies of nanomaterial preparation which involve the use of templates, reagents, precursors, mechanical changes and different chemical strategies. Some of these methods are reasonably simple and cheap and have led to scaling-up, while other are expensive, not easily scalable and require toxic reagents. Biosynthetic strategies have been explored as a greener alternative to traditional synthetic strategies by employing environmentally friendly protocols. Using such protocols, nanomaterials can be prepared using whole organisms such as bacteria, yeast and algae, cell extracts and individual biomolecules such as DNA, peptides or enzymes.

One of the most widely referenced microorganisms that naturally produce nanomaterials is **magnetotactic bacteria**. These single-cell organisms use magnetotaxis to align themselves along an external magnetic field with the help of organelles called magnetosomes (Figure 2.22).

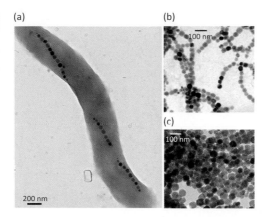

Magnetosomes are membrane enveloped nanosized crystals, either magnetite Fe_3O_4 or iron sulphide greigite Fe_3S_4. It is believed that magnetosome vesicles are first synthesised and then the nanoparticles are formed at the interface of **magnetosomes** and supersaturated solution of iron present within the vesicle (Faivre and Schüler, 2008). Supersaturation of the mineral constituents is achieved with the help of the protein pumps within the vesicle membrane, which pump iron in but do not allow it to get out, thus maintaining the biologically optimal concentration. There have been many attempts to purify and use magnetosomes, but biosynthesised nanoparticles usually have a layer of proteins and other biomolecules on their surface, which can interfere with purification and subsequent modification strategies. In addition, they are often not suitable for biomedical applications, as any traces of foreign biomaterial on the surface of nanoparticles could have a detrimental effect on the immune system.

Biosynthetic strategies have been used for the synthesis of many different nanomaterials, ranging from noble metals to quantum dots. For example, **algae** can be used for the synthesis of nanoparticles (Sheng et al., 2004), and it was shown that both algae and other microorganisms engage their bimolecular machinery to convert ions into more stable and less toxic clusters and nanoparticles, which can then be processed and excreted. Algae can be used for **biosynthesis of nanomaterials** either directly within living algal cultures or through the use of their biomass or cell extracts (Dahoumane et al., 2017). The size and shape of obtained nanomaterials can differ between algal species, but the major challenge is still the polydispersity of obtained samples within the single system (Figure 2.23).

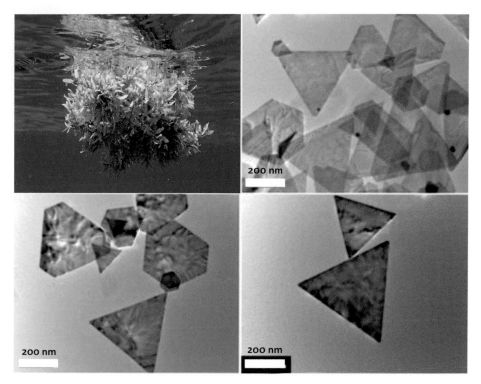

It seems that switching algae for fungi might help to tackle the issue of polydispersity, as the use of fungi, such as **yeasts**, results in monodispersed nanoparticles with tunable composition. In addition, fungi possess high intracellular metal uptake capacities, can be easily cultured for large-scale production, and afford a significant amount of enzymes useful for nanoparticle synthesis (Hulkoti and Taranath, 2014).

Indeed, **enzymes** are the key biomolecules for reduction of metal ions (more on enzyme structure in Chapter 3), the first stage of nanoparticle formation. For example, the enzyme cysteine desulfhydrase enables reduction of cadmium ions and formation of CdS quantum dots upon addition of $CdSO_4$ to the photosynthetic bacteria *Rhodoseudomonas palustris*.

Besides enzymes, reducing agents can also be sugars attached to the cell walls, peptides, vitamins, or proteins such as silk fibroin, the main constituent of silk fibres, which has been used to produce gold nanoparticles. DNA or even the whole viral capsids can also be employed as templates and will be explored in later chapters.

Key Concepts

Arc discharge: method used to vaporise the graphite electrode by use of direct-current arc voltage applied in an inert atmosphere. It was the first and it is still widely used method used to produce fullerenes and carbon nanotubes.

Biosynthesis of nanomaterials: preparation of nanosized structures with the help of whole organisms (usually microorganism but plants have been used) or biomolecules such as DNA, peptides and proteins.

Bottom up process: larger nanostructures are obtained by assembly of smaller elements (molecules and atoms).

Chemical vapour deposition (CVD): thermally induced breakdown of gaseous reagents and deposition and growth of material on the substrate surface. Commonly used for preparation of carbon nanotubes.

Graphene: an atom-thick layer of graphitic carbon prepared by graphite exfoliation.

Graphene wrapping vector: a vector that determines the wrapping and the final orientation of the carbon tubes, which in turn change the electronic properties of resulting carbon nanotubes.

Micelle-guided strategies: growth of nanocrystals at the interface of fused micelles containing reducing agent and metal precursor. Micelles are core–shell droplets composed of liquid core and soft outer shell prepared by mixing oil and water in the presence of surfactants.

Multi-walled carbon nanotubes (MWCNT): nanotubes made of many layers of curved graphene positioned within each other.

Nitrogen-vacancy (NV) centres: centres introduced to nanodiamonds by high-energy irradiation characterised by fluorescence, which is sensitive to small changes in temperature and pressure.

Polymer nanoparticles: hard nanospheres or cavity-containing nanocapsules made of man-made or natural polymers.

Porous nanomaterials: materials characterised by the presence of nanosized pores. Depending on the size of the pores they can be grouped into microporous (pores smaller than 2 nm), mesoporous (2–50 nm) and macroporous (pores larger than 50 nm).

Reducing agents: chemical reagents that can reduce metallic ions in a first stage of metallic nanoparticle preparation. They can be strong such as sodium borohydride or mild such as citrate or methanol.

Single-walled carbon nanotubes (SWCNT): carbon nanotubes composed of a single layer of curved graphene.

Sol–gel process: wet chemical route for synthesis of metal oxide nanoparticles from metal salts or metal alkoxides with addition of catalysts.

Superparamagnetism: a form of magnetism found in small magnetic nanoparticles and characterised by large magnetic susceptibility.

Top-down approach: nanostructures are prepared starting from larger structures or bulk materials using carving out, etching, printing or surface patterning.

Problems

2.1   Name two different strategies to prepare 10 nm spherical and cubic gold nanoparticles. Use chemical equation(s) to explain one of the strategies.

2.2   Platinum nanoparticles (Pt NPs) were prepared using 0.2 mm solution of $HPtCl_4$ precursor. After reduction with $NaBH_4$, 5 ml of 20 nm spherical Pt nanoparticle are obtained. Calculate the number of nanoparticles in the solution assuming a uniform size distribution. The atomic radius of Pt is 175 pm and the Avogadro number is $N_A = 6.022 \times 10^{23}$.

2.3   Silver nanoparticles can be prepared by reduction of silver nitrate with formaldehyde in aqueous solution according to the following equation:

$$Ag^+ + HCHO + OH^- \rightarrow Ag + HCOOH + \frac{1}{2}H_2$$

(a) How could you achieve the growth of larger Ag NPs and even larger agglomerates?

(b) Name at least one reaction condition that can be changed to achieve stable small nanoparticles.

(c) What can be added to the solution to enable diffusion-controlled growth?

2.4   During preparation of TiO_2 nanoparticles long nanorods are obtained using two-stage heating: first the $Ti(iPr)_4$ precursor is heated at 140 °C for 30 min and then further heating at 100 °C for 24 h is needed to obtain stable 25 nm long nanorods. Explain why.

2.5   The sol–gel process is used to prepare 50 nm SiO_2 nanoparticles. Name at least two strategies that can be employed to obtain smaller nanoparticles.

2.6   Why is a ZnS shell grown over the core of CdS quantum dots and how does the addition of the shell impact the fluorescence of such core–shell nanoparticles?

2.7 Describe how the structure of nanodiamonds differ from the structure of carbon nanotubes and fullerene taking into account the geometry of the carbon atoms. How many nearest neighbours has a single carbon atom in diamond, and how many in graphite?

2.8 The arc discharge method is used to make single-walled carbon nanotubes using graphite as a starting material. You need to use carbon nanotubes to connect two neurons, which are 1 μm apart. Until now you have only been able to make 400 nm long nanotubes. How could you improve your synthesis to obtain longer tubes?

2.9 Estimate the surface-to-volume ratio of a C_{60} fullerene by treating the molecule as a hollow sphere and using 77 pm for the atomic radius of carbon.

2.10 A single gram of highly porous MOF material can have a surface area of 5000 m^2. How does this value compare with the surface area of a 1 g cube of gold? If you could flatten out the gold into a sheet how thin does it have to be to achieve the same surface area as the MOF?

Further Reading

Metal Nanoparticle Synthesis

Koczkur, K. M., Mourdikoudis, S., Polavarapu, L. and Skrabalak, S. E. (2015). Polyvinylpyrrolidone (PVP) in nanoparticle synthesis. *Dalton Transactions*, **44**, 17883–17905.

Carbon Nanomaterials

Doherty, M. W., Struzhikin, V. V., Simpson, D. A., et al. (eds.) (2010). *Carbon Nanotubes and Related Structures: Synthesis, Characterisation, Functionalisation, and Applications*, Wiley-VCH.

Doherty, M. W., Struzhikin, V. V., Simpson, D. A., et al. (2014). Electronic properties and metrology applications of the diamond NV-center under pressure. *Physical Review Letters*, **112**, 047601.

Dresselhaus, M. S., Dresselhaus, G. and Avouris, P. (eds.) (2006). *Carbon Nanotubes. Synthesis, Structure, Properties and Applications*, Springer-Verlag.

Odom, T. W., Huang, J.-L., Kim, P. and Lieber, C. M. (2000). Structure and electronic properties of carbon nanotubes. *Journal of Physical Chemistry B*, **104**, 2794–2809.

Peng, L.-M., Zhang, Z. and Wang, S. (2014). Carbon nanotube electronics: recent advances. *Materials Today*, **17**(9), 433–442.

Prawer, S. (2014). Electronic properties and metrology applications of the diamond NV-centre under pressure. *Physical Review Letters*, **112**, 047601.

Rao, R., Pint, C., Islam, A., et al. (2018). Caron nanotubes and related nanomaterials; critical advances and challenges for synthesis toward mainstream commercial applications. *ACS Nano*, **12**, 11756–11784.

Schirhagl, R., Chang, K., Loretz, M. and Degen, C. L. (2014). Nitrogen-vacancy centres in diamond: nanoscale sensors for physics and biology. *Annual Review of Physicl Chemistry*, **65**, 83–105.

Polymer Nanoparticles

Mohammed, M. A., Syeda, J. T. M., Wasan, K. M. and Wasan, E. K. (2017). An overview of chitosan nanoparticles and its application in non-parenteral drug delivery. *Pharmaceutics*, **9**, 53–79.

Rao, J. P. and Geckeler, K. E. (2011). Polymer nanoparticles: preparation techniques and size-control parameters. *Progress in Polymer Science*, **36** (7), 887–913.

Porous Nanomaterials

Liu, Y., Zhao, Y. and Chen, X. (2019). Bioengineering of metal-organic frameworks for nanomedicine. *Theranostics*, **9**(11), 3122–3133.

Rahikkala, A., Pereira, S. A. P, Figueiredo, P., et al. (2018). Mesoporous silica nanoparticles for targeted and stimuli responsive delivery of chemotherapeutics; a review. *Advanced Biosystems*, **2**(7), 1800020.

Biosynthesis

Chen, L., Bazylinski, D. A. and Lower, B. H. (2010). Bacteria that synthesize nano-sized compasses to navigate using Earth's geomagnetic field. *Nature Education Knowledge*, **3**(10), 30.

Gahlawatt, G. and Choudhury, A. R. (2019). A review on the biosynthesis of metal and metal salt nanoparticles by microbes. *RSC Advances*, **9**, 12944–12967.

References

Achee, T. C., Sun, W., Hope, J. T., et al. (2018). High-yield scalable graphene nanosheet production from compressed graphite using electrochemical exfoliation. *Scientific Reports*, **8**, 14525.

Alphandéry, E. (2014). Applications of magnetosomes synthesized by magnetotactic bacteria in medicine. *Frontiers in Bioengineering and Biotechnology*, **2**(5).

Ando, T. (2009). The electronic properties of graphene and carbon nanotubes. *Asia Materials*, **1**, 17–21.

Brust M., Walker M., Bethell D., Schiffrin D. J. and Whyman R. (1994). Synthesis of thiol-derivatised gold nanoparticles in a two-phase liquid–liquid system. *Journal of the Chemical Society, Chemical Communications*, **7**, 801–802.

Courtney, C. M., Goodman, S. M., Nagy, T. A., et al. (2017). Potentiating antibiotics in drug-resistant clinical isolates via stimuli-activated superoxide generation. *Science Advances*, **3**(10), E1701776.

Dahoumane, S. A., Mechouet, M., Wijesekera, K., et al. (2017). Algae-mediated biosynthesis of inorganic nanomaterials as a promising route in nanobiotechnology: a review. *Green Chemistry*, **19**, 552–587.

De France, K. J., Xu, F. and Hoare, T. (2018). Structured macroporous hydrogels: progress, challenges and opportunities. *Advanced Healthcare Materials*, **7**(1), 1700927.

Duff, D. G., Edwards, P. P. and Johnson, B. F. G. (1995). Formation of a polymer-protected platinum sol: a new understanding of the parameters controlling morphology. *Journal of Physical Chemistry*, **99**, 15934–15944.

Eatemadi, A., Daraee, H., Karimkhanloo, H., et al. (2014). Carbon nanotubes: properties, synthesis, purification, and medical applications. *Nanoscale Research Letters*, **9** (1), 393.

Faivre, D. and Schüler, D. (2008). Magnetotactic bacteria and magnetosomes. *Chemical Reviews*, **108**, 4875–4898.

Hulkoti, N. I. and Taranath, T. C. (2014). Biosynthesis of nanoparticles using microbes: a review. *Colloids and Surfaces B*, **121**, 474–483.

Hung, C.-Y., Tu, W.-T., Lin, Y.-T., Fruk, L. and Hung, Y.-C. (2015). Optically controlled multiple switching operations of DNA biopolymer devices. *Journal of Applied Physics*, **118**, 235503.

Iijima, S. and Ichihashi, T. (1993). Single-shell carbon nanotubes of 1-nm diameter. *Nature*, **363**, 603–605.

Izquierdo-Barba, I., Ruiy-Gonzaley, L., Doadrio, J. C., Gonzaley-Calbet, J. M. and Vallet-Regi, M. (2005). Tissue regeneration: a new property of mesoporous materials. *Solid State Science*, **7**, 233–237.

Kamali, A. R. and Fray, D. J. (2015). Preparation of nanodiamonds from carbon nanoparticles at atmospheric pressure. *Chemical Communications*, **51**, 5594–5597.

Krätschmer, W., Lamb, L. D., Fostiropoulos, K. and Huffman, D. R. (1990). Solid C60: a new form of carbon. *Nature*, **347**, 354–358.

Kresge, C. T., Leonowicz, M. E., Roth, W. J., Vartuli, J. C. and Beck, J. S. (1992). Ordered mesoporous molecular sieves synthesised by a liquid-crystal template mechanism. *Nature*, **359**, 710–712.

Kroto, H. W., Heath, J. R., O'Brien, S. C., Curl, R. F. and Smalley, R. E. (1985). C60: buckminster fullerene. *Nature*, **318**, 162–163.

Kucsko, G., Maurer, P. C., Yao, N. Y., et al. (2013). Nanometre-scale thermometry in a living cell. *Nature*, **500**, 54–58.

Matijevic, E. (1977). The role of chemical complexing in the formation and stability of colloidal dispersions. *Journal of Colloid and Interface Science*, **58**, 374–389.

Mazzatenta, A., Giugliano, M., Campidelli, S., et al. (2007). Interfacing neurons with carbon nanotubes: electrical signal transfer and synaptic stimulation in cultured brain circuits. *The Journal of Neuroscience*, **27**(26), 6931–6936.

Mochalin, V. N., Shenderova, O., Ho, D. and Gogotsi, Y. (2011). The properties and applications of nanodiamonds. *Nature Nanotechnology*, **7**, 11–23.

Mojica, M., Alonso, J. A. and Méndez, F. (2013). Synthesis of fullerenes. *Journal of Physical Organic Chemistry*, **26**, 526–539.

Motta, M., Moisala, A., Kinloch, I. A. and Windle, A. H. (2007). High performance fibres from 'dog bone' carbon nanotubes. *Advanced Materials* **19**, 3721–3726.

Murray, C. B., Norris, D. J. and Bawendi, M. G. (1993). Synthesis and characterisation of nearly monodiscperse CdE (E=S, Se, Te) semiconductor nanocrystallites, *Journal of American Chemical Society*, **115**, 8706–8715.

Ramirez, E., Erades, L., Philippot, K., Lecante, P. and Chaudret, B. (2007). Shape control of platinum nanoparticles. *Advanced Functional Materials*, **17**, 2219–2228.

Reibold M., Paufler P., Levin A. A., et al. (2006). Carbon nanotubes in ancient Damascus sabre. *Nature*, **444**, 286.

Rezvantalab, S., Drude, N. I., Moraveji, M. K., et al. (2018). PLGA-based nanoparticles in cancer treatment. *Frontiers in Pharmacology*, **9**, 1260.

Sheng, P. X., Ting, Y. P., Chen, J. P. and Hong, L. (2004). Sorption of lead, copper, cadmium, zinc, and nickel by marine algal biomass: characterisation of biosorptive capacity and investigation of mechanisms. *Journal of Colloid and Interface Science*, **275**, 131–141.

Skrabalak, S. E., Chen, J., Sun, Y., et al. (2008). Gold nanocages: synthesis, properties and applications. *Accounts of Chemical Research*, **41**(12), 1587–1595.

Stöber, W., Fink, A. and Bohn, E. (1968). Controlled growth of monodisperse silica spheres in the micron size range. *Journal of Colloids and Interface Science*, **26**, 62–69.

Tao, A., Sinsermsuksakul, P. and Yang, P. (2006). Polyhedral silver nanocrystals with distinct scattering signatures. *Angewandte chemie*, **45**(28), 4597–4601.

Usmani, S., Aurand, E. R., Medelin, M., et al. (2016). 3D meshes of carbon nanotubes guide functional reconnection of segregated spinal explants. *Science Advances*, **2**, e1600087 (10 pages).

Van Bemmelen, J. M. (1894). Das Hydrogel und das krystallinische Hydrat des Kupferoxyds. *Zetischrift für anorganische Chemie*, **5**(1), 466–483.

Werner, D. and Hashimoto, S. (2013). Controlling the pulsed laser induced size reduction of Au and Ag nanoparticles via changes in the external pressure, laser intensity and excitation wavelength. *Langmuir*, **29**(4), 1295–1302.

Wu, S.-H., Mou, C.-Y. and Lin, H.-P. (2013). Synthesis of mesoporous silica nanoparticles. *Chemical Society Reviews*, **42**, 2862–3875.

Xu, G., Zeng, S., Zhang, B., et al. (2016). New generation cadmium-free quantum dots for biophotonics and nanomedicine. *Chemical Reviews*, **116**, 12234–12327.

Yang, F., Wang, X., Zhang, D., et al. (2014). Chirality-specific growth of single-walled carbon nanotubes on solid alloy catalysts. *Nature*, **510**, 522–524.

Zeng, H., Rice, P. M., Wang, S. X. and Sun, S. (2004). Shape-controlled synthesis and shape-induced texture of $MnFe_2O_4$ nanoparticles. *Journal of the American Chemical Society*, **126**(37), 11458–11459.

Zhang, X., Zeng, D., Li, N., et al. (2016). Functionalised mesoporous bioactive glass scaffolds for enhanced bone tissue regeneration. *Scientific Reports*, **6**, 19361–19374.

3 Biomolecules and Scales of Biological Systems

Before we start looking into modification of nanomaterials and nanostructuring of biomolecular elements for various applications in biomedicine and material design, we need to get a glimpse into the structure of biomolecular building blocks and the way they interact and assemble.

The cell, a basic unit of living organisms, is a self-containing functional system driven by complex cellular processes aimed at producing energy and building blocks to maintain functioning balance. Nobody has ever been able to measure the number of reactions that occur in a single cell per second, but depending on the cell that number might be well above a billion. All of these reactions, like any regular chemical reactions, involve an exchange of energy and conversion of reagents into products using water as a universal solvent. A cell is a dynamic system capable of adapting to a changing environment, and reactions are performed simultaneously through coordination of multiple functional modules distributed across different cell compartments known as **organelles**. As illustrated in Figure 3.1, there is plenty of diversity down at the cellular bottom not only in terms of structure and function, but also the size of individual molecular species and their larger assemblies.

Figure 3.1

Scales down at the cellular bottom. Dimensions of the red blood cell compared to some molecule species and structures found in living cells.

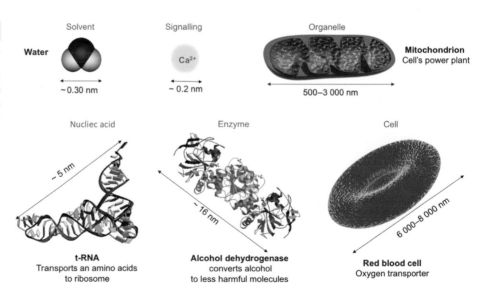

3.1 Cell Compartments

The basic architecture of a eukaryotic cell is given in Figure 3.2 and Back to Basics 3.1 describes differences between prokaryotic and eukaryotic cells.

A phospholipid **membrane** surrounds the cell creating a natural boundary between intracellular space (cytoplasm) and the extracellular matrix. Intracellular membranes divide a cell into compartments characterised by their own structure, biochemical composition and function. By regulating free diffusion, membranes act as physical and chemical boundaries, and the molecules embedded within the phospholipid layer play an important role in cell recognition and signalling.

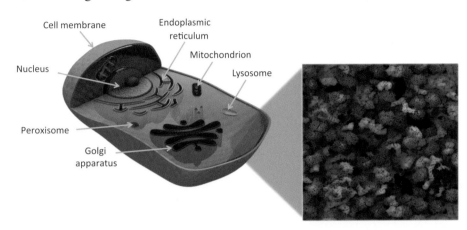

Figure 3.2

Eukaryotic cell and its organelles. A cell's interior (cytoplasm) is crowded and filled with (bio)molecules. Courtesy of Adrian H. Elcock and Sean R. McGuffe, University of Iowa, USA, McGuffe and Elcock (2010).

The interior nuclear membrane, often referred to as the nuclear envelope, protects the **nucleus**. The nucleus is the cell compartment which contains deoxyribonucleic acid (DNA), the carrier of genetic information, as well as the complete machinery needed for expression of genes (see later for more details). Three major functions are performed in the cell nucleus: (i) replication of DNA, (ii) transcription of DNA into messenger ribonucleic acid (mRNA) and (iii) assembly of ribosomes, protein-making machines. After assembly, ribosomes are transported out of the nucleus to enable translation of mRNA information into protein structure. Ribosome-controlled protein production as well as the synthesis of phospholipids, membrane building blocks, is performed in the **endoplasmic reticulum (ER)**. The endoplasmic reticulum contains chaperone proteins that help to fold linear polypeptide chains into complex three-dimensional protein structures. It also serves as a principal storage space for calcium ions (Ca^{2+}), a major signalling ion involved in the regulation of muscle contraction and many other cellular processes. Spread over a large area and containing more than 50% of the total amount of cell membrane lipids, ER also serves as an internal communication network, like a very fast intracellular internet. Similar to ER, but containing only 15% of the total membrane lipids and much smaller is the **Golgi apparatus**, which plays a crucial role in post-synthetic processing of proteins and lipids such as addition of sugar molecules (glycosylation).

All of the processes that take place in various organelles require energy, and that energy is supplied by **mitochondria**. Mitochondria are surrounded by their own membrane and unlike other compartments, have small amounts of their own DNA. It is presumed they originated from invading bacteria, which developed symbiotic relationship with eukaryotic cells in early stages of life development. As crucial organelles involved in cell metabolism and the control of cell suicide, a natural mechanism for removal of faulty or old cells, they have been the subject of many studies aiming to decipher diseases such as Alzheimer's disease or different types of cancer.

Energy needed for cells to thrive and reproduce can be produced in sufficient amounts only if there is a continuous supply of nutrients, and an efficient removal of cellular garbage and toxins. Cell compartments such as **endosomes** are responsible for the organisation of a robust nutrient supply chain. Endosomes are vesicles involved in early transport and sorting of compounds entering a cell. In short, they are a conveyer belt and a sorting operator in one. If an endosome perceives a compound entering the cytosol as useful, it will deliver it to the organelle responsible for further processing. However, if it is perceived as faulty or inactive, it will be digested. The protein sorting mechanism is still full of unknowns, but what we know is that, for example, the decision on the proteins to be used further or digested is made on the basis of subtle differences in the protein's charge, concentration, shape and curvature. As a common entry route for viruses, endosomes have extensively been studied to find new strategies to protect cells from pathogen invasion. They are also involved in transport of drugs (see Chapter 9), and understanding their mechanism of action will aid formulation of drugs and drug nanocarriers and avoid premature deactivation.

Back to Basics 3.1   Prokaryotic vs Eukaryotic Cells

Cells are grouped in two broad categories: **prokaryotic** and **eukaryotic**. **Prokaryotes** (from Greek πρό (pro) 'before' and κάρυον (karyon) 'nut' or 'kernel') are single-cell organisms that are divided into two domains: bacteria and archaea. Many prokaryotes are extremophiles, which thrive in extreme environments (high level of radioactivity, high or low pH/temperature, absence of light, extreme dryness). Prokaryotic bacteria are very common and also play an important role in the human digestive system.

Eukaryotes (from Greek εὖ (eu) 'well' or 'true' and κάρυον (karyon) 'nut' or 'kernel') have cells with defined compartments (organelles), which have specialised functions. Eukaryotes include animals, plants, fungi and protists, such as algae. The main differences between prokaryotes and eukaryotes are given below, but it should be noted that there are always exceptions to the rule.

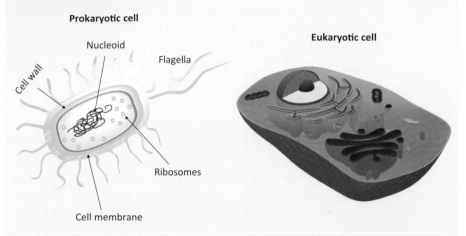

Prokaryotic cell	Eukaryotic cell
• Cell size: 1–10 µm	• Cell size: 10–100 µm
• Chemically complex, rigid cell wall, may contain peptidoglycan	• Chemically simple, flexible phospholipid membrane surrounded by cellulose in plants
• No defined organelles nor cytoskeleton	• Several defined organelles and network of tubules and filaments (cytoskeleton)
• Nucleus is not well defined; DNA is found in a form of irregularly shaped nucleoid	• Nucleus is well defined, surrounded by a membrane
• No mitochondria; metabolic enzymes bound to the membrane	• Mitochondria full of metabolic enzymes
• Asexual reproduction (binary fission)	• Sexual reproduction (meiosis and mitosis)
• Small ribosomes	• Large ribosomes in cytosol/nucleus, small ribosomes in organelles
• DNA transcription and mRNA translation occur simultaneously in cytosol (liquid found inside cells)	• DNA transcription in nucleus, and mRNA translation in cytosol

Compounds deemed unsuitable for further cellular use are transferred from endosomes to **lysosomes** or **peroxisomes** (sometimes called microbodies), vesicles with diameter ranging from 0.1 to 1.2 μm (peroxisomes tend to be slightly smaller than lysosomes). Lysosome's interior is very acidic (pH 4–5) and contains many enzymes that help recycling and disposal of cell garbage or anything that is considered undesirable. Similar to endosomes, the mechanism of lysosome- and peroxisome-mediated garbage disposal is not entirely clear, which poses a huge problem for drug design. It has often been observed that carefully formulated drugs, having successfully crossed the cell membrane, end up in lysosomes where they are quickly deactivated or degraded, and therefore become ineffective. The same happens in peroxisomes, which are named after the large amount of hydrogen peroxide (H_2O_2) they contain. Peroxide is a common product of molecular oxidation and one of the regulatory compounds involved in various enzymatic and signalling processes. Approximately hundreds of peroxisomes can be found in a single cell, with liver and other organs involved in metabolism even containing specialised cells laden with peroxisomes. Although the main role of digestive vesicles is to destroy and remove (bio)molecules, they also act as manufacturers of cell building blocks. Peroxisomes, for example, produce cholesterol and phospholipids found in brain and heart tissue.

It is clear that compartments within a cell have evolved to perform distinct functions, and this compartmentalisation of functions is crucial for the preservation of a cell's robustness while ensuring damage containment and control. Cell membranes protect cells from the environment, but also ensure that there is control over intercellular communication, nutrient uptake and garbage removal. Containment of digestive enzymes within lysosomes and peroxisomes stops them from damaging the cell's integral components needed to perform vital functions. Energy production is contained and finely tuned within the mitochondria and genetic information and a complete read-out machinery are safely tucked into the nucleus. A small amount of damage within compartments can be contained and not immediately spread to the whole cell, allowing for provisions to be made to bring the dynamic system into functioning equilibrium. Of course, serious dysfunction of individual compartments ultimately leads to cell death and its removal, but not before all fail-safe mechanisms are deactivated. Although crucially important, such compartmentalisation also means that a drug or a nanocarrier has to overcome many barriers not only on the way to a cell, but also once the membrane is crossed. Luckily, as we will see later, various nanocarriers with drug cargo have been successfully delivered into the cell, even though the design of cell-targeting systems is still a huge challenge. Studies of biological compartments enable us to compile a set of design rules needed to prepare efficient bionano systems, which can be used either to repair and improve cellular machinery or to mimic its activity.

The following sections are meant to provide a general overview of major biomolecular classes, which play important roles in the design of bionano systems and hybrid materials within the field of bionanotechnology. The description of different classes is simplified and generalised to provide basic information needed to understand subsequent chapters, which provide more details on a particular design or application.

3.2   Carbohydrates

Let us start our overview of molecules crucial for the production of energy. One of the definitions of the living system states that they are living because of their ability to transform and use energy to ensure growth and reproduction. The principal source of energy for most cells in higher organisms is a carbohydrate, D-glucose. Carbohydrates are a large family of compounds composed of carbon, hydrogen and oxygen, and often referred to as sugars. They can be classified according to size into mono- or polysaccharides (saccharide is a chemical name for a sugar unit). Sugar structure is characterised by asymmetric carbons, which determine their **chirality** or orientation in space and result in the formation of isomers.

| Back to Basics 3.2 | Isomers and Molecular Mirror Images |

Isomers are compounds with the same molecular formula, but a different arrangement of atoms. We distinguish **structural** (constitutional) **isomers**, with atoms and functional groups joined together in different ways, and **stereoisomers**, which differ in positions of atoms and functional groups in space. Pairs of stereoisomers that are mirror images of each other are known as **enantiomers**. Enantiomers have identical physical properties (melting point, boiling point, density), but differ in how they interact with polarised light and with other stereoisomers such as proteins.

L- and D-alanine cannot be superimposed: they are molecular mirror images

Enantiomers are **chiral** (from the ancient Greek χεῖρ (cheir) 'hand') molecules. Like the left and right hand, their mirror images are non-superposable and they have no plane of symmetry. Chiral molecules contain one or more asymmetric carbon centres usually referred to as chiral centres (marked by *), such as tetrahedral carbons with four different substituents.

Carbohydrates and amino acids are designated as D- or L- according to the stereochemistry of the highest numbered carbon in a Fischer projection (simplified 2D representation of a 3D molecule named after Emil Fischer in 1891). If the hydroxyl or amino group is pointing to the right in the Fischer projection, the sugar or amino acid is designated as a D isomer (from the Latin dexter, 'right'). If the hydroxyl or amino group is pointing to the left in the Fischer projection, the sugar or amino acid is designated as an L isomer (from Latin laevus, 'left').

Simple sugars such as glucose can have two **stereoisomers** referred to as L- and D-, which have identical chemical composition but two different orientations in 3D space (see Back to Basics 3.2 for more on isomers). The presence of this distinct stereochemical character is important for interactions of sugars with other biomolecules involved in their metabolism and recognition. However, one of the still unexplained structural mysteries of biological world is the predominant presence of **D-sugars and L-amino acids** in nature. Reverse L-sugars and D-amino acids are much less prominently featured. Some microorganisms have been found that can digest L-sugars, and D-amino acids have been identified in some marine invertebrates, bacteria and plants, mainly as a structural component of the cell wall, but not the protein building block. Sugar metabolism is a major source of energy for all organisms except for some microorganisms, which use other energy sources such as hydrocarbons, lipids, amino acids or single carbon molecules. Complex sugars such as starch are first digested into smaller glucose units, which can then enter the cell's metabolic cycles.

In vertebrates, blood transports glucose throughout the body. When the cellular energy is low, glucose is used as a fuel for **glycolysis**, a process that results in release of two **adenine triphosphate (ATP)** molecules, the bitcoins of chemical energy (see Back to Basics 3.3 for more).

Glycolysis is believed to be among the oldest biochemical pathways. It occurs in almost every living cell and it is a first step of both the aerobic (in the presence of oxygen) and the anaerobic (in the absence of oxygen) respiration by which a molecule of glucose is degraded into carbon dioxide, water and energy.

When levels of glucose are high and no more glucose is needed, it can be stored in the liver or muscle in a form of glycogen through the process of **glycogenesis**.

| Back to Basics 3.3 | It Is an ATP World |

Adenosine triphosphate (ATP) is a nucleotide (triphosphate of the nucleoside adenosine) and the molecular currency of intracellular energy. It is mainly produced by processes of glycolysis and oxidative phosphorylation.

Hydrolysis of anhydride bonds in ATP generates enough energy to drive movement of all muscles, transport of nerve signals and, basically, all chemical reactions within the cell. Cleavage of one phosphate anhydride bond releases about $30.6\,\text{kJ}\,\text{mol}^{-1}$ of energy while producing adenosine diphosphate (ADP) and a phosphate molecule. Double dephosphorylation of ATP into adenosine monophosphate (AMP) releases about $45.6\,\text{kJ}\,\text{mol}^{-1}$.

The human body uses $\sim 2 \times 10^{26}$ transient molecules of ATP in a single day (mass of the body's own weight). Additionally, ATP serves as a phosphate donor for the synthesis of nucleic acids as well as an important modulator of signalling cascades.

The balance between all of these processes is crucial and glucose metabolism is closely regulated by the hormone insulin, which is responsible for activation of different pathways depending on glucose levels and cell needs. For example, brain and red blood cells rely exclusively on glucose as the energy source and irregularities in the glucose level can have serious consequences. It should be noted that glucose is not only obtained from complex sugars such as starch, but also from non-carbohydrate sources such as lactate (from skeletal muscle), amino acids (from proteins) or glycerol (from fat). Besides glucose, other sugars such as monosaccharide fructose, or disaccharides sucrose and lactose from milk can directly be used as metabolic energy sources.

In addition to its role in energy production, glucose can be used to synthesise other monosaccharides, fatty acids and even some amino acids, and it is a major component of polysaccharides cellulose, chitin and lignin. Cellulose and chitin are being extensively used to prepare biocompatible nanofibres with the width in nanometre range. Cellulose is a particularly interesting material; as a main building block of the plant cell walls it is the most abundant molecule on Earth, and has been one of the most important materials that helped development of civilised societies. There would not be books without paper, shelters without wooden building blocks, cooked food and warm houses without the fire. In a nano-form, cellulose continues to play an important role for the design of modern materials.

Nanocellulose, both fibres and crystals, which can be obtained from plant and microbial sources, is characterised by high strength and stiffness, a large surface area and contains a large number of hydroxyl groups for additional modification. Due to its excellent mechanical properties and biocompatibility, it is used in applications ranging from material design to electronics and tissue engineering (Back to Basics 3.4).

Back to Basics 3.4   Nanocellulose

Nanocellulose, the term which encompasses cellulose nanofibres and nano-crystals, is mostly obtained from **lignocellulosic biomass**, through mechanical and chemical treatment. Plant lignocellulosic biomass is considered to be one of the most promising sustainable sources of carbon materials and a feedstock for production of biochemicals and biofuel (Jensen et al., 2017).

Cellulose fibrils in the plant cell walls are made of fibres composed of highly ordered crystalline and disordered amorphous regions. Depending on the shape, size and structure we distinguish three main types of nano-cellulose: longer **nanofibres** with length (l) up to 2000 nm, rod-shaped **nanocrystals** with length from 100 to 500 nm and **bacterial nanocellulose**, which usually comes in the form of twisted ribbons with diameter (d) from 20 to 100 nm (Phanthong et al., 2018). Bacterial nanocellulose is obtained in a bottom-up process from glucose monomers. Nanocellulose is characterised by excellent mechanical properties such as high tensile strength (eight times higher than that of stainless steel), and high stiffness of up to 220 GPa, which is greater than Kevlar fibre. Nanocellulose is also transparent and contains a large number of hydroxyl (OH) groups, which can be additionally modified. Together with high biocompatibility, these properties make nanocellulose particularly useful for applications ranging from biodegradable material design (biopackaging, water cleaning filters) to electronics (foldable displays) and medicine (nanocomposites discussed in Chapter 9) and engineered tissues (Chen et al., 2018).

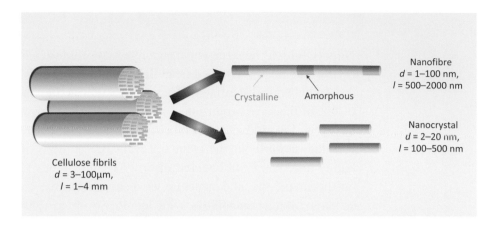

In mammalian cells, most proteins and many lipids contain covalently bound sugars, which increase the hydrophilic character of lipids and proteins and contribute to stabilisation of membrane protein structure. **Glycoproteins** and **glycolipids** also play an integral role in cell–cell and cell–matrix interactions by regulating cell adhesion, tracking and signal transduction. Cells often contain sugar-binding receptors, which aid cell recognition, particularly important for proper functioning of the immune system, and immune cell docking by which unwanted cells can be removed. Numerous studies have shown that formation of tumour cells is often related to complex alteration in glycosylation of molecules, making this process one of the potential targets for cancer therapies (Chen et al., 2018).

3.3 Lipids

Lipids are the family of macromolecules (very large molecules) made of a head group and fatty acid chain, which can differ in length and the level of saturation (saturated or unsaturated based on the presence of saturated single or unsaturated double carbon–carbon bonds).

They not only build cell membranes, but act as precursors for synthesis of steroid hormones (for example, cortisol and testosterone), engage in signalling and, in the form of fat or triglycerides (glycerol bound to three fatty acids), are used for long-term energy storage in animals. Due to their structure and the presence of fatty acid chains, lipids are generally hydrophobic (water repelling), non-polar and immiscible with water.

An important class of lipids are **phospholipids**, components of the eukaryotic cell membrane. Composed of two fatty acid chains and glycerol–phosphate head, phospholipids can also contain additional functional groups, such as choline or serine (R in Figure 3.3), which determine their charge and the way they interact with neighbouring molecules. Presence of structural elements of opposing charge gives phospholipids an **amphiphilic character** meaning that they can be both **hydrophilic** (water loving) and **hydrophobic** (water repelling). In cell membranes, the phospholipid bilayer is arranged in a such way that the hydrophilic heads are exposed to the exterior and interior of the cell, and hydrophobic tails are facing the membrane's inner space. Such organisation ensures low energy, a stable state in which any breakage is energetically unfavourable and the system has self-healing properties. If a hole is formed within the bilayer, it will reseal quickly to cover exposed hydrophobic tails.

Figure 3.3

Structure of phospholipid bilayer that comprises a cell membrane. The water-loving (hydrophilic) and water-repelling (hydrophobic) characteristics of phospholipids guide the cell membrane assembly into two adjacent layers of phospholipids, forming a bilayer.

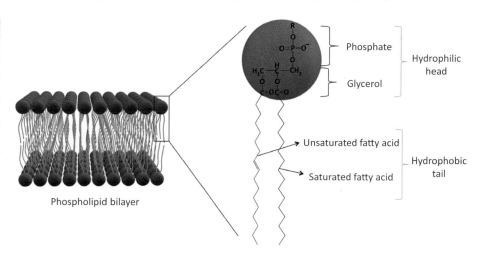

Far from being homogeneous assemblies, cell membranes contain a large number of proteins. It was long believed that no protein could penetrate a membrane and that the main role of the lipid bilayer is to separate extracellular from intracellular proteins. Today we know that this is not the case and that **transmembrane proteins** span the cell membrane and act as molecular gateways for control of molecular trafficking. Contrary to proteins, which can be found on the exterior and interior of the cell membrane, sugars present in the form of **glycolipids** are mostly exposed to the cell exterior. They play an important role in cell–cell interactions and also have a stabilising effect through formation of hydrogen bonds with surrounding water molecules.

Due to their high self-assembling ability (more on self-assembly in Chapter 4), lipids can form small droplets or micelles in water. A variation of such micelles are **liposomes**, nanosized spherical vesicles with a bilayer membrane, which are often used in bionanotechnology as carriers of therapeutic cargo into the cells (Figure 3.4).

Figure 3.4

Common lipid-based architectures. From left to right; bilayer vesicles called liposomes, single-layer micelles and a planar bilayer.

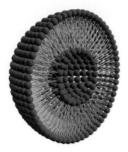

3.4   Nucleic Acids

Code that determines the structure and function of each cell, ultimately affecting the health and longevity of every organism, is written within two types of nucleic acids, **deoxyribonucleic (DNA)** and **ribonucleic (RNA)** acid. Both are polymeric species made of repeating chains of basic elements composed of *sugar* (deoxyribose or ribose), *base* (adenine, thymine, guanine, cytosine and uracil) and *phosphate* groups (Figure 3.5 and Back to Basics 3.5).

Figure 3.5

Structure of nucleic acid chain. Bases linked to sugars (nucleosides) are joined into a polymeric chain through phosphate linkage. A nucleic acid polymer unit, composed of a base, sugar and at least one phosphate, is referred to as a nucleotide.

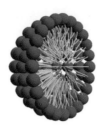

Ribose (in RNA)

Uracil (in RNA)

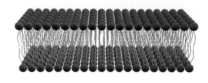

Nucleic acids perform two primary biological functions related to coding and transfer of biological information; one is the storage of genetic information, which determines the structure and function of every protein within a cell (this is usually the role of DNA, although some simple organisms such as viruses store their genetic information within RNA), and the other is the transcription of this coded information into the language of protein-making machines (this is mediated by RNA). Although it was long believed that nucleic acids can be found exclusively in the nucleus, it has been shown that there are also small DNA structures found in the extracellular space of microorganisms. **Extracellular DNA (eDNA)** has been discovered in cultures of numerous species of bacteria, archaea and fungi, in particular in multi-cellular microbial communities known as biofilms. The exact role of eDNA is yet to be determined, but it is known that it is important for biofilm formation and defence, can be used as a nutrient (it is an excellent source of nitrogen and phosphorus), and is involved in DNA damage repair and gene transfer (Okshevsky and Meyer, 2013).

Back to Basics 3.5	Nucleic Acid Glossary
Nucleoside:	structural subunit of nucleic acids, consisting of a molecule of sugar (deoxyribose in DNA, and ribose in RNA) linked to a nitrogenous base (nucleobase thymine, adenine, guanine, cytosine, uridine).
Nucleotides:	monomers which form DNA and RNA polymers. A nucleotide consists of sugar, a nitrogenous base and at least one phosphate group. The nucleotide can also be termed as 'nucleoside monophosphate' (e.g. adenosine monophosphate).
Base pairs (bp):	a pair formed between complementary bases. Adenine pairs with thymine (AT pair) forming two hydrogen bonds, guanine with cytosine (CG pairs) forming three hydrogen bonds. This is referred to as a conventional Watson–Crick base pairing.
Base stacking:	also called π–π stacking refers to an attractive, non-covalent interaction between aromatic nucleobases. Base stacking interactions are hydrophobic and electrostatic in nature and depend on the aromaticity of the bases and their dipole moments. Base stacking interactions can occur within a single or between different strands, but are much more prevalent in duplexes and in the presence of high salt concentration.

Hybridisation:	formation of a non-covalent, sequence-specific bond between mainly two (high-order complexes are possible, see Chapter 7) complementary single DNA or RNA strands. Although the DNA double helix is generally stable under physiological conditions, high temperature or basic conditions can split or 'melt' the double helix into single complementary strands.
DNA melting temperature (T_m):	the temperature at which 50% of DNA has denatured from double-stranded DNA (dsDNA) to single-stranded DNA (ssDNA). T_m depends on the length of DNA, the nucleotide sequence composition, salt concentration (ionic strength of the added salt) and, generally, lies between 50 °C and 100 °C.
Gene:	a segment of DNA or RNA that codes for a specific polypeptide sequence/protein involved in cellular processes. Often multiple genes at different positions of nucleic acids work in synergy to control particular function or a process. Human genes vary in size from a few hundred (i.e. the gene for histone proteins involved in DNA packing has ~500 bp) to more than two million DNA bases (the *DMD* gene coding for the protein dystrophin involved in muscle movement has ~2.5 million bp). Humans have between 20 000 and 25 000 genes.
Chromosome:	a thread-like structure of packed DNA stored in the cell nucleus. Each chromosome is made up of DNA coiled many times around histone proteins, ensuring tight packing. Different species have a different number of chromosomes, for example, ants have 2, mice 40, humans 46, potatoes 48 and some butterflies more than 250.
Genome:	a complete set of genes or genetic information present in a cell or an organism. Genomes contain all the information needed to build and maintain a functioning, living cell.

3.4.1 Deoxyribonucleic Acid

Native deoxyribonucleic acid (DNA) consists of two single polymeric chains, which pair up to form a structure often referred to as a double helix. The stability of the double helix stems from hydrogen bonding between complementary base pairs, two hydrogen bonds for A–T and three for G–C (Figure 3.6). It also depends on base stacking within the interior of the helix to shield hydrophobic bases from water molecules surrounding the exterior of the double helix.

Formation of base pairs in a double-stranded DNA. There are two hydrogen bonds between T–A and three between G–C.

Both complementary single strands within the double-stranded structure are negatively charged due to the presence of phosphate groups. They require positively charged cations such as Mg^{2+} to act as bridging ions, enabling the strands to come close enough to engage in short-range hydrogen bonding. The complementary strands form a double helix in an antiparallel fashion: they run next to each other but in the opposite directions meaning that the 'head' of one strand is always laid against the 'tail' of the other. Directions of the strands are indicated by writing $5'$ (five prime) and $3'$ (three prime) in front of the base sequence. The numbers 5 and 3 refer to the carbon numbers within the sugar with $5'$ indicating the position at which phosphate is bound, while $3'$ is a carbon with attached OH group. If we take the $5'$-ATT GCC TTA TGC-$3'$ strand, the sequence of the complementary strand which runs in an antiparallel fashion would be $3'$-TAA CGG AAT ACG-$5'$ (as a convention, sequences are noted down using only one prime number and usually starting with $5'$ on the left-hand side).

A double helix formed of two antiparallel single strands has distinct structural features such as **major and minor grooves**, which play important roles in the control of DNA–protein interactions, and a **pitch** which is a measure of the vertical distance separating two points on a helix after one complete 'turn' (Figure 3.7). There are three known forms of DNA double helix, referred to as **A-, B- and Z-DNA**. Our genetic information carrier is **B-DNA**, a right-handed helix with pitch of 10.4 bases (3.32 nm) and diameter of approximately 2 nm.

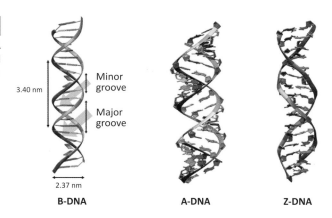

Figure 3.7

Dimensions of B-DNA and structures of A- and Z-DNA forms.

Water molecules play an important role in the stabilisation of the helix by enforcing base stacking, and there are at least 12–15 water molecules associated with each nucleotide in B-DNA. When the humidity conditions change, the B-helix collapses into the A-DNA form, bringing the phosphate groups closer together and changing the geometry of the structure. Unlike A- and B-DNA, Z-DNA, another form discovered in 1979, is left handed, has a pitch of 12 bases, which makes it slimmer than B-DNA, and it lacks major grooves. Due to its structure, Z-DNA is less stable than other DNA forms and it needs to be stabilised with lots of salt. It is also considered a transient structure, which can occasionally be induced by certain biological processes, but disappears quickly. Although its function has not been fully explained, it is clear that Z-DNA plays a role in replication and DNA information read-out (Rich and Zhang, 2003) as well as immune response (D'Ascenzo et al., 2016).

DNA is a remarkable biopolymer, characterised by high physiochemical stability. It is more stable than proteins so it can survive hours in a boiling water and thousands of years if the conditions are right (the oldest sample of DNA was extracted from a 700 000-year-old horse). DNA is also programmable, which means that a single-stranded DNA can be made with desired sequence of bases, can be cut at the precise positions with the help of restriction enzymes, joined together by ligases, and copied using polymerases. The breakthrough that ultimately led to the development of the DNA nano-technology field (explored in Chapter 6) was chemical synthesis of small single strands of DNA (up to 80 bases) and introduction of non-native functional groups to various positions within the strand.

Unlike eukaryotic DNA, DNA in most prokaryotes and many viruses, which have smaller genomes (see Back to Basics 3.5 for the definition of genome), is circular, which makes it more stable and eases the replication, both traits important for fast replicating organisms. Such DNA is also found in almost all plant chloroplasts involved in photosynthesis and eukaryotic mitochondria. Therefore, it is believed that it originated from bacteria that were engulfed by early eukaryotic cells. One type of DNA particularly important for molecular biology is a **plasmid DNA**, small circular DNA that usually contains one or few genes. Plasmid DNAs are used in molecular biology to introduce genes for specific non-native proteins to fast-growing organisms such as bacteria, which then act as protein-making factories (see Back to Basics 3.9).

3.4.2   Ribonucleic Acid

The primary structure of ribonucleic acid (RNA) is similar to DNA with two notable differences: deoxyribose is replaced by ribose, which has an additional hydroxyl group at the $2'$ position, and thymine (T) base by uracil (U) (see Figure 3.5). Due to the intramolecular reaction in which additional hydroxyl oxygen from ribose sugar can cleave a phosphate backbone, RNA is less stable and not as suitable for information storage as DNA. The presence of the hydroxyl group and particular shape are responsible for catalytic activity of some RNA structures known as ribozymes, short for ribonucleic acid enzymes.

Like DNA, RNA can be single or double stranded, linear or circular, but unlike natural DNA, RNA comes in many shapes and lengths, adapting to the different roles it plays in the cell. There have been more than 25 different types of RNA identified so far, and possibly there are many more. These RNA molecules are involved in regulation of cell processes ranging from gene expression to protein trafficking. The three most prominent and best understood types of RNA are messenger RNA (mRNA), ribosomal RNA (rRNA) and transfer RNA (tRNA) (Figure 3.8), involved in transcription of DNA code into the language of the protein-making machines.

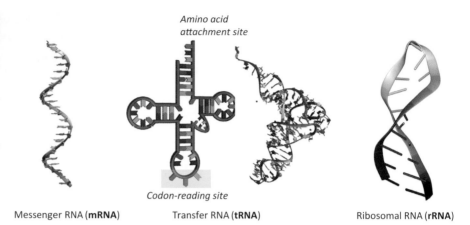

Figure 3.8

Different types of RNA.
Whereas mRNA is a
single strand of
nucleotides of varying
lengths, tRNA and rRNA
are composed of various
structural elements such
as loops and bulges. To
simplify the depiction of
complex structures,
schematic 2D
representations have
been developed.

Messenger RNA **(mRNA)**   Transfer RNA **(tRNA)**   Ribosomal RNA **(rRNA)**

mRNA are linear RNA molecules, whereas tRNA and rRNAs form heterogeneous structures characterised by 'hairpins' made of double-stranded stems and terminal, single-stranded loops. Hairpin sequence, size and number vary across different RNA types, and it has been shown that hairpins are crucial for regulation of gene expression, serve as binding sites for proteins, and can act both as centres of intrinsic catalytic activity and the substrates for enzyme catalysed reactions (Svoboda and Di Cara, 2006).

3.5   From DNA to Protein: Central Dogma of Molecular Biology

DNA is made of nucleotides, proteins are made of amino acids. Figure 3.9 shows the 20 naturally occurring amino acids that can be combined to build millions of proteins, all of which vary in shape, size and the function they perform. To illustrate the diversity of proteins, let us just consider their size. The smallest protein Trp-cage contains a mere 20 amino acids, whereas more than 40 000 amino acids are needed to build the protein titin, the largest human protein found in muscle.

Amino acids are covalently linked through peptide bonds, and their sequence is encoded in nucleotides. Specifically, a triplet of nucleic acid bases corresponds to a single amino acid. There are 4 nucleotides meaning that there are 4^3 or 64 triplet combinations called **codons**. There are 61 codons that encode for 20 natural amino acids, while the remaining 3 represent STOP signals responsible for arrest of amino acid chain formation. Since there are more codons than amino acids, often there is more than one codon for a particular amino acid. Only a tryptophan (Trp) and methionine (Met) are encoded by a single triplet. Such degeneracy of the code minimises

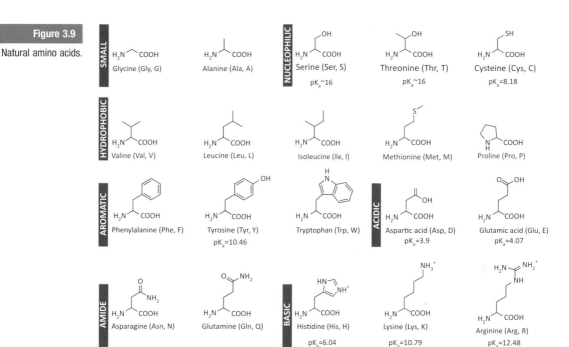

Figure 3.9

Natural amino acids.

detrimental effects of DNA mutations by ensuring that even if a base changes, an amino acid chain with a correct sequence can still be synthesised. If there were only one codon per amino acid, 20 codons would be responsible for coding, whereas 44 would signal the STOP action, arresting the synthesis and leading to faulty and inactive proteins.

The principle that describes the transformation of genetic information stored in DNA into a protein is called the **central dogma of molecular biology** and it consists of two distinct steps: **transcription** and **translation** (Figure 3.10).

Figure 3.10

Central dogma of molecular biology. Information on amino acid sequence is stored in DNA, transcribed into mRNA and then translated into a polypeptide chain, which folds into 3D protein structure.

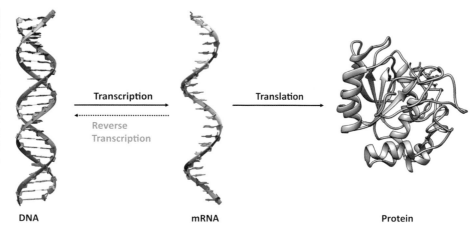

During transcription, mRNA is obtained which is complementary to a DNA region encoding for a protein of interest. Once synthesised and often additionally modified, mRNA leaves the nucleus and interacts with a **ribosome**, a protein-making machine in the cytoplasm (Back to Basics 3.6).

The mRNA binding to a ribosome initiates translation, which ultimately results in formation of an amino acid chain. A ribosome moves along the mRNA, reading the transcribed code, and at the same time, it captures tRNAs, which carry amino acids, and incorporates them into the growing chain by peptide bond formation. It is important to note that each amino acid is enzymatically bound to its own tRNA. There are two distinct regions within tRNA: one contains the bound amino acid, and another nucleotide triplet complementary to the codon of the bound acid. For example, phenylalanine will be bound to the tRNA specific for phenylalanine (tRNA^{Phe}), which contains the AAA triplet complementary to the UUU codon, one of the phenylalanine coding nucleotide triplets.

Back to Basics 3.6   Ribosomes: True Biological Machines

Ribosomes are protein machines, catalytic centres for the synthesis of polypeptide chains from the mRNA code template. Eukaryotic cells assemble approximately 20 amino acids per second (the mRNA that brings the message is degraded within 2 min so the ribosome needs to be fast), and the ribosomes are composed of between 55 and 80 different proteins and four types of ribosomal RNAs (rRNAs) (prokaryotic ribosomes contain three rRNAs).

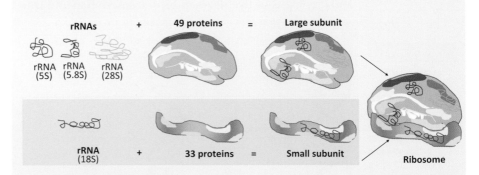

A recent study has shown that ribosomes are composed of many small protein units, rather than one large protein, to ensure that proteins, including those that make up the ribosome, are made quickly and are readily available whenever a new species has to be made (Reuveni et al., 2017).

Eukaryotic cells contain around 10 million ribosomes. Assembly of ribosomes starts in the nucleus, with the synthesis of rRNA. Three rRNAs (28S, 5.8S and 5S) then assemble with 49 proteins to form the large subunit, referred to as 60S subunit (S is a Svedberg unit, a non-metric unit for the sedimentation coefficient). The fourth rRNA (18S) assembles with 33 proteins to form a small 40S subunit. Finally, both subunits assemble as a functional ribosome in the cell cytoplasm.

Prokaryotic ribosomes, as well as those found in chloroplasts and mitochondria, are smaller in size (70S ribosomes) and made of the small 30S subunit (16S rRNA and 21 proteins) and a large 50S subunit (5S rRNA, 23S rRNA and 31 proteins).

rRNA is an important part of the ribosomal machine, it constitutes 60% of its mass. It plays a role in the recognition of certain parts of mRNA and tRNA to ensure the correct read-out, and it is involved in catalysis for both the ribosome assembly and protein synthesis.

3.6   Proteins

Ribosome-aided translation results in a linear polypeptide chain of amino acids. Such a chain comprises a protein skeleton, which folds, or it is folded into complex 3D structure after synthesis.

Protein structure determines its function, and we distinguish four levels of structural complexity: primary, secondary, tertiary and quaternary structure. **Primary structure** describes amino acid sequence within the polypeptide chain. **Secondary protein structure** takes into account hydrogen bonding between different amino acids present in the primary sequence and it can be divided into α-helices and β-sheets (see Back to Basics 3.7).

Back to Basics 3.7	Secondary Protein Structure Motifs

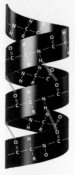

α-helix

α-helices result from hydrogen bonding between the backbone amides resulting in the right-handed helices containing 3.6 amino acids per turn. Most helices are based on heptad (7) sequence repeats (abcdefg). The first and fourth position (a and d) are usually hydrophobic residues while others tend to be polar. The whole heptad measures 1 nm, but longer sequences (20–30 amino acids) are required to achieve α-helical structures. α-helices are important components of fibrous proteins found in water-rich environments.

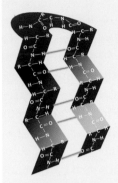

β-sheet

β-sheets are planar structures composed of two or more β-strands, which are organised perpendicular to the fibril axis and connected through a dense hydrogen-bonding network between amide and carboxyl groups in the protein backbone. Individual β-strands are short and usually composed of 5–8 residues. In many proteins, β-sheets form the floor of the reaction pocket, while in structural proteins, multiple layers of sheets are responsible for toughness. Silk fibres consist almost entirely of stacks of antiparallel β-sheets.

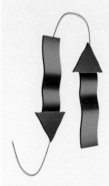

β-hairpin

β-hairpin is composed of two antiparallel β-sheets. The loop sequence usually contains alternating hydrophobic (such as valine) and hydrophilic (lysine) amino acids. Hairpin structures can be found in high-order fibres and peptide hydrogels. They have also been shown to exhibit inherent antibacterial activity against bacteria probably due to disruption of the bacterial cell membrane (Salick et al., 2007).

Interactions between helices and sheets result in more complex 3D **tertiary protein structure**, and finally, **quaternary structure** refers to assemblies of distinct amino acid chains (domains) into multi-domain proteins (Figure 3.11). The mass of protein is reported in **daltons** (a dalton, Da, is an atomic mass unit), which is directly related to its molecular weight (MW, dimensionless number). Given that the average amino acid has a molecular mass of 100 Da, a protein that is made of 60 amino acids will have a mass of 6000 Da or 6 kDa. The size of the protein can be considered both in terms of its geometrical parameters (how much space it takes up) and in terms of its sequence size (measured in Da). Determination of how much space the protein takes up (its geometrical size) is much more complex than determining its amino acid sequence and structure. It usually relies on the determination of size through sedimentation and diffusion of proteins, taking into account the number of bound water molecules (hydration) and applying different mathematical algorithms to obtained parameters (Erickson, 2009). In some cases, the size can be determined by electron microscopy (Chapter 5). However, such measurements do not take into account the hydration and do not reflect the physiological reality, so that electron microscopy data need to be used in combination with other methods.

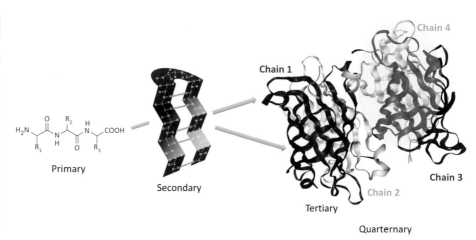

Figure 3.11

Protein architecture. Primary structure showing peptide bond, β-sheet formed through interactions between amino acids (secondary), and tertiary structure composed of β-sheets and α-helices. Quarternary structure represents multiple distinct peptide chains (protein domains) joined together.

Based on the assumption that all proteins have approximately the same density of $1.37\,\mathrm{g\,cm^{-3}}$, a simplified formula can be deduced, which states that $M\,(\text{in Da}) = 825\,V\,(\mathrm{nm^3})$ (Erickson, 2009). For spheric proteins, protein radius can be calculated from the volume, but such calculations are less straightforward for proteins of other shapes.

Besides amino acids, proteins often contain metals, small nucleic acids or organic molecules such as flavin or heme within their structure. Many of those belong to a family of enzymes, biomolecular catalysts that speed up chemical transformations in the cell. **Enzymes** are characterised by high specificity and efficiency. For example, enzymes involved in cleavage of the peptide bond (proteases), a process crucial for protein recycling, make this reaction 10^{13} times faster than it would be in the absence of a catalyst. As a result, a reaction which would take 300 to 600 years to complete without any help is completed within 1 ms in the presence of an enzyme. As far as the enzymes go, this is still relatively slow; one of the fastest enzymes known is carbonic anhydrase, which aids transport of metabolically produced CO_2 from cell to the lungs by hydrating 10^6 molecules of CO_2 per second. It is not surprising that the use of enzymes as well as the design of bionano hybrids that mimic their function, is considered one of the solutions to the ongoing goals of sustainable development.

But let us go back to proteins in general. Due to their remarkable structural and functional diversity there are different ways of grouping protein into families or classes (see Back to Basics 3.8).

Back to Basics 3.8   Protein Classification

There are many approaches to protein classification, and more details can be found in biochemistry textbooks. The groups given here illustrate the variety of their functions and structures.

According to their source:

Animal proteins: sometimes referred to as higher-quality proteins, as they contain an appropriate amount of essential amino acids. Examples are egg protein ovalbumin, milk protein κ-casein, or meat and fish proteins such as oxygen transporter myoglobin.

Plant proteins: also called lower-quality proteins, as they contain a lower amount of one or many essential amino acids. Such is biotechnologically important horseradish peroxidase enzyme.

According to their shape:

Globular or **corpuscular proteins:** their axial ratio (length:width) is less than 10 (usually not over 3 or 4) and therefore have a relatively spherical/ovoid shape. Complex in terms of conformation, they also have a great range of biological functions compared to fibrous or membrane proteins (i.e. antibodies, enzymes).

Fibrous or **fibrillar proteins:** with an axial ratio greater than 10 and shaped as fibres that can further assemble into ribbons and fibrils. They are characterised by exceptional mechanical properties (collagen, elastin, keratin, fibroin).

Integral membrane proteins: permanently attached to a cell membrane (i.e. calcium ATPase, aquaporin, permease).

According to solubility and composition:

Simple proteins or holoproteins: contain only amino acids as structural elements.

Conjugated or complex proteins/heteroproteins: contain distinguishable non-protein molecule (metal or small functional molecule) called *prosthetic group*. Depending on the role of the prosthetic group they can be metalloproteins, chromoproteins glycoprotein, phosphoproteins and lipoproteins.

Derived proteins: protein derivatives formed as a result of a chemical reaction, heat or enzymatic treatment (i.e. coagulated proteins).

According to biological function:

Enzymic proteins: biological catalysts (amylase, catalase, alcohol dehydrogenase).

Structural proteins: maintain biological structures (collagen, keratin).

Transport proteins: transport ions and small molecules (haemoglobin).

Nutrient and storage proteins: provide nutrition and store ions (ferritin, casein).

Contractile or motile proteins: components of the contractile system (myosin, tubulin, actin).

Defence proteins: defend organism from injury/pathogens and toxic agents (antibodies, thrombin).

Regulatory proteins: regulate cellular and metabolic activity (insulin, growth hormone).

Those of known structure are included in the **protein data bank (PDB),** which currently has more than 100 000 entries, although the function of around 40% of those has still not been elucidated. The PDB, an open and freely accessible protein archive, was established in 1971 at Brookhaven National Laboratory in the USA, and originally contained only seven protein entries, expanding into a worldwide protein data bank in 2003.

In bionanotechnology, proteins can be roughly classified into four groups, depending on the distinct role they play in either the build-up of hybrid materials, devices or biosensors. These are:

1. **Interfacing proteins**, which can be used to design biocompatible interfaces, and either facilitate attachment of other molecular species or act as biorecognition elements.
2. **Labelling proteins/protein tags**, genetically fused to proteins of interest to enable their identification, purification or in vivo visualisation.

3. **Catalytic proteins or enzymes**, which catalyse specific reactions useful either for preparation and modification of nanomaterials or used for the design of biosensors.
4. **Structural proteins,** which can be used for preparation of hybrid materials by either acting as templates or active building blocks.

Often groups 1 and 2 can be used interchangeably as there are proteins such as streptavidin (STV) that can be classified both as an interfacing and labelling protein.

3.7   Proteins in Bionanotechnology: Interfacing Proteins

Proteins can act as biomolecular glue for modification of the nanomaterial surface or for binding two distinct components of a hybrid material. They can stabilise the surface and prevent aggregation of nanocomponents, but also act as recognition components, for example to ease the interaction with other (bio)molecules on the cell surface.

3.7.1   Streptavidin

The most extensively used 'protein glue' in bionanotechnology are proteins from the avidin family. **Avidin**, a tetrameric protein (composed of four distinct domains), is a major component of egg white, characterised by its antibiotic properties; it sequesters biotin (also known as vitamin B7 or vitamin H), and in such a way, it helps prevent bacterial growth within an egg. Binding of biotin is so efficient that the avidin–biotin bond is considered the strongest known non-covalent interaction and it is unaffected by extremes of pH, high temperature, presence of organic solvents and other denaturing agents, all of which have damaging effects on biomolecules. Studies have shown that the force of 257 pN is needed to destroy streptavidin–biotin bonds, while 40 pN is sufficient to impair other typical protein–protein and protein–small molecule interactions. Streptavidin is an avidin protein obtained from the bacterium *Streptomyces avidinii* (Figure 3.12), but unlike avidin, it does not contain surface sugars so it is much less prone to non-specific interactions, which is advantageous for use in hybrid systems. Although there are around 180 different proteins in the avidin family, streptavidin remains the most widely used interfacing protein in molecular biology and bionanotechnology.

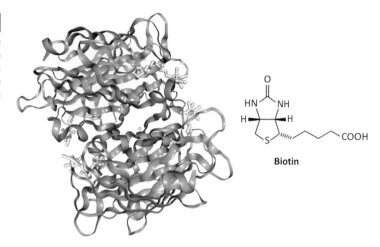

Figure 3.12

Streptavidin protein with four bound biotin molecules shown in yellow (PDB structure 4GJV; Zimbron et al., 2013).

Biotin

Other proteins that interact with small molecular species or biomolecules such as various protein tags (see Section 3.8) have also been used for building block assembly, but none are so specific and versatile as antibodies.

3.7.2 Antibodies and Nanobodies

Antibodies or immunoglobulins are produced by the immune systems of vertebrates to neutralise dangerous pathogens or (bio)molecules. Antibodies circulate through the blood in search of unfamiliar structures, called **antigens**, bind to their surface and alert the immune system to initiate their removal. This action is facilitated by antibodies' distinct structure. They are composed of two arms attached to the central body (Y-shape) through thin and flexible chains, allowing for an adaptive binding to the unknown molecular species (Figure 3.13 shows the antibody crystal structure). The Y-shaped antibody contains two distinguishable protein parts: two long heavy chains (grey in Figure 3.13) typically 50–70 kDa in size, and two shorter light chains (red in Figure 3.13) of 25 kDa. Sometimes researchers talk about Fc (Fc stands for crystallisable fragment) and Fab (Fab stands for binding site containing fragments), stemming from the characteristic profile of antibody breakage in the presence of enzyme papain. When exposed to papain antibody can be cleaved into one Fc and two Fab fragments.

Antibodies can have up to 10 sites for antigen binding, which can vary in strength, but still enable tight overall binding. These are found at the tips of

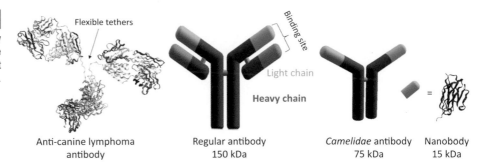

Figure 3.13

Structures of antibody and nanobody. Flexible tethers join different structural units.

Anti-canine lymphoma antibody

Regular antibody
150 kDa

Camelidae antibody
75 kDa

Nanobody
15 kDa

the two arms, in a pocket formed between light and heavy chain, and have very different lengths and amino acid composition.

Our blood contains more than a hundred million different antibodies, and each binds to a specific antigen. This exceptional specificity makes them excellent recognition elements for cell targeting. They have also shown promise for cancer research and therapy (Research Report 3.1), as they can be designed to specifically bind to the cancer cells and inhibit their signalling pathways and growth (Scott et al., 2012).

Research Report 3.1   Antibodies in Cancer Therapy

More than 350 antibodies are currently in clinical trials, and in 2018 around 70 intact antibodies or fragments received approval for clinical applications as anti-cancer therapeutics. Three monoclonal antibodies, which specifically bind to one particular target, and are made in the lab, bevacizumab, rituximab and trastuzumab (Herceptin), are bestselling protein therapeutics.

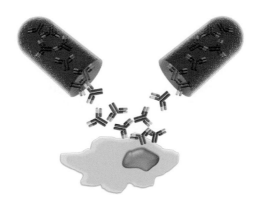

In cancer therapy, **antibodies** can be used either to directly induce cell death by binding to the cell surface and interfering with cell signalling, or by changing the tumour environment, for example, by inhibiting blood vessel growth. Once attached to the cancer cells, they can also flag down the immune system cleaner cells to help with their removal. In bionanotechnology, they are often employed as targeting molecules aiding delivery of drugs or nanoparticles. Despite the potential of antibody therapies, there are still a few challenges such as difficult target access, large variations in individual response to therapy and the lack of control over penetration and distribution of antibodies within the tumour tissue.

Some of these challenges have been tackled by use of **nanobodies**. Due to their small size, a nanobody can penetrate tumours easier than regular antibodies. In addition, they have a high degree of sequence identity with human antibodies and can be easily expressed in microbial hosts, and readily cloned to form fusions with other therapeutic proteins. Nanobodies targeting various growth factors and other membrane proteins have been developed and successfully used in model studies. They have also been linked to toxins such as diphtheria toxin, and numerous drugs to induce cancer cell death, and have been labelled with radionuclides such as ^{68}Ga, ^{111}In, ^{64}Cu and ^{18}F to be used for combined imaging and targeted radiotherapy. They seem to be particularly promising for the treatment of solid tumours, and the next decade might result in effective therapies targeting both extracellular and intracellular pathways leading to cancer cell death and reprogramming (Hu et al., 2017).

Antibodies are large proteins (~150 kDa), which hampers their handling and purification, complicates modification and often hinders delivery of antibody-modified cargo to a particular cell.

Interestingly, smaller antibodies (75 kDa) containing only heavy chains have been found in nature. They are produced by animals from the Camelidae family such as camels, llama and vicuña. Evolved over thousands of years, these antibodies have a 15 kDa single antigen-binding domain (single-domain antibody, sdAb) referred to as a **nanobody** (Muyldermans, 2013). Besides their size, advantageous features of nanobodies include high solubility, stability and a low ability to induce immune response in humans (low immunogenicity). All of these make them particularly well-suited for attachment to various nanomaterial surfaces, and the use for cell targeting.

3.8   Proteins in Bionanotechnology: Labelling Proteins/Protein Tags

To study a particular protein, it needs to either be directly explored in its natural environment or isolated from a melting pot of biomolecules present in cells. Taking into account the vast number of different yet structurally similar proteins, and the range of fast biological and chemical transformations they are involved in, this is not a small feat. A fitting comparison would be looking for a needle in a haystack. Thankfully, biotechnological tools were developed that allow the design of fusion proteins composed of a peptide chain or a whole protein attached to the protein of interest. Some of these bio-tags can bind radioactive or optically active molecules (chromophores), easing detection of the protein. Others, such as **fluorescent proteins**, already have embedded chromophores and do not require additional labelling. Use of fluorescent protein fusions was a game changer (more details in Back to Basics 3.9), not only for exploration of the protein fate within a cell, but also for development of advanced fluorescent microscopy.

Back to Basics 3.9	Recombinant DNA and Fusion Proteins

Recombinant DNA is a chimeric DNA (made of DNA molecules from different sources) constructed in vitro (out of the cell), then reproduced in a host cell or organism. The process of producing recombinant DNA is frequently called DNA cloning or gene cloning, and it was first reported by Peter Lobban and Armin Dale Kaiser in 1973 (Lobban and Kaiser, 1973), followed by insertion of the fully functional recombinant DNA into bacteria by researchers at Stanford University and University of California (Cohen et al., 1973).

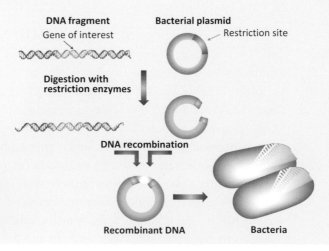

Typically, a recombinant DNA construct contains the gene of interest (i.e. gene for insulin production) fused to a vector, a small circular double-stranded DNA (bacterial plasmid). This is done first by cutting the vector using restriction enzymes and fusing two DNAs together with the help of ligases. The ligated recombinant DNA is then introduced into fast-growing organisms, such as bacteria (*Escherichia coli* is widely used) where it can be replicated.

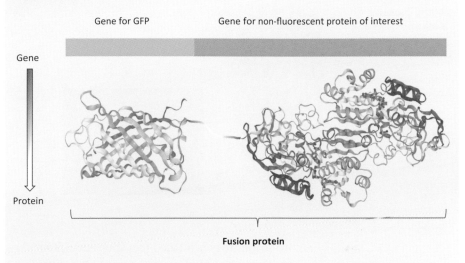

Fusion proteins are chimeric proteins created by recombination of two or more genes that originally coded for separate proteins. Fusion proteins can be used to aid the purification of cloned genes, report on a success of an expression and to visualise proteins in cells. Luciferase, β-galactosidase and the **green fluorescent protein (GFP)** are the most often used proteins as fusion partners for the construction of reporter systems. The GFP emits green light under blue or UV light excitation and can be used to study living cells, and even whole organisms.

3.8.1   Fluorescent Proteins

The first fluorescent protein, green fluorescent protein (GFP), was isolated from the jellyfish *Aequorea victoria* in the 1960s, but its potential was only recognised 30 years later when GFP–protein fusions were made (see Back to Basics 3.9). In the meanwhile, fluorescent proteins have been found in a number of other marine organisms, and shown to play an important role in bioluminescence. Recent studies have shown that they can also act as electron transfer facilitators in a process that resembles photosynthesis in plants. All of the fluorescent proteins have a unique **barrel-shaped structure**, evolved to protect the inner core, which contains a chromophore. The GFP is 27 kDa barrel-shaped protein comprised of 238 amino acids, three of which (serine, tyrosine and glycine) form a fluorescent chromophore buried within the protein's core (Figure 3.14).

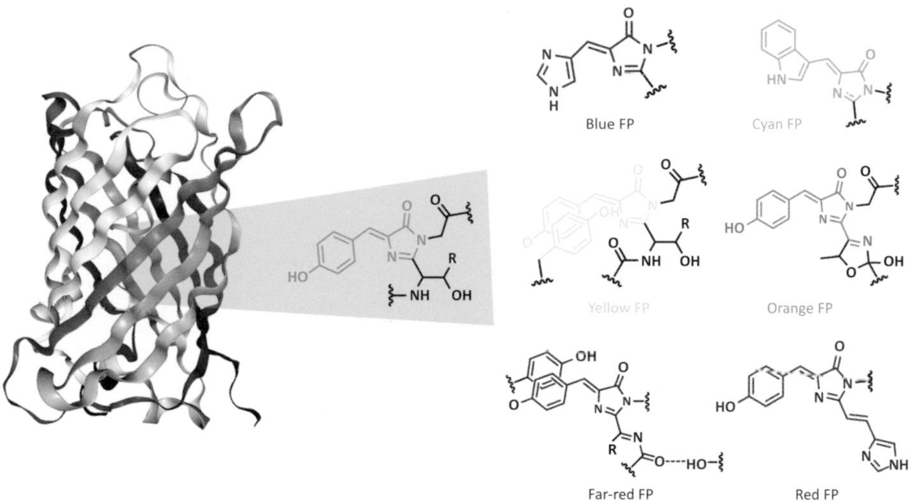

Figure 3.14

Fluorescent protein structure. Chromophore is composed of amino acids and positioned within the barrel structure interior. Fluorescence emission will differ depending on a chromophore's composition.

This chromophore is produced in a series of chemical reactions catalysed by the protein itself (autocatalysis) and its optical properties are affected by the protein's microenvironment. Depending on their emission wavelength, fluorescent proteins are divided into seven distinct classes: blue (440–470 nm), cyan (471–500 nm), green (501–520 nm), yellow (521–550 nm), orange (551–575 nm), red (576–610 nm) and far-red (611–660 nm) (Sample, 2009). Currently there are around 50 different fluorescent proteins available, either isolated from various organisms or designed through amino acid exchange within or in close proximity of the chromophore. The GFP gene was first cloned in 1992 and introduced to *E. coli* bacteria and nematode *Caenorhabditis elegans*, and the resulting protein was fluorescent despite being in a foreign host. After this initial success, fluorescent protein fusions quickly became an indispensable tool for molecular biology, complementing and often surpassing the quality of data obtained from small, chemically coupled fluorescent labels.

3.8.2 Protein Tags

Not all proteins can be fused with fluorescent proteins. They need to be made fluorescent using other strategies such as the chemical coupling of organic fluorophores to amino acids on the protein's surface, interaction with fluorescently labelled antibodies and specific binding of fluorescent species to protein tags. **Protein tags** are peptide chains or small proteins fused genetically to the protein of interest. Originally, they were developed to aid protein purification and are also known as affinity tags. They bind to various molecular species, which can often (but not always) be reversibly removed by treatment with a stronger binding competitor.

The first affinity tags used in the 1980s, such as protein A (binds to IgG antibody) or β-galactosidase known as LacZ (binds to *p*-amino-phenyl-β-D-thio-galactosidase) were large proteins (280 to 1000 amino acids) exclusively used for purification of proteins from *E. coli*. Smaller tags developed later were either whole proteins (maltose-binding protein, MBP), parts of the natural protein (calmodulin-binding peptide), mutated proteins (HALO tag) or short peptides (His tag). Some of the most common affinity tags are given in Table 3.1.

During the purification of proteins, protein tag affinity towards particular molecular species is used to attach the tagged protein to solid surfaces such as resins or silica gels. Specific competitive or bond-cleaving compounds are then employed to cleave the bound protein from the surface (Figure 3.15).

Table 3.1 Common affinity tags for protein purification

Protein tag, size and date first used	Affinity to	Tag removal
His tag 6–8 histidines, 1991	Nitrilotriacetic acid (NTA) in presence of cations such as Ni^{2+}	Imidazole solution
Glutathione-S-transferase (GST tag) 26 kDa, 1988	Glutathione	Urea or guanidium hydrochloride solution
Maltose-binding protein (MBP tag) 45 kDa, 1988	$n = 300\text{–}600$ Amylose	Maltose solution

Table 3.1 (*cont.*)

Protein tag, size and date first used	Affinity to	Tag removal
Calmodulin-binding peptide (CBP tag) 26 amino acids (4 kDA), 1995	Calmodulin protein	Egtazic acid or EGTA
Intein–chitin binding domain, 1997	Chitin	Dithiothreitol (DTT) solution
STREP tag 8–9 amino acids, 2000	Native or modified streptavidin	Biotin
SNAP tag 182 amino acids, 19.4 kDa, derived from an enzyme involved in DNA damage repair, 2003	Benzylguanine Covalent bond formed	Cleavage with the help of protease enzyme
Halo tag 33 kDa modified hydrolase enzyme, 2008	Chloroalkane ligand Covalent bond formed	Cleavage with the help of protease enzyme

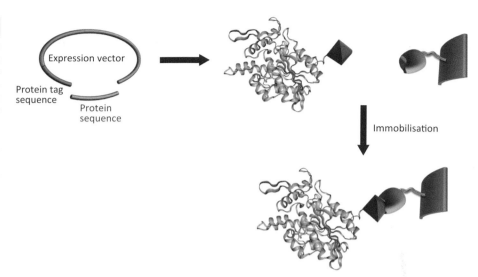

Figure 3.15

Principle of protein immobilisation using protein tag strategy. The tag is introduced to the protein genetically using expression vector containing information for both structures. The tag specifically (reversibly or irreversibly) binds to a molecular species attached to solid carriers enabling protein attachment.

Expression vector

Protein tag sequence

Protein sequence

Immobilisation

Such a strategy, originally employed for purification of protein of interest after expression, is now extensively used in applications which require protein immobilisation, for example the design of biosensors or biofunctionalisation of nanomaterials (see Chapter 4).

3.9   Proteins in Bionanotechnology: Enzymes

Enzymes are a class of proteins that speed up and facilitate chemical transformations in cells, without being affected in the process. They act by lowering the activation energy of the reaction by stabilising the transition state. This can be achieved by formation of stable enzyme–substrate bonds, by bringing multiple substrates close to each other, by bending the substrate just enough to enable the bond breakage, or by creating a more favourable environment for reaction to occur (for example making it more acidic or hydrophilic).

Back to Basics 3.10   Six Enzyme Families

There are around 75 000 enzymes in our body and they are usually grouped into six main families depending on the type of reaction they catalyse.

1. **Oxidoreductases:** catalyse reactions in which electrons are transferred from one molecule to another. They are also known as dehydrogenases that catalyse the removal of hydrogen atoms, or oxidases that remove electrons from their substrates.

$$A_{\text{oxidant}} + B_{\text{reductant}} \Leftrightarrow A_{\text{reductant}} + B_{\text{oxidant}}$$

The enzyme **alcohol dehydrogenase** (ADH1A) catalyses the oxidation of ethanol to acetaldehyde in the liver.

2. **Transferases:** catalyse the transfer of various chemical groups (other than hydrogen, i.e. amine, methyl, phosphate) from one compound to another.

$$A + BX \rightarrow AX + B$$

The enzyme **glutathione S-transferase** is an important detox enzyme that catalyses the addition of glutathione group to xenobiotic substrates, which are usually not naturally produced within an organism.

3. **Ligases:** catalyse the joining of two molecules, usually deriving needed energy from cleavage of an energy-rich phosphate bond through conversion of adenosine triphosphate (ATP) to adenosine diphosphate (ADP).

$$A + B + \text{ATP} \rightarrow AB + \text{ADP} + \text{P}_i$$

The enzyme **DNA ligase** catalyses the joining of two pieces of DNA with matching ends into a single, unbroken molecule of DNA.

4. **Hydrolases:** catalyse the cleavage of chemical bonds with the help of water, usually cleaving one large molecule into two small ones. These large molecules can be lipids (lipases), nucleic acids (nucleases), sugar molecules (glucosidases), proteins/peptide bonds (proteases/peptidases).

$$A + \text{H}_2\text{O} \rightarrow B + C$$

The enzyme **human gastric lipase** is responsible for hydrolysis of triglycerides (fats) into their component fatty acid and glycerol molecules.

5. **Lyases:** catalyse the removal of various groups from a substrate usually through the formation of double bonds or ring structures. For example, this family includes decarboxylase (removal of –COOH) and dehydratase (removal of H_2O) and a range of synthetases, involved in the synthesis of important biomolecules (i.e. threonine synthetase).

$$A \rightarrow B + C$$

The enzyme **carbonic anhydrase** catalyses the interconversion of carbon dioxide (CO_2) and carbonic acid (H_2CO_3) and plays an important role in respiration and CO_2 transport.

6. **Isomerases:** catalyse structural rearrangement of molecules. Such as, for example, alanine racemase, which catalyses the conversion of L-alanine into is mirror image form D-alanine, or tautomerases, which interconvert keto and enol groups.

$$A \Leftrightarrow A'$$

The enzyme **glucose 6-phosphate isomerase** catalyses the conversion of glucose 6-phosphate into fructose 6-phosphate. It is involved in the process of glycolysis and also in the growth and survival of developing and mature neurons.

Enzymes are either named after a type of reaction or after their substrate (Back to Basics 3.10), and can be recognised by the suffix **-ase**. For example, DNA polymerase catalyses synthesis of DNA polymer from deoxyribonucleotides, and maltase cleaves maltose sugar into glucose units.

Unlike some families of proteins such as antibodies, which have a characteristic structure, enzymes are structurally diverse. They are also characterised by high reaction rates, specificity and selectivity towards one substrate or a small family of chemically similar substrates. Such selectivity and specificity is one of the features that differentiate enzymes from a typical small molecule catalyst. Another feature is their sensitivity to pH and temperature. Most enzymes, with the exception of those found in extremophiles – microorganisms thriving in extreme environments – operate within moderate pH and temperature range, which limits their industrial application.

The substrate specificity is controlled by a structural fit between the enzyme and its substrate in the enzyme's active site. The active site consists of amino acid groups that form temporary bonds with the substrate (**binding site**) and the amino acids that catalyse a reaction (**catalytic site**). The sequence and three-dimensional arrangement of amino acids determine the physiochemical properties of the active site making it uniquely suited for a particular reaction (Figure 3.16).

Figure 3.16

Principle of enzyme action. Enzymes contain an active site that binds the substrate. Once bound, catalysis is performed after which the product is released freeing the active site for another catalytic cycle.

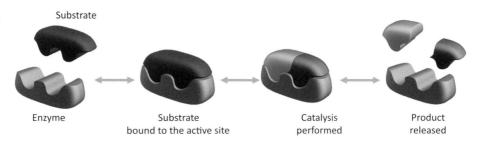

Substrate

Enzyme   Substrate   Catalysis   Product
              bound to the active site   performed   released

Many enzymes, known as **enzyme cofactors**, also contain organic molecules or metal ion cofactors, which are either directly responsible for substrate binding or electron transfer necessary for reactions to occur. **Organic cofactors**, such as widely found haem and flavin, can be covalently or non-covalently bound to the enzyme (Figure 3.17). For example, haem, an iron-containing porphyrin ring, can be non-covalently coordinated within oxygen-transporting protein haemoglobin, and covalently bound to a number of metabolic P450 enzymes. Metabolic flavin-containing enzymes (Figure 3.17b) involved in a range of detox reactions are the most prominent class of enzymes used in the chemical industry, in particular for production of polymers and pharmaceuticals (Joosten and van Berkel, 2007). Due to specific optical properties of flavin, flavoenzymes are also explored as potent photocatalysts.

Figure 3.17

Common organic cofactors. (a) Haem b found in myoglobin (Scouloudi and Baker, 1978). (b) Flavin mononucleotide from bacterial monooxygenase (Cho et al., 2011).

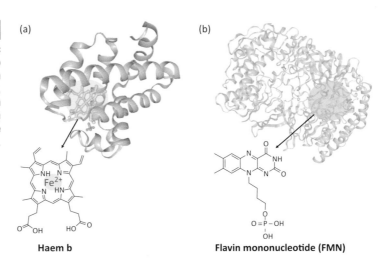

(a)

(b)

Haem b

Flavin mononucleotide (FMN)

Inorganic cofactors are usually metals (metalloenzymes) and clusters such as iron–sulphur clusters found in numerous enzymes such as NADH dehydrogenase and cytochrome bc_1 complex used in the electron transport chain that results in generation of ATP (see Back to Basics 3.3).

In fact, roughly 40% of proteins crystallised to date contain a protein shell-bound metal. In enzymes, these metals are involved in oxidation–reduction reactions, and assist in positioning and activation of substrates within the active site. Enzymes are usually very selective to which metals they use, and replacing one metal for another can lead to their deactivation. For example, all DNA polymerases involved in synthesis of DNA require two divalent cations, commonly magnesium (Mg^{2+}) and manganese (Mn^{2+}). One of these can be replaced with cobalt (Co^{2+}) or nickel (Ni^{2+}) ions, but use of other metal induces the enzyme malfunction, and as a result, damaged or incomplete DNA (Vashishtha et al., 2016). In some cases, however, exchange of cofactors can be an interesting route to development of artificial enzymes with improved activity or containing features absent in native enzymes (Research Report 3.2).

Research Report 3.2	Cofactor Exchange and Reconstitution

Native cofactors can be exchanged for slightly modified or entirely new cofactors. Such attempts to make modified enzymes have been done first to explore structure and function of the enzymes, and later to enhance their activity or introduce new functionalities, such as ability to attach to a particular surface.

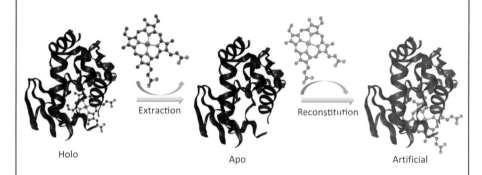

Enzymes with non-covalently bound cofactors are generally good candidates for **cofactor reconstitution** as it is easier to remove native cofactor (an enzyme in which a cofactor is absent is usually referred to as an **apo-enzyme**), while leaving the protein shell intact.

Artificial catalytic systems were designed by reconstitution of modified flavin or haem cofactors, or by exchanging the coordinated metal (Fruk et al., 2009). For example, flavin has been attached to gold nanoparticles, and allowed to reconstitute into apo-glucose oxidase (GOx) resulting in sevenfold enhancement of electron transfer between the enzyme and the electrode used in the design of glucose sensing system (Katz et al., 2004). DNA-modified haem was used to prepare protein–DNA conjugates and led both to the significant enhancement of enzyme activity and the development of a strategy for reversible immobilisation using DNA hybridisation (Fruk and Niemeyer, 2005). In fact, modified haem was one of the most prominent examples of cofactor reconstitution resulting in hybrid enzymes with various biopolymers for enzyme stabilisation, design of enzyme wires, or entirely novel activity profile by exchanging iron in haem with another metal. In this way, new enzyme-based catalytic systems can be designed that perform catalysis of industrially relevant organic reactions. One such example was demonstrated in 2016, when researchers replaced native Fe with iridium (Ir) in the P450 group of detox enzymes, and subjected this modified enzyme to additional directed evolution to obtain artificial metalloenzymes with the kinetic profile of the native enzyme (Dydio et al., 2016).

The activity of many enzymes also depends on the presence of **coenzymes**, free organic molecules, which can bind loosely to the protein during the reaction, get transformed and be regenerated and reused after the reaction is completed. All of the water-soluble and two of the fat-soluble vitamins (A and K) function as coenzymes involved in the fine-tuning of biochemical reaction cascades that drive the cell cycle. For example, thiamine pyrophosphate (TPP), active coenzyme form of vitamin B1, is involved in decarboxylation (removal of COOH groups), an important step in breakdown of sugars. On the other hand the enzymes involved in sugar synthesis are usually assisted by nicotinamide adenine dinucleotide (NAD) and nicotinamide adenine dinucleotide phosphate (NADP).

An animal cell contains between 1000 and 4000 different types of enzymes, each of which catalyses a particular reaction or a set of similar reactions. Some enzymes can be found in all of the cells as they are responsible for vital reactions such as synthesis of cell components or production of energy, whereas others are confined to particular cells such as liver or nerve cells. Some enzymes are secreted in the blood or digestive tract, where they help to break down complex nutrients or pathogenic molecules. But no matter where they are, these tiny chemists are crucially important for the health and longevity of our cells. Their dysfunction may cause havoc and lead to cell damage and death. A large proportion of bionano activities is devoted to finding new ways to diagnose diseases through monitoring enzyme activity, design enhanced or novel, artificial enzymes, and find new nanotechnological applications of existing enzymes (Research Report 3.3).

Enzymes are exquisite chemists: precise, specialised, fast and produce little if any waste and side products. Irreplaceable within living systems, they are also playing an increasingly important role in industrial manufacturing. Significant research efforts are dedicated to finding new ways to stabilise enzymes and make them suitable for industrial batch processes, and to provide new enzymes which can catalyse reactions not found in nature.

Without doubt, by combining biological and nanotools and strategies enhanced enzymes and enzyme-like materials can be designed with high medical and industrial relevance.

Research Report 3.3 | An Enzyme Degrades Graphene

Graphene has been hailed as an ideal component for flexible biomedical electronic devices, implants or drug delivery vehicles. However, before it can be taken from the lab to the clinic, it is important to check its biocompatibility and bio-degradation profile. Analysing single layer and few layer graphene (SLG and FLG) in the presence of **neutrophils**, the most abundant types of white blood cells, researchers found that an enzyme excreted from those cells can degrade large sheets into smaller fragments.

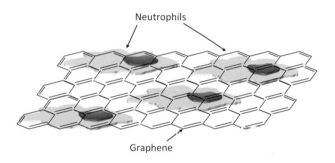

The responsible enzyme is human myeloperoxidase (MPO), a haem protein usually found in the lysosomes of neutrophils responsible for production of hypohalus acid (HO–X, where X can be Cl, F or Br) with high antimicrobial activity. Degradation of graphene sheets in the presence of isolated enzyme and whole neutrophils was followed using Raman spectroscopy and depending on the graphene type degradation was completed either within 24 hours or 5 days, with the presence of defects or oxygen in the graphene structure speeding up degradation. These results demonstrated that our immune system has strategies to remove carbon nanomaterials, which makes it even more attractive for biomedical applications (Kurapati et al., 2018).

3.10   Proteins in Bionanotechnology: Structural Proteins

Structural proteins are the most abundant proteins in nature, and also make up 30% of all proteins in our body, building up structural and connective tissues such as bones, skin and blood vessels. Although their main role is to act as structural elements providing mechanical support, strength and elasticity, they are also crucial for protein transport and inter- and intracellular communication.

Seventy-five per cent of all structural proteins in humans are found in skin, with **collagen** being the most prominently featured. Collagen is composed of three interwoven polypeptides that form triple helices of different lengths, some of which are up to 420 nm. Triple helices further assemble into collagen fibres, which provide tensile strength to ligaments, bones and dense connective tissue and as such, reinforce most organs. Fibrillary collagen is widespread in nature, mainly in vertebrates, although its existence has been confirmed in some marine invertebrates such as sponges. Besides fibrils, collagen can also form sheets, which are commonly found as structural elements around muscles and nerve cells, and cross-linking collagen, which acts as a connector between the fibres and sheets.

Due to its structure, collagen fibre is mechanically strong and can sustain extensive force, but it is not particularly extendible. Tissue elasticity is mainly provided by **elastin fibrils** found throughout the body, but most prominently in connective tissue, walls of arteries and in the lungs. Major components of elastin fibrils are 60 kDA proteins called tropoelastins, which are heavily cross-linked into insoluble and highly elastic structures. The most suitable comparison to elastin fibres is rubber, and the elasticity is achieved by combining rigid cross-linked and flexible linear regions. As a result, rigid and flexible regions coil into random structures, which can be readily extended (Figure 3.18). These fibrils are exceptionally resilient. For example,

Figure 3.18

Examples of common structural proteins. Collagen is the most abundant structural protein in the human body, keratin is a main structural component of nails, and elastin is often found in connective tissue.

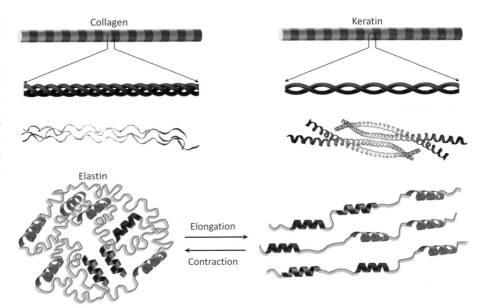

elastic fibres that build arteries are capable of withstanding more than 2 billion cycles of stretching and recoiling during a lifetime.

Unlike elastin, the protein **keratin** is a hard structural component found in humans and across the animal kingdom. α-keratin, a helical, fibrillary form of keratin, is a structural element of skin, hair, nails, horns and claws, whereas sheet-forming β-keratin can be found in birds' feathers and claws as well as in most reptiles. It is also present in all epithelial cells (cells that line the surfaces of the organs) both in those covering external body surfaces, and internal surfaces such as the lining of the digestive tract. Some invertebrates, such as crustaceans, also contain keratin, although often in combination with the polysaccharide chitin.

All of these proteins are insoluble, which complicates their isolation and structural analysis by traditional X-ray diffraction (Chapter 5). Their structure and the ability to form fibrils is a result of their amino acid composition and polypeptide sequence. For example, keratin has a high content of cysteine, which can form strong covalent bonds through sulphur–sulphur interactions (formation of disulphide bridges), leading to exceptionally robust structures. Characteristic collagen triple helices contain a high percentage of glycine, proline and hydroxyproline, and the elasticity of coiled elastin regions stems from glycine–valine–proline triplets. As we will see in Chapter 7, such structural insights can be used to tune the mechanical properties of designer materials, in particular various bionano hybrids.

A structural protein not found in humans, but produced by insects is fibroin, and another is the slightly different relative produced by spiders known as spidroin. In addition to a sticky protein sericin, fibroin is the main structural component of silk (Figure 3.19), material produced by *Bombyx mori* larvae.

Figure 3.19

Structural components of silk. Silk is composed of silk fibroin fibrils that contain distinct crystalline regions composed of mixed helices and sheets, and amorphous, flexible chains.

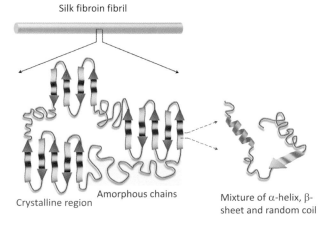

Silk fibroin fibril

Crystalline region   Amorphous chains   Mixture of α-helix, β-sheet and random coil

The remarkable properties of silk are equally valued by the fashion and electronic industries, and lately by medicine. Recent years have seen development of recombinant fibroins and design of hybrid nanosilk structures for applications in tissue engineering (see Chapter 9) and electronics. Similar to other structural proteins, silk fibroin also has a high glycine content. However, the similarity stops here since the fibroin fibres are composed entirely of protein sheet layers and lack any helical regions.

Collagen, elastin, keratin and fibroin are structural proteins responsible for the structural integrity of the organism and also act as structural components to build protective external layers. An integral structural part of the cell's interior is a cytoskeleton, a complex and dynamic system of filaments spread throughout the cell. A cytoskeleton supports the cell shape (and cells come in different shapes and sizes), guides the organisation of organelles, acts as an internal cellular highway for transport of various building blocks and signalling molecules, and it is also involved in cell adhesion and tissue organisation. The main components of this important cell structure are three long filament structures: microtubules, linear actin filaments and intermediate filaments.

These filaments are usually cross-linked with motor proteins, which enable their assembly, disassembly and contraction. **Microtubules** are composed of 50 kDA protein **tubulin**, which self-assembles into long filaments (Figure 3.20; more on self-assembly in Chapter 4). Structurally, microtubules are multimeric filaments with a diameter of about 25 nm and composed of 13 to 16 protofilaments assembled around a hollow core. In mammals, they also build larger structures such as cilia and flagella, important for propelling materials out of the respiratory passages and the movement of the sperm towards an egg. Long linear filaments are composed of **actin**, a helix-forming protein involved in the control of cell dynamics. In skeletal muscle, actin forms a large spiral filament, which slides along the motor protein myosin causing the muscle cells to contract. In other types of cells, actin filaments tend to be less organised and not coupled to myosin to such an extent as in muscle cells. With

Figure 3.20

Proteins that build the cytoskeleton. (a) Tubulin dimer forms microtubuli composed by coiling of tubulin filaments, while actin (b) forms linear filaments.

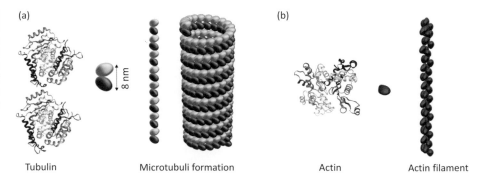

(a)

8 nm

Tubulin   Microtubuli formation

(b)

Actin   Actin filament

a diameter of around 6 nm actin filaments are much thinner than microtubules (around 25 nm) and are often found on the inner side of the cell membrane, where they act as a cell-shape and membrane modulator during cell movement.

Both microtubules and actin filaments are dynamic structures characterised by plus (+) and minus (−) ends, which refer to the rate of addition of a single protein unit at both ends of a filament. The end that grows more rapidly is called the plus end, as opposed to a slowly growing minus end.

Intermediate filaments, such as laminin, vary in the type of protein subunits, and their size lies in between microtubule and actin filaments. They are generally strong, resemble ropes and play less of a dynamic but more of a mechanical role.

Structural proteins are particularly interesting in the design of novel nano-materials and nanocomposites suitable for medical applications. Understanding their structure and assembly could ultimately lead to dynamic materials and adaptable, self-healing artificial structures. Collagen is already extensively used to build hydrogels (Back to Basics 2.5, Chapter 2) for tissue engineering (Chapter 9) whereas mimicking nanostructured keratin surfaces in birds' feathers led to the development of structural colours and optically active biomaterials (Chapter 7).

Structural proteins will continue to play an increasingly important role as building blocks in bionanotechnology, in particular within the bionano hybrids capable of transforming chemical into mechanical energy, or responding to environmental cues.

Key Concepts

Amphiphilic molecules: molecules such as phospholipids from cell membranes composed of distinct regions with different affinity for polar (such as water) and non-polar solvents.

Antibodies/nanobodies: large proteins or small protein units that bind molecular species (antigen) with high specificity in non-covalent fashion. In bionanotechnology they are used for biofunctionalisation and cell targeting.

Chirality: property of some molecules (and larger systems such as nanoparticle assemblies), which have the same elemental composition and structural elements but different orientation in space: they are mirror images of each other. Many biomolecules are chiral, most notably sugars and amino acids.

Enzyme cofactor: organic molecule or inorganic species such as metallic ion that ease the substrate binding and conversion within a catalytic protein.

Most prominent organic cofactors are iron-containing haem and photosensitive flavin.

Fluorescent proteins: barrel-shaped proteins with fluorescent chromophore made by cyclisation of natural amino acids within the core of the protein. They can be genetically fused to other proteins and are an exceptionally useful tool to study biomolecules within cells.

Glycoproteins and glycolipids: proteins and lipids found in cell membranes with covalently bound sugar molecules. They stabilise the membrane, but also play a big role in cell signalling, and cell–cell and cell–matrix interactions.

Interfacing proteins: in bionanotechnology these are proteins, such as streptavidin, used for the design of biocompatible surfaces and biofunctionalisation of nanomaterials.

Liposomes: nanosized vesicles composed of an aqueous core enveloped by a phospholipid membrane, used as drug delivery systems.

Organelles: compartments within eukaryotic cell usually surrounded by their own membrane, which perform distinct and coordinated functions within the cell. Such as, for example, a nucleus, mitochondria and endosomes.

Plasmid DNA: small DNA molecules that can carry foreign genetic material, which can be expressed and replicated into fast-replicating host organisms such as bacteria. Plasmids are commonly made of circular, double-stranded DNA and are also used as vectors to prepare genetically altered proteins such as various fusion proteins.

Protein tags: small peptides or proteins that can be genetically fused to the protein of interest to aid its identification, purification and immobilisation. Often used in bionanotechnology to enable biofunctionalisation of nanosurfaces.

Structural proteins: proteins characterised by specific peptide motifs that result in exceptional mechanical properties, which makes them particularly interesting for the design of bionano hybrids for tissue engineering and biosensor design.

Problems

3.1 Describe the molecular components that make up the cell membrane.

3.2 Explain the three components of the cytoskeleton, including their composition and functions.

3.3 Which organelle produces large quantities of ATP when both glucose and oxygen are available to the cell?

3.4   Compare and contrast lysosomes with peroxisomes: name at least two similarities and one difference.

3.5   Translate the following RNA sequences (reading from 5′) into amino acid sequences and classify resulting peptides as hydrophilic, hydrophobic or intermediate.
(a) GUCGUCCUAAUG
(b) AACCACAAA
(c) GCCACAUGG

3.6   Which amino acids have only one codon? Are they hydrophilic or hydrophobic?

3.7   Using the relationship between molecular weight and the volume of a protein, calculate the radius of a globular protein with molecular weight of 50 kDa.

3.8   Where are active sites in an antibody located?

3.9   Antisera are produced by inoculating animals (such as sheep) with a toxin (such as the tetanus toxin) and then purifying the produced antibodies. The antiserum can then be administered to treat a person suffering acute symptoms of the toxin. Unfortunately, some people have a strong immunological reaction to an injected antiserum. What is the reason behind such reaction? Why do antisera sometimes induce the same reaction as the foreign antigens?

3.10 Collagen is a filamentous protein with a repetitive structure, composed of a sequence of three repeating amino acids. In general, collagen has very low antigenicity. Why would this be expected?

3.11 Alcohol dehydrogenase is an enzyme involved in degradation of alcohol and contains Zn ion as a metal cofactor. What is a cofactor and what is the typical role of cofactors in enzyme catalysed reactions?

3.12 Compare and contrast the structure of keratin, collagen and silk fibroin.

3.13 Describe the difference between A-, B- and Z-DNA.

Further Reading

Anal, A. K. (2018). *Bionanotechnology: Principles and Applications*, CRC Press, Taylor and Francis Group.

Cuesta, S. M., Rahman, S. A., Furnham, N. and Thornton, J. M. (2015). The classification and evolution of enzyme function. *Biophysical Journal*, **109**, 1082–1086.

Ernster, L. and Schatz, G. (1981). Mitohondria: a historical review. *Journal of Cell Biology*, **91**(3), 227–255.

Galadon, T. and Pittis, A. A. (2015). Origin and evolution of metabolic sub-cellular compartmentalisation of eukaryotes. *Biochimie*, **119**, 262–268.

Ingram, J. R., Schmidt, F. I. and Ploegh, H. L. (2018). Exploiting nanobodies' singular traits. *Annual Review of Immunology*, **36**, 695–715.

Ratledge, C. and Kristiansen, B. (eds.) (2012). *Basic Biotechnology*, Cambridge University Press.

Rodriguez, E. A., Campbell, R. E., Lin, J. Y., et al. (2017). The growing and glowing toolbox of fluorescent and photoactive proteins. *Trends in Biochemical Sciences*, **42**, 111–129.

Sercombe, L., Veerati, T., Moheimani, F., et al. (2015). Advances and challenges of liposome assisted drug delivery. *Frontiers in Pharmacology*, **6**, 286.

Valdez, C. E., Smith, Q. A., Nechay, M. R. and Alexandrova, A. N. (2014). Mysteries of metals in metalloenzymes. *Accounts of Chemical Research*, **47**(10), 3110–3117.

References

Chen, J., Liu, T., Gao, J., et al. (2016). Variation in carbohydrates between cancer and normal cell membranes revealed by super-resolution fluorescence imaging. *Advanced Science*, **3**, 1600270.

Chen, W., Yu, H., Lee, S.-Y., et al. (2018). Nanocellulose: a promising nanomaterial for advanced electrochemical energy storage. *Chemical Society Reviews*, **47**, 2837–2872.

Cho, H. J., Cho, H. Y., Kim, K. J., et al. (2011). Structural and functional analysis of bacterial flavin-containing monooxygenase reveals its ping-pong-type reaction mechanism. *Journal of Structural Biology*, **175**, 39.

Cohen, S. N., Chang, A. C. Y., Boyer, H. W. and Helling, R. B. (1973). Construction of biologically functional bacterial plasmids in vitro. *Proceedings of the National Academy of Sciences of the USA*, **70**(11), 3240–3244.

D'Ascenzo, L., Leonarski, F., Vicens, Q. and Auffinger, P. (2016). Z-DNA like fragments in RNA: a recurring structural motif with implications for folding, RNA/protein recognition and immune response. *Nucleic Acid Research*, **44**(12), 5944–5956.

Dydio, P., Key, H. M., Nazarenko, A., et al. (2016). An artificial metalloenzyme with the kinetics of native enzymes. *Science*, **354**, 102–106.

Erickson, H. P. (2009). Size and shape of protein molecules at the nanometer level determined by sedimentation, gel filtration and electron microscopy. *Biological Procedures Online*, **11**(1), 32–51.

Fruk, L. and Niemeyer, C. M. (2005). Covalent hemin-DNA adduct for generating a novel class of artificial haem enzymes. *Angewandte Chemie International Edition*, **44**, 2–5.

Fruk, L., Kuo, C.-H., Torres, E. and Niemeyer, C. M. (2009). Apoenzyme reconstitution as a chemical tool for structural enzymology and biotechnology. *Angewandte Chemie International Edition*, **48**, 1550–1574.

Hu, Y., Lie, C. and Muyldermans, S. (2017). Nanobody-based delivery systems for diagnosis and targeted tumour therapy. *Frontiers in Immunology*, **8**, 1442.

Jensen, C. U., Guerrero, J. K. R., Karatzos, S. and Olofsoon, G. (2017). Fundamentals of hydrofaction™: renewable crude oil from woody biomass. *Biomass Conversion and Biorefinery*, **7**(4), 495–509.

Joosten, V. and van Berkel, W. H. J. (2007). Flavoenzymes. *Current Opinion in Chemical Biology*, **1182**, 195–202.

Katz, E., Sheeny-Haj-Ichia, L. and Wilner, I. (2004). Electrical contacting of glucose oxidase in a redox-active rotaxane configuration. *Angewandte chemie*, **43**(25), 3292–3300.

Kimple, M. E., Brill, A. L. and Parker, R. L. (2013). Overview of affinity tags for protein purification. *Current Protocols in Protein Science*, **73**, 9.9.1–9.9.23.

Kurapati, R., Mukherjee, S. P., Martin, C., et al. (2018). Degradation of single-layer and few layer graphene by neutrophil myeloperoxidase. *Angewandte Chemie*, **57**, 11722–11727.

Lobban, P. E. and Kaiser, A. D. (1973). Enzymatic end-to end joining of DNA molecules. *Journal of Molecular Biology*, **78**(3), 453–471.

McGuffe, S. R. and Elcock, A. H. (2010). Diffusion, crowding and protein stability in a dynamic molecular model of a bacterial cystoplasm. *PLos Computational Biology*, **6**(3), e10000694.

Muyldermans, S. (2013). Nanobodies: natural single-domain antibodies. *Annual Reviews in Biochemistry*, **82**, 775–797.

Okshevsky, M. and Meyer, R. L. (2013). The role of extracellular DNA in the establishment, maintenance and perpetuation of bacterial films. *Critical Reviews in Microbiology*, **41**(3), 341–352.

Phanthong, P., Reubroycharoen, P., Hao, X., et al. (2018). Nanocellulose: extraction and application. *Carbon Resources Conversion*, **1**(1), 32–43.

Reuveni, S., Ehrenberg, M. and Paulsson, J. (2017). Ribosomes are optimized for autocatalytic production. *Nature*, **547**, 293–297.

Rich, A. and Zhang, S. (2003). Z-DNA: the long road to biological function. *Nature*, **4**, 566–572.

Salick, D. A., Kretsinger, J. K., Pochan, D. J. and Schneider, J. P. (2007). Inherent antibacterial activity of a peptide-based beta-hairpin hydrogel. *Journal of American Chemical Society*, **129**, 14793–14799.

Sample, V., Newman, R. H. and Zhang, J. (2009). The structure and function of fluorescent proteins. *Chemical Society Reviews*, **38**, 2852–2864.

Scott, A. M., Wolchock, J. D. and Old, L. J. (2012). Antibody therapy in cancer. *Nature Reviews Cancer*, **12**, 278–287.

Scouloudi, H. and Baker, E. N. (1978). X-ray crystallographic studies of seal myoglobin. The molecule at 2.5Å resolution. *Journal of Molecular Biology*, **126**, 637–660.

Svoboda, P. and Di Cara, C. (2006). Hairpin RNA: a secondary structure of primary importance. *Cellular and Molecular Life Sciences*, **63**, 901–908.

Vashishtha, A. K., Wang, J. and Konigsberg, W. H. (2016). Different divalent cations alter the kinetics and fidelity of DNA polymerases. *Journal of Biological Chemistry*, **291**(40), 20869–20875.

Zimbron, J. M., Heinisch, T., Schmid, M., et al. (2013). A dual anchoring strategy for the localisation and activation of artificial metalloenzymes based on the biotin–streptavidin technology. *Journal of the American Chemical Society*, **135**, 5384–5388.

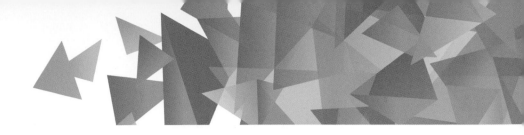

4 (Bio)functionalisation of Nanomaterials

As discussed in Chapter 1, unique features of nanomaterials such as size-dependent optical and magnetic properties, and high surface-to-volume ratio make them particularly interesting for applications in electronics and biomedicine. Biomedical applications are a powerful driver of the development of bionano hybrids, and novel preparation strategies have already enabled manufacturing of high-quality nanomaterials such as carbon nanotubes at scales that can satisfy market demands. Although the size of nanomaterials brings numerous advantages, working with them can be challenging. Due to their high surface energy, nanoparticles can form random aggregates, or non-selectively bind various molecular species, which impacts their physiochemical properties. This can be prevented by the functionalisation of nanomaterials' surface with known molecules in a controllable way. Surface modification not only improves the stability of nanomaterials, but enables introduction of various functional groups that can change their properties and make them more adaptable to a broad range of applications.

In this chapter we will look into strategies for nanomaterial modification and discuss the structural components of surface-stabilising linkers. However, to understand the functionalisation, we first need to explore the process of **self-assembly**, which is not only involved in formation of self-replicating and self-healing biological systems, but plays an important role in the design of large molecular structures and bionano hybrids.

4.1 Self-Assembly

Self-assembly refers to a spontaneous organisation of small elements or building blocks into larger structures (Back to Basics 4.1).

Back to Basics 4.1 Concept of Self-Assembly throughout History

Philosophers throughout history have debated the concept of self-assembly without directly using this term. In the seventeenth century, French philosopher and mathematician Rene Descartes (1596–1650) talked about the Universe arising out of chaos and smaller parts joining together into larger structures according to mathematical laws.

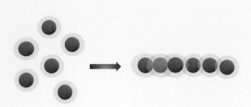

Later on, at the beginning of the twentieth century, bio-mathematician D'Arcy Wentworth Thomson (1860–1948), while studying the formation of large organic forms from smaller cells using mathematical/geometrical principles, coined the term morphogenesis. With this he tried to explain the self-assembly of living organisms and the formation of complex shapes through an assembly of smaller elements.

Self-assembly was the basis of the work of Katherine B. Blodgett (1898–1979) and Irving Langmuir (1881–1957) in the 1930s. They investigated the self-assembly of amphiphilic molecules, which resulted in the invention of closely packed monolayer films known today as Langmuir–Blodgett films.

Self-assembling strategies fully came to life through the study of chemisorption of alkanethiol molecules at the beginning of the 1980s (Nuzzo and Allara, 1983). The term was fully embraced in the 1990s with the development of the lithographic methods and the use of self-assembled monolayers (SAMs) to design nanostructured surfaces pioneered by Harvard chemist George Whitesides and his team.

If we consider molecular self-assembly, molecules organise into larger structures due to non-covalent interactions and without any external input of energy through, for example, heating or magnetic force. The exact origin of the self-assembly process at the small scales, in particular in **stochastic systems** such as whole cells, is still a subject of debate (more on the meaning of stochastic in Back to Basics 4.2).

Back to Basics 4.2   Stochastic Processes

Originating in the Greek word *stokhos* (aim, guess), a **stochastic process** has a random probability distribution or pattern, which can be analysed statistically but not precisely predicted. That means that even with the full knowledge of the state of a particular system (and also of its past), its value at future times cannot be precisely determined. Contrary to a stochastic process, a **deterministic process** implies that identical initial conditions always lead to the same future dynamics.

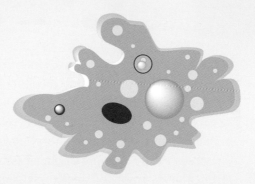

The term stochastic was first used in mathematics, but in the past 20 years, stochastic processes have become the basis of mathematical and physical modelling in cellular biology. To a large extent this is due to the increase in the understanding of cell dynamics and the availability of data at the single molecule level. Mathematical stochastic models help us to understand different biological paths and processes, and have been used to study events ranging from the growth of bacterial colonies and spread of infections to the impact of signalling proteins.

To produce a reliable outcome, eukaryotic cells need to develop different strategies to integrate many stochastic events. One such strategy is the evolution of cell compartments (Chapter 3) within which stochastic processes are segregated and continuously screened to provide a reliable output, not affected by fluctuations of individual events. Such segregation enables a level of control that can compensate for the failure of individual events. As a consequence, an error in one compartment might lead to new pathways being activated such that the activities in the other compartments are not disturbed. The balance of stochastic processes and damage control accounts for the unique adaptability and self-repair properties of living systems.

Intuitively it seems that self-assembly violates the second law of thermodynamics, which states that the entropy of an isolated system always increases until the entropy attains its maximum value in the equilibrium (check Back to Basics 1.4 for more on laws of thermodynamics). If this is the case, clearly there is something unusual about self-assembled systems, which spontaneously form ordered structures decreasing the local entropy. However, the resolution of this contradiction lies in the term 'local'. The second law is very much in action if the self-assembled system is considered as a subsystem of a larger entity. Even though entropy decreases within the subsystem undergoing the self-assembly, somewhere else within the large system entropy increases enough to compensate for that local decrease. For example, it has been shown that the entropy of nanoparticles in solution increases even when the particles form ordered, string-like structures. The reason for this is the occurrence of small 'rattlesnake movements' within the nanoparticle assemblies, which create disorder on a larger scale (Termonia, 2014).

An important feature of self-assembly is that it is a reversible process, and the assembled species are held together by weak forces (Table 4.1). For example, hydrogen bonding has a bond dissociation energy in the range 10–$50\,\mathrm{kJ\,mol^{-1}}$, whereas the values obtained for the covalent bonds are in the range 200–$600\,\mathrm{kJ\,mol^{-1}}$. Although hydrogen bonds are weak, they act collectively resulting in a stable large structure. As a consequence, it is much easier to repair damage and correct structural errors in self-assembled systems than within the covalently bound structures. For that reason, self-assembly is essential for the evolution of adaptable, self-healing and growing biological systems, and highly desired in the design of larger functional assemblies from nanosized elements.

Table 4.1 Forces involved in molecular self-assembly processes

Type of interaction	Features	Strength
Ion–ion interaction Repulsive force Attractive force	Non-directional force Long-range interactions Highly dependent on the dialectic constant of the medium. In terms of solvents, high dielectric constant means higher polarity, for example, *water,* *NaCl crystal lattice (Na$^+$ and Cl$^-$ ions)*	250 $\mathrm{kJ\,mol^{-1}}$
Ion–dipole interaction	Non-directional force Medium-range interaction ($1/r^2$) Significantly weaker than ion–ion interaction Commonly found in solutions, such as *the solution of ionic compounds, for example, salt NaCl in polar solvents; hydration of ions in water*	50–250 $\mathrm{kJ\,mol^{-1}}$

Table 4.1 (*cont.*)

Type of interaction	Features	Strength
Dipole–dipole interaction	Somewhat directional force Short-range interaction ($1/r^6$) Occur between molecules that have permanent net dipoles (*polar molecules such as hydrochloric acid*) $H^{\delta+} - Cl^{\delta-} \cdots H^{\delta+} - Cl^{\delta-}$	Up to 5 kJ mol^{-1}
π–π interaction Displaced Edge-to-face Sandwich	Weak electrostatic interaction between aromatic rings *Stacking of DNA bases* *Interactions of carbon nanotubes*	Up to 50 kJ mol^{-1}
Hydrophobic effects	Burial of hydrophobic groups or amino acid residues in the core of the micelle/protein to stabilise the system in aqueous solution *Micelle formation* *Protein folding*	Difficult to assess
Hydrogen bonding	Directional force and short-range interaction (0.24–0.35 nm) Forms when a hydrogen atom is positioned between two electronegative atoms, mainly oxygen and nitrogen It is considered a special case of a dipole–dipole interaction, but it can be much stronger *Water, DNA double helix*	10–50 kJ mol^{-1}

Guidelines on how to prepare nanoelements that can be self-assembled into larger structures stem from the exploration of natural self-assembled systems, and the field of **supramolecular chemistry**.

In supramolecular chemistry, the instructions on how to assemble larger structures are encoded in the structural motifs within individual molecules (Menger, 2002), and supramolecular structures are assembled from molecular building blocks through highly selective, structure-specific interactions. These interactions are enabled by the presence of specific functional groups or structural features that can engage in hydrogen bonding, or formation of metal-ligand and host-guest systems through ion–dipole, dipole–dipole or π–π interactions (see Table 4.1).

These interactions are crucial also for the self-assembly of biological systems, although individual building blocks tend to be more complex than those in supramolecular chemistry. A protein-making biological machine, a ribosome (Back to Basics 3.6, Chapter 3), is made by assembly of tens of small proteins and several RNA molecules. The shape and charge of both types of building blocks is controlled by the presence of particular features and motifs on the surface or within the structure. For example, proteins might contain amino acids that can engage in hydrogen bonding, and RNA loops and stems that ease the interaction with the protein surface. The self-assembly of man-made nanoelements explored within bionanotechnology often relies on the self-assembly of the motifs present on their surface. For example, the self-assembly of two different nanoparticles containing complementary strands of DNA will be driven by interactions between these DNA and the double helix formation.

In some cases, the structural motifs are introduced and shaped by the action of enzymes, which can transform individual components to fit into a larger structure in the same way a good tailor transforms a piece of material to make it into a dress. For example, several enzymes are involved in the production of microtubule networks in muscles by facilitating reactions that modulate the cross-linking and orientation of individual fibres before they assemble into larger muscle components (Volker et al., 1995). Such enzyme-instructed self-assembly is particularly interesting for the design of greener materials for tissue engineering (Chapter 9) or new generation of bioinspired therapeutics (Research Report 4.1). Unlike the assembly of supramolecular structures and nanoelements, self-assembly on the macroscale is not restricted to the short-range interactions, but can also proceed on a larger scale with the help of van der Waals, electric, magnetic and elastic forces, and shear.

| Research Report 4.1 | Enzyme-Instructed Self-Assembly |

Enzyme-instructed self-assembly (EISA) employs enzymes to cleave substrates, usually peptides, and in such a way affords smaller elements suitable for assembly into larger structures. Such EISA strategy can be used to induce cancer cell death by directly employing enzymes present in cancer cells. One of the enzymes present in cancer cells in large amounts is alkaline phosphatase (ALP). However, it is very difficult to design drugs for ALP as those that are effective usually cannot be transported through the cell membrane.

Phosphotyrosine: APL cleavage site

This could be overcome by the design of cell-penetrating peptides that contain a phosphotyrosine group. Phosphate groups contained within phosphotyrosine are cleaved by the ALP enzyme, and resulting hydroxyl (–OH) groups ease the self-assembly of peptides into large fibril structures. Such fibrils significantly impair the function of the cancer cell and ultimely lead to cell death (Feng et al., 2017).

Enzyme-instructed self-assembly is an excellent example of rational drug design, which relies on the use of the cancer cells' resources to induce their death. Such an approach, which relies on a natural process, avoids the use of toxic drugs that can have detrimental side effects and also helps to circumvent the common problem of drug resistance, often encountered with chemotherapeutics.

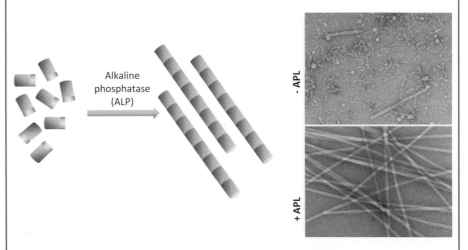

Source: Feng et al. (2017). https://pubs.acs.org/doi/10.1021/jacs.7b07147. Permission to reuse this material should be directed to the ACS.

Large-scale, complex assemblies such as whole cells are considered non-equilibrium systems and the process by which they are made is referred to as **dynamic self-assembly** (Whitesides and Grzybowski, 2002). Dynamic self-assembly differs from **static self-assembly** based on the needed energy input and the final energy of a system.

Static self-assembly refers to a formation of ordered structures, which reach an equilibrium state and do not change further following the assembly. An example of static self-assembly is protein folding, during which a polypetide chain folds into a specific three-dimensional structure (Figure 4.1). Once assembled, proteins will remain in an equilibrium state and stable until energy is supplied externally, usually in the form of heat that disrupts their form. Contrary to static self-assembly, dynamic self-assembly results in a non-equilibrium state and requires a continuous input of energy to maintain a steady state once the structure is formed. In the absence of this energy, the system falls apart. Energy is supplied either as heat, through irradiation or by application of a magnetic or electric field. As mentioned earlier, most of larger self-assembled systems are made by such a dynamic process. Dynamic self-assembly has some crucial advantages over static self-assembly. First, dynamically assembled systems such as our cells are **adaptable**; they are far from equilibrium and need to constantly maintain themselves to respond to environmental changes. In addition, they have the ability to **self-heal**; this property is closely related to adaptability. Self-healing means that a perturbed 'wounded' system will return into its stable configuration and 'heal' provided that the perturbance is not so large as to cause the dissipation of the whole system.

Figure 4.1

An example of static self-assembly. Folding of a polypeptide chain into ferritin protein responsible for iron storage.

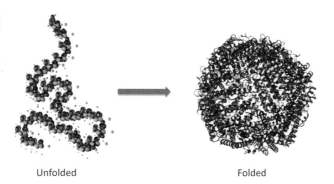

Unfolded   Folded

Let us use the example of a school of fish to illustrate what we mean: if some fish decide to go their separate way, the school will reform and continue moving as a dynamic unit – the school will 'heal'. However, if a certain critical number of fish is eaten by a predator, the school will likely dissipate. Finally, dynamic self-assemblies such as cells have the ability to **self-replicate**. However, such a process requires a significant energy input, which in living organisms is supplied through the metabolism of nutrients (Fialkowski, 2006).

One of the biggest scientific and engineering challenges is to design an artificial 'living' system that can acquire energy, respond to the environment, and produce and recycle its own components. As more knowledge on self-assembly is acquired, the closer we will get to the design of intelligent, self-repairing structures, and possibly artificial living cells made entirely from man-made bionano elements. To achieve that we need to develop ways to tune the surface properties of nanostructures, which can be done by using different functionalisation strategies.

4.2   Modification of the Nanomaterial Surface

4.2.1   Self-Assembled Monolayers

Self-assembled monolayers (SAMs) play an important role in modification of nanomaterials; densely packed surface layers not only stabilise the material but also influence the surface properties and enable or arrest further functionalisation. In general, SAMs are considered to be ordered and closely packed molecular assemblies driven into the formation of two-dimensional crystal-like structures by electrostatic forces, hydrophobic interactions and chemisorption.

In bionanotechnology, SAMs have been widely used to affect the surface properties of nanomaterials and to enable attachment of additional molecules. Typical SAM-forming species, as well as other **surface-binding linkers** used for functionalisation of nanomaterials are composed of three distinct parts; a **surface-binding group**, a **spacer** and a **functional group** (Figure 4.2). Some ligands can engage in a very strong interaction with the surface known as **chemisorption**. In chemisorption, a group is first adsorbed to the surface and then engages in a covalent bond with the surface atoms. One of the most studied chemisorption processes important for bionanotechnology is that of the gold and sulphur-containing thiol groups (Au–SH) (Research Report 4.2).

Figure 4.2

Structure of a typical
linker involved in the
formation of a self-
assembled monolayer on
the surface of
nanomaterials.

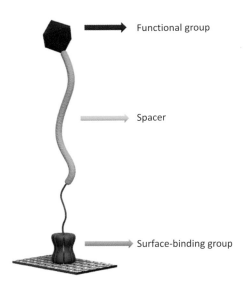

Figure 4.2

Structure of a typical
linker involved in the
formation of a self-
assembled monolayer on
the surface of
nanomaterials.

As a result of the exothermic interaction of the head group with the surface, molecules tend to occupy every available binding site and create a densely packed layer (Figure 4.3). Alkanethiols, which contain a number (a few to tens) of repeats of alkane chains ($-CH_2-$), result in stable mono-layers, and for more ordered films, the longer is the chain. This is a result of the stronger van der Waals interactions between the larger number of alkane groups. The van der Waals forces prevent the alkanethiols from collapsing and keep monolayers sticking up. This is an important feature of monolayer films as it enables the introduction of various functional groups to the surface, which are not sterically hindered and, consequently, can engage in further reactions.

Research Report 4.2	Gold–Thiol Self-Assembled Monolayers

The surface chemistry of alkanethiols on gold, which is widely used for formation of self-assembled monolayers on Au nanomaterials, has been a topic of heated debate from the first publication in the 1980s. Two main mechanisms have been postulated to explain the thiol–gold interaction. One is based on the chemisorption of thiol to gold surface and formation of H–S–Au bonds, and the other considers the interaction as an oxidative addition whereby the thiol S–H bond is cleaved at the gold surface with the release of a small amount of hydrogen. Thiol species are also prone to formation of disulphide (–S–S–) bonds, and initially it was not clear how this process impacts the formation of a monolayer. We know today that both –SH and S–S species can be successfully used to modify gold surfaces.

Interestingly, studies have shown that once the Au–S bond is formed, it can diffuse along the surface causing monolayer restructuring. This can be explained by differences in the strength of the Au–Au and Au–S bonds. Weaker Au–Au bonds, with dissociation energy of $24\,\text{kcal mol}^{-1}$, can be broken once Au–S is formed (dissociation energy of $40\,\text{kcal mol}^{-1}$), resulting in the movement of Au–S species over the surface. This was beautifully shown by scanning microscopy studies of the surface done in 2003 (Ramachandran et al., 2003).

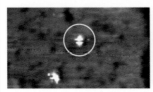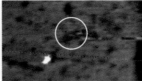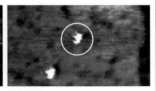

Source: Ramachandran et al. (2003). Reprinted with permission from AAAS.

Shown here are electron microscopy images of a thiol monolayer on a planar gold surface. The circled region focuses on the disappearance and appearance of alkanethiols on the gold surface due to the cleavage of Au–Au bonds and movement of the molecular species within the monolayer.

Surface properties of SAM-coated materials will depend on the nature of the functional group. For example, surfaces can be made either hydrophilic by use of charged functional groups such as carboxylic acid (–COOH), hydroxyl groups (–OH) or amines (–NH$_2$), or hydrophobic by the addition of methyl (CH$_3$ shown in Figure 4.3), or other hydrophobic functional groups such as fatty acids.

Figure 4.3

Self-assembled monolayer of alkane–thiols on gold. The thiol-binding group is shown in blue and alkyl spacer containing the methyl (–CH^3) end group in yellow.

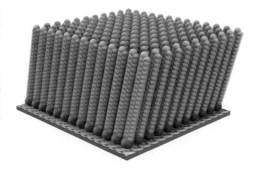

The choice of a functional group is also crucial for further modification of material, in particular for the addition of biomolecules. When we consider a route to be taken to achieve (bio)functionalisation of a particular nanomaterial, several aspects need to be taken into account. First, we need to consider the ultimate fate of the modified nanomaterial; what is it going to be used for? When we require materials to be stable in harsh conditions, the linkers and functional groups we employ will need to sustain high temperatures or, maybe, low pH values. Second, we need to decide at what point during the synthesis of nanomaterial are we going to perform the functionalisation. There are two possibilities: the addition of the appropriate surface linkers can be done either directly during synthesis, this is often referred to as the **one-pot synthesis**, or by **post-modification**, once a material is prepared and isolated. For example, preparation of thiol-coated gold nanoparticles by the Brust–Schiffrin method (Chapter 2) involves the addition of alkane–thiols during the synthesis. However, such a strategy cannot be used if the temperature, ionic strength or solvents damage the molecules used for functionalisation, as is the case with the synthesis of quantum dots. Common classes of quantum dots require temperatures which often exceed 100 °C and can go up to 370 °C, which makes the addition of biomolecules during synthesis unfeasible. Instead, biofunctionalisation is achieved post-synthetically by exploiting the process of **ligand exchange**. During ligand exchange, the initial stabilising ligands, such as TOPO or oleic acid, are replaced by other strongly binding ligands such as alkanethiols added to the solution of quantum dots in excess amounts to ensure efficient replacement.

The choice of appropriate surface ligand is an important step in preparation of nanomaterials. Composed of three distinct components, a surface ligand can either be used to tune the surface character by determining the charge or hydrophobicity, or it can be employed for further modification.

Let us now have a closer look at the distinct components of the surface ligand.

4.2.2 Surface-Binding Groups

The two most common ways to attach functional molecules to nanosurfaces are chemisorption and physio-sorption by complexation of ions present at the surface. Coordination chemistry is usually a valuable source of surface binding groups, particularly for metal or metal oxide nanomaterials. For example, benzotriazole (Figure 4.4a) has been known as a copper and silver coordinating ligand and anti-corrosion agent long before it was used for modification of silver and copper nanoparticles.

Figure 4.4

Some of the common surface binding groups for modification of nanomaterials (a), and different ways of carboxylate–metal coordination (b).

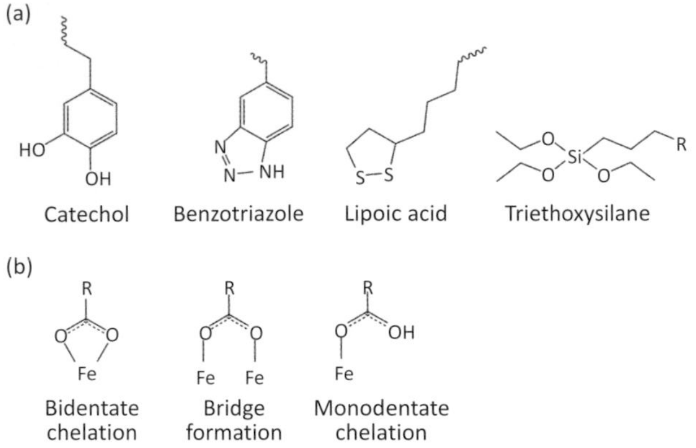

(a)

Catechol   Benzotriazole   Lipoic acid   Triethoxysilane

(b)

Bidentate chelation   Bridge formation   Monodentate chelation

Exploration of thiol chemisorption on gold nanosurfaces led to an understanding of the self-assembled monolayers discussed here, and ligands rich in carboxylic acid groups such as citric acid have traditionally been used for the preparation of various metallic nanoparticles. Due to their availability, carboxylic acids have been particularly popular **chelating agents** for metal oxides and metal oxide nanoparticles. Chelating agents are compounds that can form bonds with a single metal ion and aid formation of metal complexes. Monodentate, bidentate or bridging chelates can be formed, and their properties can be tuned either by changing the carboxylic acid substituents (R in Figure 4.4b) or by adjusting pH.

As iron oxide-based magnetic nanoparticles have been the first metal-based nanoparticle class to be approved by the US Food and Drug Administration (FDA) for applications in magnetic resonance imaging (more on that in Chapter 9), it is not surprising that lots of effort was put into exploration of various surface binding groups for stabilisation of that particular class of nanomaterials (Figure 4.5).

Figure 4.5

Common surface binding groups used for modification of iron oxide magnetic nanoparticles. Adapted by permission of Springer Nature: Boyer et al. (2010).

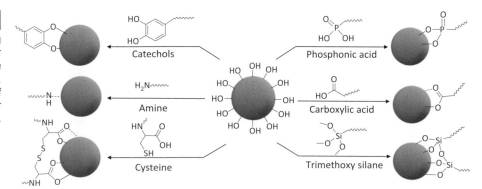

Catechols are particularly interesting as they exhibit strong binding to metal oxide surfaces, and binding can even be enhanced by the presence of electron withdrawing groups such as nitro groups ($-NO_2$) on the benzene ring. In fact, for some nitro-catechols, binding was shown to be so strong that individual iron ions were pulled from within the particle, leading to the dissolution of the whole system. With some ions, such as titanium ions present on the surface of titanium oxide (TiO_2) nanomaterials, catechols can form a strong charge transfer complex (Research Report 4.3).

Research Report 4.3   Catechol–Titanium Dioxide Charge Transfer Complex

Catechol molecules are an interesting class of surface ligands used for stabilisation and functionalisation of titanium oxide (TiO_2) nanomaterials. Such nanomaterials are employed extensively in the design of solar cells and other photovoltaic devices, in particular artificial photosynthetic devices, but also in cosmetics and medicine. Titanium oxide nanomaterials are semiconducting and like quantum dots can also form exciton pairs (see Research Report 2.1) under irradiation with appropriate wavelength, which can then recombine with water molecules and be used for activation of enzymes or for water splitting (Bai et al., 2014).

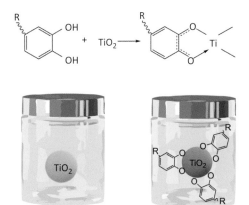

Catechol molecules in aqueous solutions are adsorbed onto the surface of TiO_2 nanomaterials by chelation to surface titanium (Ti^{4+}) ions. Such chemisorption induces strong absorption of light in the visible region due to charge transfer (CT) from catechol to the conduction band of TiO_2 (Murata et al., 2015). Depending on the conditions, the colour of these complexes can range from yellow to orange and dark brown.

The bond between catechols and titanium ions is very strong and it has been shown that it could reach half of the covalent bond strength. For example, strength of a silicon–carbon covalent bond is measured to be 2.0 nN (nano-newtons), gold–sulfphur 1.4 nN, and single catechol on wet TiO_2 surface 0.8 nN.

However, unlike a covalent bond, the catechol–TiO_2 bond is reversible under certain conditions, and therefore interesting for biofunctionalisation of TiO_2 nanomaterials. For example, catechol linkers containing different functional groups were synthesised to enable attachment of DNA and fluorescent dyes to the surface of TiO_2 nanoparticles for use in biosensing (Geiseler and Fruk, 2012).

Phosphonic acid is a preferred surface-binding group in the design of TiO_2 and Fe_3O_4 biomedical devices such as bone grafts. It readily forms SAMs but does not require prior surface treatment as in the case of widely used silanes.

Although there are surface binding groups with a particular affinity towards a specific nanomaterial, many groups can often be used interchangeably. For example, although catechols are preferred for modification of metal oxide nanostructures, they have been shown to effectively coat gold nanoparticles and carbon nanodiamonds. However, for some nanostructures, additional surface treatments are required prior to the addition of linkers containing surface binding groups. In the case of silica (SiO_2) nanostructures the exposure to strong acids prior to modification affords hydroxyl (–OH) a rich surface and facilitates subsequent reaction with silanes. Acid treatment is also used in modification of carbon nanotubes, as it introduces carboxylic groups to the surface on nanotubes, which can then be used for further modification.

4.2.3   The Space Between: The Spacer

The molecular chain between the surface binding and functional group not only determines the thickness of the surface layer, but also contributes to its stability. One of the most common spacers, widely used in the design of biologically compatible and stable nanoparticles and nanomaterials is **polyethylene glycol (PEG)**, and the process of PEG addition to nanomaterials is known as PEGylation (Figure 4.6).

Figure 4.6

PEGylation of nanosurfaces. Structure of ethylene glycol monomer which composes the polyethylene glycol (PEG) polymer often employed as a spacer in linkers used for nanomaterial functionalisation. The process of PEG addition is often referred to as PEGylation.

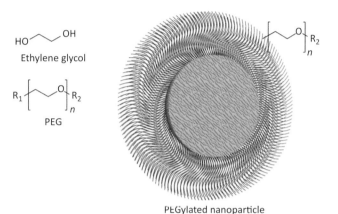

PEGylated nanoparticle

Currently, there are around 35 FDA approved nanoparticle formulations that are either entirely based on PEG or contain PEG linkers (Jonerst et al., 2011). PEG has proven to be exceptionally good for stabilisation of nanomaterials in biological fluids, preventing their agglomeration and increasing hydrophilicity of the whole system. PEG polymers can be modified to contain various functional groups on either ends and length can be tuned to contain n number of ethylene glycol units (n can be anything from 5 to 20 000 and more).

In both the drug delivery and imaging applications discussed in more detail in Chapter 9, PEGylation is used to increase the circulation time and the probability of reaching the biological target and to reduce the uptake by the **reticuloendothelial system (RES)**. The reticuloendothelial system is the part of our immune system responsible for nanomaterials being shuttled into liver, spleen or bone marrow and out of circulation soon after administration. Such fast removal minimises the circulation time, lowering the probability that the material will reach the desired biological target. PEG increases the 'stealth' of the nanomaterials by preventing binding of opsonin proteins, a process known as **opsonisation**. The biological role of opsonins, which can be antibodies or other types of binding proteins, is the recognition of foreign structures. They are bivalent proteins, meaning that they can bind both to the surface of the nanomaterial and interact with receptors on the surface of white blood cells (Figure 4.7).

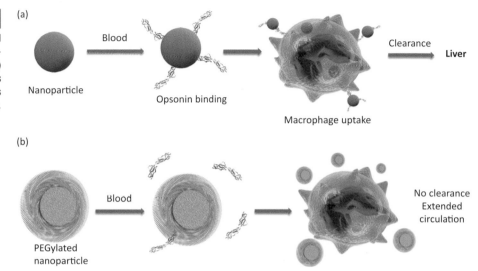

(a)

Nanoparticle   Blood → Opsonin binding   Macrophage uptake   Clearance → **Liver**

(b)

PEGylated nanoparticle   Blood →   No clearance Extended circulation

In general, opsonins make foreign species more susceptible to phagocytosis, a process of removal of foreign compounds by engulfment by white blood cells. When a nanoparticle is associated with opsonin, it can be recognised by cleaner white cells called macrophages and transported to the liver. Macrophages in the liver known as Kupffer cells are then recruited to afford nanoparticle scavenging (more on Kupffer cells in Back to Basics 4.3). However, if the binding of opsonins to nanoparticles is prevented, macrophages do not perceive them as biological garbage or dangerous species, and they are able to circulate through the blood until they reach the target.

Back to Basics 4.3   Kupffer Cells

First described by Karl Wilhelm von Kupffer (1829–1902) in 1876 as 'Sternzellen' (star cells or stellate cells), Kupffer cells were shown to be macrophages in 1898 by Tadeusz Browicz (1847–1928). Kupffer cells are macrophages found in liver. They comprise the largest population of resident tissue macrophages in the body and play an important role in the innate immune response. Due to their localisation in a particular part of liver called the hepatic sinusoid, Kupffer cells efficiently scavenge and phagocytise pathogens such as protein complexes, small and large particles and aged (senescent) red blood cells. As a response to injury, Kupffer cells release inflammatory signals including cytokines, reactive oxygen species, chemokines and growth factors. Depending on which mediator is released, this response leads to progression or attenuation of liver damage.

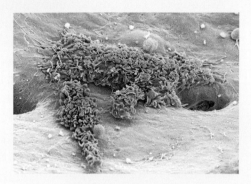

Source: Thomas Deerinck. NCMIR/Science Photo Library.

Human Kupffer cells specifically bind monoclonal antibodies CD14, CD16 and CD68; Kupffer cells from rat with CD68 or CD163 and from mouse with F4/80, all of which have been used to identify and target these specific cells.

Prior to PEGylation of a surface, special attention needs to be given to the amount of PEG used. Namely, the behaviour of the surface layer strongly depends on the density of individual PEG linkers. If the density of PEG is low, the layer takes on a collapsed 'mushroom' conformation (Figure 4.8a), and a 'brush' conformation (Figure 4.8b) with PEG chains extending away from the nanoparticle surface is taken when the density is high.

Figure 4.8

(a) Collapsed 'mushroom' and (b) 'brush' conformation of PEG groups on the surface of nanoparticles. Which conformation will be taken depends on the density of PEG layer.

(a)

(b)

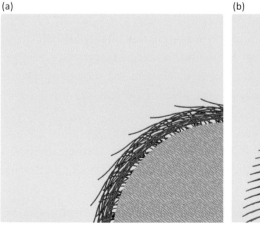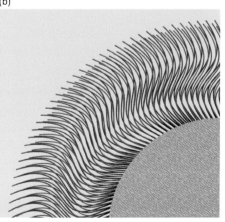

Nanomaterials with brush conformation generally have longer circulation time since dense packing prevents the protein adsorption. In addition, any functional groups present at the end of the PEG linker will be less sterically hindered and more available for any further modification.

Although PEGylation has many advantages such as biocompatibility and low toxicity, which helped to take some nanomaterials from the lab bench into the clinic, PEG is not biodegradable, thereby it can accumulate in cells. Furthermore, it can be degraded into smaller fragments under the influence of light, heat or shear stress, which limits the shelf life of modified nanomaterials and the resulting degradation products might affect the properties of nanomaterials, and cause tissue damage. Alternative coatings based on biomolecules such as polysaccharides chitosan and hyaluronic acid (see Chapter 2), various sugars or short polypeptide chains are being explored to make nanomaterials more suitable for medical applications.

4.2.4   Functional Groups

The choice of the functional group is primarily determined by the type of species that needs to be attached to a nanostructure and the strength of the required attachment. If a covalent binding of a protein to the **carboxylic group**-rich surface of nanomaterials is desired, simple amide coupling can be employed through **amine**-rich lysine groups on the protein surface (Figure 4.9a). When a modification through amine group is not possible, but the protein contains cysteines, Michael addition, covalent bond formation between **thiols** and **maleimides**, can be employed (Figure 4.9b).

Covalent attachment results in formation of strong bonds, which are not suitable for applications in which the attached species needs to be released from the surface under favourable conditions. In that case, a reversible binding is required which can, for example, be achieved by electrostatic interaction and facilitated by the introduction of negatively or positively charged ligands to the nanomaterial surface. When the non-covalent binding is considered too weak, and the properties or the structure of attached species, particularly biomolecules, change by covalent bond formation, milder **antibody–antigen** (Figure 4.9c) or **protein–tag**-mediated functionalisation can be employed (Figure 4.9d).

(Bio)functionalisation strategies can roughly be grouped into non-covalent and covalent, both of which can be further divided into distinct routes depending on the type of interacting species and employed reagents and conditions.

The surface of gold nanoparticle modified with ligands containing different functional groups for further modification with biomolecules. (a) Amide coupling to the protein's lysines; (b) Michael addition of maleimide to the protein's cysteines; (c) an antibody for specific protein binding; and (d) streptavidin modified nanoparticles for biotin–DNA conjugation.

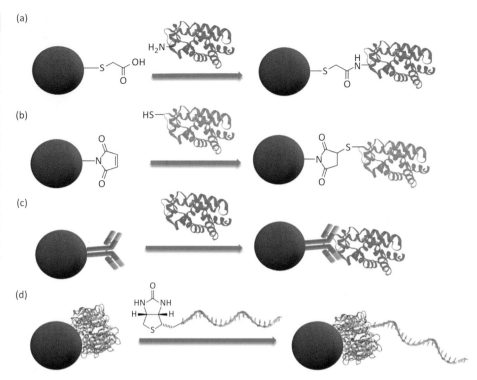

4.3 Non-Covalent Biofunctionalisation Strategies

4.3.1 Physical Adsorption

Biomolecules can be attached to the surface of nanomaterials using direct adsorption facilitated either by electrostatic or hydrophobic interactions. For example, a negatively charged surface modified with carboxylic or hydroxyl groups can directly be modified by positively charged biomolecules (Figure 4.10). Electrostatic interactions result in weakly bound surface species, which can be easily removed by addition of competitive, stronger binding ligand or change in pH. Sometimes they are used simply for the stabilisation of the surface so that they can be modified at a later stage, and sometimes to provide a simple and cheap strategy to afford design of useful bionano hybrids using sensitive proteins. However, many proteins do not possess a significant net charge.

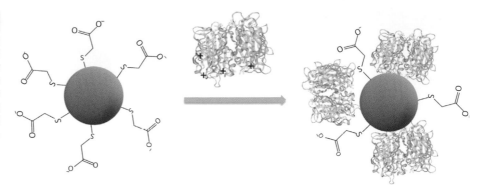

If this is the case, and no other alternative for their attachment exists, positive or negative charges can be engineered into proteins through fusion of peptides containing charged amino acids. It is often easier and cheaper to introduce the charges to the surface of the nanoparticles, using various charged ligands, for example cationic and anionic surfactants (Figure 4.11). Cationic surfactants, such as cetyl-trimethyl sodium bromide (CTAB), are often used in preparation and modification of nanomaterials, and commonly used in synthesis of gold nanorods.

Figure 4.11

An example of cationic (CTAB) and anionic (DBS) surfactants used to prepare charged nanomaterial surfaces.

CTAB

DBS

Anionic surfactants such as 4(5-dodecyl)benzenesulfonate (DBS) usually contain carboxylic or sulfonate (SO_3^-) groups. Using surfactant coatings, nanomaterials can be rendered more stable in desired solvents, but also more prone to bind target biomolecules. Such nanoparticles can then be used for preparation of hybrid enzyme systems that catalyse reactions in organic solvents, which would not be efficient in the presence of the enzyme only (Research Report 4.4).

A larger number of charged or hydrophobic groups can be introduced to the surface by use of polymers, in particular branched structures, which afford uniform distribution of desired groups over the surface. The advantage of polymers is that they can also be designed to change properties under the action of light, temperature or pH resulting in a modular surface that can be adapted on demand. For example, the hydrophobicity of a polymer layer can be controlled by a light-triggered cleavage of a particular functional group embedded within the structure (Lin et al., 2008), and the density by changing the temperature. Taking into account that the number of such materials is continuously increasing, they play an important role in design of adaptable bionano hybrids for biosensing and other biomedical applications.

| Research Report 4.4 | Improving Stability of Lipase Enzyme |

Lipases are an important class of enzymes, which catalyse many enantiomeric reactions resulting in chiral products (see Chapter 3 for more on chirality), and therefore have huge potential for drug synthesis. However, their catalytic activity decreases significantly in organic solvents, which limits their practical application for organic synthesis. In addition, it is not easy to remove them from the reaction mixture and reuse them in subsequent catalytic cycles. One route to increase the catalytic performance of an enzyme's stability and storage time, as well as recyclability, is to immobilise them onto solid surfaces (encapsulation is the other commonly employed route).

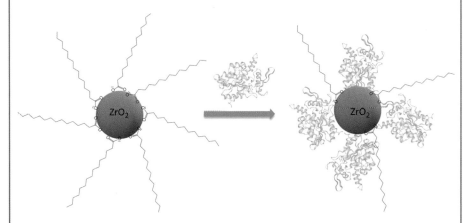

Nanoparticles are particularly suitable for immobilisation due to high surface area, which enables attachment of a large number of enzymes. For example, lipase enzymes can be immobilised onto stable and non-toxic zirconia (ZrO_2) nanoparticles. However, chemical modification strategies need to be avoided as they lead to deactivation of the enzyme. The mildest route to prepare ZrO_2 NP–lipase conjugates is an adsorption of lipases onto a hydrophobic layer on the surface of a nanoparticle. Such a layer is achieved by addition of ligands that contain long alkyl chains and carboxylic acid groups for coordination onto ZrO_2 surface. This is not only a simple and cheap surface modification strategy, but also results in favourable lipase orientation, which facilitates substrate binding and higher catalytic activity (Chen et al., 2008).

4.3.2   DNA-Directed Functionalisation

Short single-stranded DNAs can be synthesised using solid phase synthesis and reagents such as phosphoramidites (more on that in Chapter 6). During the process of DNA synthesis, different functional groups such as amine, thiol, carboxylic acid, biotin, various fluorophores can be added to either $3'$ or $5'$ end of the strand. The presence of such groups means that such modified DNA strands can be conjugated to other biomolecules or immobilised onto various surfaces. Once attached, single-stranded DNAs can be hybridised with their complementary strands to form a stable double helix, which is the basic principle of the surface modification strategy known as **DNA-directed immobilisation** or **DDI** (Figure 4.12). Developed in the mid 1990s (Niemeyer et al., 1994), DDI has been extensively used for applications in biosensing, in particular to precisely position proteins or nanoparticles onto various surfaces. There are a number of advantages of this DNA-based strategy compared to other methods. DDI is chemically mild, meaning that it does not involve use of harsh conditions or catalysts, and it proceeds readily in aqueous solutions. This makes it particularly well-suited for immobilisation of other

Figure 4.12

Surface modification with proteins using DNA-directed immobilisation of DNA-modified protein to complementary strands on the surface.

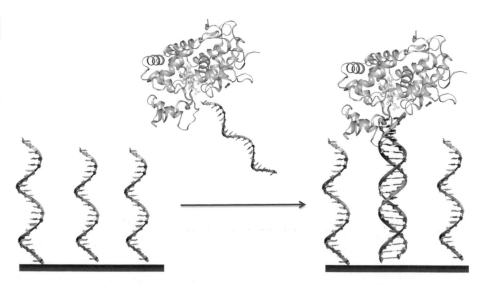

biomolecules. In addition, DNA hybridisation is a reversible process (Chapter 3), and the double helix can be unwound (or melted) into two single strands using heat or increasing pH. These single strands can reassemble and hybridise again when the conditions become favourable. Finally, DNA sequences are highly programmable: there is a vast number of possible base sequences. Together with the high specificity of hybridisation, sequence diversity means that the immobilisation of multiple species can be achieved in one go.

DNA-directed immobilisation is not only successfully used for biofunctionalisation of nanomaterials, but has been shown to aid the immobilisation of whole cells, and to guide assembly of large structures from man-made nanomaterials (Research Report 4.5).

Research Report 4.5	DNA-Directed Assembly of Nanoparticles

Thiol containing single-stranded DNAs can be attached to the surface of gold nanoparticles using chemisorption. Controlled assembly of a number of such nanoparticles can be achieved by using carefully programmed DNA sequences. Using DNA hybridisation four nanoparticles of different size were assembled into R and S enantiomers: mirror-image structures of same chemical composition but different orientation in space (check Chapter 3 for more). Such chiral nanoparticle assemblies interact differently with light depending on their orientation (Mastroianni et al., 2009). Nano-sized systems that can be designed to interact with light in a particular manner are interesting for the field of nanophotonics, in particular for construction of quantum circuits for quantum-information processing and the development of quantum computers (Lodahl et al., 2017).

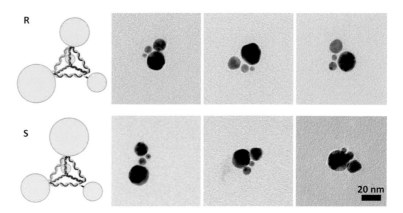

Source: Reprinted with permission from Mastroianni et al. (2009). © 2009 American Chemical Society.

We will talk more about DNA nanotechnology and design of hybrid DNA structures in Chapter 6.

4.3.3   DNA Aptamers

Besides short single-stranded DNAs, more complex DNA structures called aptamers can be used for biofunctionalisation of nanomaterials (Figure 4.13). DNA aptamers are short DNA strands with usually 20 to 80 nucleotides. They bind to target molecules with high affinity and specificity, which stems from their characteristic structure composed of loops and bulges (similar to some RNAs, Chapter 3). Aptamers are identified and isolated from a large sequence pool based on their binding to a specific target molecule using interactive enrichment techniques such as SELEX (Back to Basics 4.4).

Back to Basics 4.4	Systematic Evolution of Ligands by Exponential Enrichment

Systematic evolution of ligands by exponential enrichment (SELEX) is employed for selection of specific DNA aptamers (or RNA aptamers) from a pool of sequences. Such a selection is usually achieved through several SELEX rounds. A typical round consists of a few distinct steps:

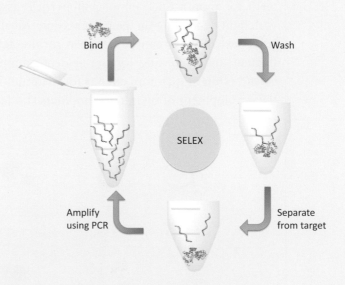

1. The library of DNA sequences is first generated by changing the position and type of bases within the sequence.

2. The library is then incubated with the selected target (bio)molecule or exposed to a particular surface. Those DNAs that bind to the target are potential aptamers.
3. After removal of unbound sequences, bound sequences are separated from the target and purified. Different techniques such as filtration, gel electrophoresis, use of magnetic beads and affinity chromatography can be used for separation of unbound and bound DNA.
4. Bound sequences are amplified using the polymer chain reaction (PCR) strategy, creating a more specific library with fewer candidate sequences. This library is then used for a new selection round for further optimisation.

The procedure is generally repeated 10–15 times.

Attachment to the nanomaterial surface can be achieved either through DNA-directed hybridisation or through a linker that contains a surface binding group (Figure 4.13). It is important that during the process of attachment, the three-dimensional structure is left undisturbed so it does not interfere with further binding of other species. One can think of aptamers as DNA-based antibodies, although they have a few advantages over antibodies. They are smaller, more stable in harsher environments and have higher flexibility, and, therefore, generally regarded as excellent substitutes for antibodies (Proske et al., 2005). However, they also have a relatively short half-life,

Figure 4.13

DNA aptamer immobilisation onto nanoparticles. Surface immobilisation can be achieved either through capture of DNA complementary to DNA aptamer or directly through a chemical linker containing surface binding group.

(a)

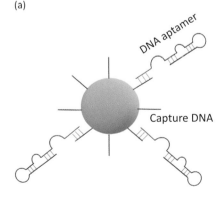

(b)

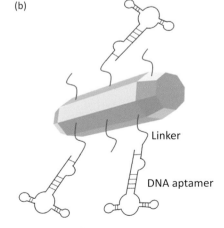

and in many cases, lower specificity and weaker target binding than antibodies, which can complicate their use in complex environments such as biological fluids. Strategies are continuously being developed to overcome these drawbacks, and afford aptamers to be used not only for nanomaterial functionalisation, but also for cell targeting and design of novel therapeutics (Zhou and Rossi, 2014).

4.4   (Bio)functionalisation Using Proteins and Protein Tags

4.4.1   Streptavidin–Biotin Interaction

Streptavidin–biotin interaction (Chapter 3) is one of the most widely used strategies for biofunctionalisation and assembly of nanomaterials. This is due to the strong and specific binding between protein streptavidin and the small molecule biotin. Modified nanomaterials can be obtained using two strategies. One strategy involves preparation of streptavidin-coated surface by attachment or adsorption of STV, which is then followed by binding of the target molecule (DNA, protein, sugar, small molecule) conjugated with biotin (Research Report 4.6).

Research Report 4.6	STV–Gold Nanoparticles to Study Cell Receptor Geometry

Epidermal growth factor receptor (EGFR) is a transmembrane receptor that plays an important role in the progression of different types of cancers. However, it is difficult to image the EGFR in an intact cell. Techniques such as cryogenic transmission electron microscopy (cryo-TEM) and super-resolution fluorescence microscopy (Chapter 5), commonly used to explore proteins in cells, do not have the required resolution. To overcome that drawback and visualise the receptor in an intact cell, gold nanoparticles (Au NPs) were coated with a single streptavidin protein and allowed to bind biotinylated-EGF (epidermal growth factor). Such Au NP construct was attached to the EGFR receptor on the surface of the cancer cell through specific interaction with EGF on the surface of the nanoparticle. Cells were then fixed and imaged with scanning transmission electron microscopy (STEM) enabling the localisation of EGFRs with a resolution of 3 nm. Distinct dimers (bright Au NP spots in the STEM images) can clearly be observed and the distance between two Au NPs of 19 nm corresponds to the native configuration of the EGFR dimers (Peckys et al., 2013).

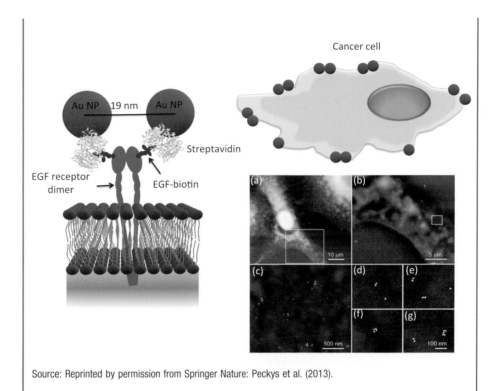

Source: Reprinted by permission from Springer Nature: Peckys et al. (2013).

Imaging receptors on the cell surface with such precision is important for exploration of cell–cell interactions, but also for design of cell-targeting species or drugs.

An alternative strategy is based on preparation of biotinylated nanomaterials, and fusing streptavidin to the target. If the target is a protein, such an approach requires design of fusion proteins, which, due to the size of streptavidin, is not easy and can significantly change the properties of the target. Attaching DNA to streptavidin is much easier and can be done using covalent coupling (see Section 4.5) or binding through protein tags (see Section 4.4.3). Naturally occurring streptavidin, usually referred to as the wild type streptavidin, is a tetrameric protein and has four biotin-binding sites. Variants have been engineered which are smaller and contain only one biotin-binding domain, increasing their specificity. In addition to biotin, streptavidin-binding peptide sequences (STREP tactin or STREP tag) have been developed that can be genetically inserted into target proteins and employed for binding onto streptavidin-coated nanomaterials.

4.4.2 Antibody–Antigen Interactions

Antibody interactions with antigens such as proteins or small molecules are highly specific and widely used for functionalisation of nanomaterial surfaces, in particular in the design of biosensors (Research Report 4.7 and Chapter 8), for targeted drug delivery and tissue imaging. For example, iron oxide nanoparticles used for magnetic resonance imaging can be coated with antibodies specific for a particular cancer cell receptor, and in such a way ease their detection.

Despite their extensive application in bionanotechnology, antibodies are proteins sensitive to modification. Their unique structure is responsible for specific binding of antigens, and any structural changes, no matter how minute, can impact their binding ability. To ensure that they are immobilised onto the surface of nanomaterials in an active form, the choice of the anchoring strategy is crucial.

Research Report 4.7	Carbon Nanotube Biosensor for Lyme Disease

Antibody–antigen interactions have been used to help detect Lyme disease, also known as *Lyme borreliosis*, which is a bacterial infection that can be spread to humans by infected ticks. It is treatable if diagnosed early, but if patients are treated too late they suffer tiredness and chronic fatigue that lasts for years. Late detection of Lyme disease can also lead to further complications including arthritis and permanent neurological disorders. Diagnosis of Lyme disease is severely hindered by the lack of reliable diagnostic tools. To address this problem, a sensor for Lyme disease bacteria was developed based on carbon nanotube field effect transistor (FET). FET is an electronic device composed of a gate, drain and source and uses an electric field to control the flow of current (Chapter 8). Flow of current is controlled by application of a voltage to the gate terminal, which in turn alters the conductivity between the drain and source terminal. When carbon nanotubes are used as gates, changes on their surface induce easily detected change of conductivity.

To design carbon nanotube FET for detection of Lyme disease bacteria, carbon nanotubes were modified with an antibody specific to the bacterial flagellar antigen p41. Amide coupling was employed to attach the antibody's lysines to carboxylic groups introduced to the surface of the carbon nanotube.

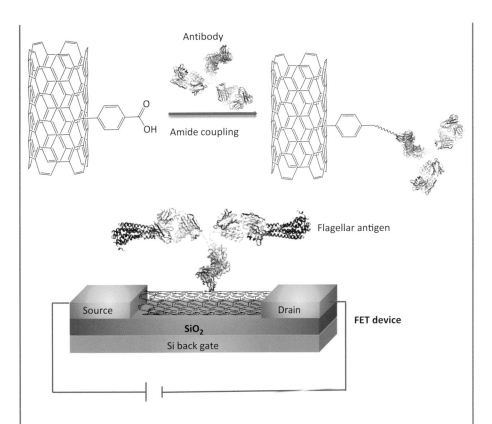

Antibody

Amide coupling

Flagellar antigen

Source

Drain

FET device

SiO$_2$

Si back gate

The presence of the bacterial antigen in solution was detected using measurements of the current as a function of a gate voltage resulting in detection of upto 1 ng ml^{-1} of antigen, which is much lower than that diagnostically relevant of 12–15 ng ml^{-1} (Lerner et al., 2013).

4.4.3 Protein Tags

Protein tags were originally developed to aid purification and identification of proteins (developments and types of protein tags were covered in Chapter 3). Namely, with the development of molecular biology and the ability to prepare large quantities of proteins in bacterial (and later eukaryotic) cells, the challenge that needed to be overcome was the purification of proteins from the melting pot of biomolecules within the cell. The solution was a tag fusion; tags are either small peptides, parts of or whole proteins characterised by an ability to bind to particular small molecules.

Historically first and still the most widely used tag is the **His tag**, which contains up to 7–8 histidine (His) amino acids added to one of the protein ends. Coordination chemistry has already shown that certain metals such as zinc (Zn) and nickel (Ni) can coordinate molecules rich in nitrogen and oxygen, such as imidazoles contained within histidine. By using histidine-tag on a protein and another chelating agent such as nitrilotriacetic acid (NTA) on the surface, chelating complex can be formed in the presence of coordinating ions (Figure 4.14).

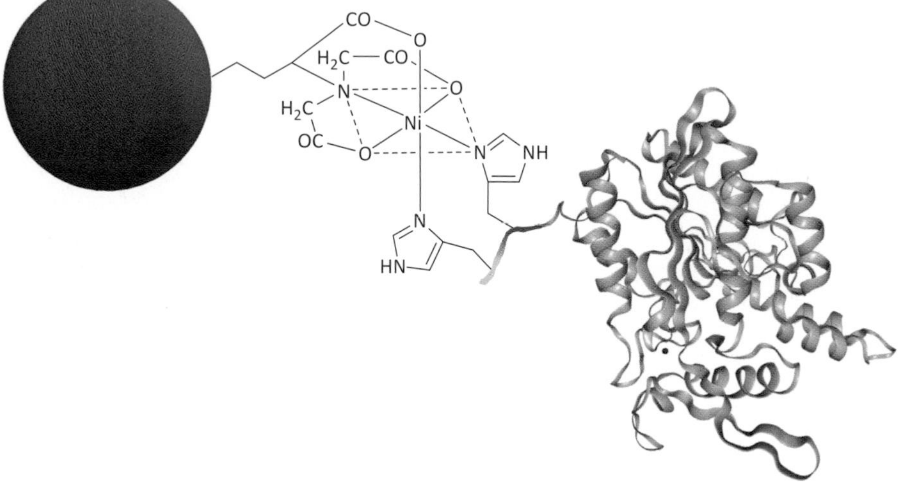

Figure 4.14

Biofunctionalisation of nanoparticle using His tag strategy. A nanoparticle is modified with nitrilotriacetic acid (NTA) and a complex is formed with His tag containing protein in the presence of nickel ions (Ni^{2+}) ions.

Due to its small size, a His tag is usually the first choice when tagging is required. Like other tags in use, it does not work with all proteins and it has its limitations. For example, the His–NTA complex can be easily disassembled in the presence of nitrogen-containing species such as urea, which has a higher binding affinity than NTA.

Other protein tags, predominantly SNAP and CLIP tags (Back to Basics 4.5), are also employed for biofunctionalisation of nanomaterials. Both SNAP and CLIP tags are based on the formation of a covalent bond with benzyl guanine (SNAP) or benzyl cytosine (CLIP) groups, meaning that protein remains attached to the nanomaterial and can be cleaved only by use of enzymes that can digest the peptide bond between the protein and the tag. The SNAP-tag strategy has been employed to modify a range of nanomaterials through immobilisation of benzylguanine groups onto the surface of the nanomaterial and addition of SNAP-tagged protein of interest (Figure 4.15).

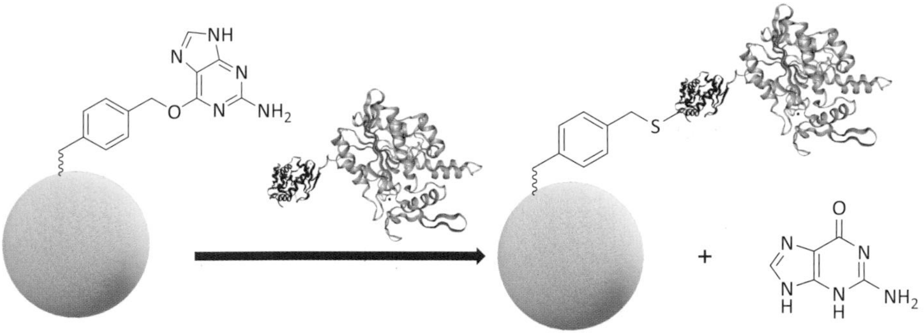

Figure 4.15

Biofunctionalisation of nanoparticles using the SNAP-tag strategy. A nanoparticle is first modified with benzyl guanine and then allowed to react with SNAP tag (blue) fused to a protein of interest. A covalent bond is formed between SNAP tag and benzyl moiety with the release of guanine.

Back to Basics 4.5   SNAP, CLIP and Halo Tags for Protein Conjugation

Both SNAP and CLIP tags are small proteins engineered from a particular domain of DNA methyl-transferase enzymes, and are characterised by covalent binding to benzyl guanine (SNAP) or benzyl cytosine (CLIP).

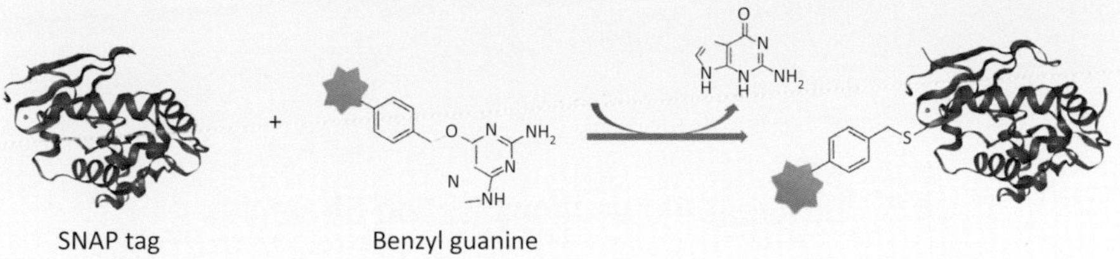

SNAP tag   Benzyl guanine

SNAP tag is a small protein (20 kDa) derived from the human DNA repair protein O6-alkylguanine-DNA-alky-transferease (AGT). The function of AGT is the repair of alkylguanine in DNA by transfer of alkyl group to a reactive cysteine in AGT. In this process the protein is irreversibly deactivated as a strong covalent thioether bond is formed.

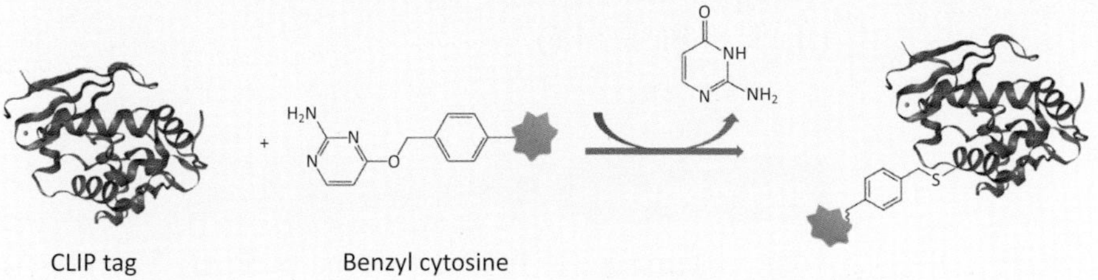

CLIP tag   Benzyl cytosine

CLIP tag is a mutant of SNAP tag specifically developed to react with benzyl guanine. SNAP and CLIP tags are orthogonal (they do not cross-react) and can be used for simultaneous labelling of multiple proteins at the same time.

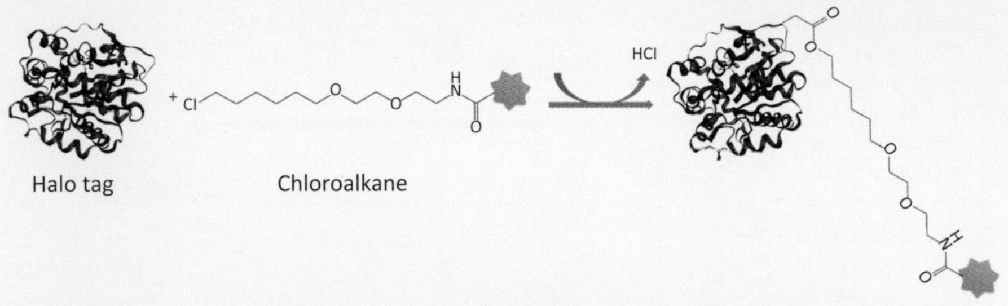

Halo tag   Chloroalkane

Halo tag is a mutant of haloalkane dehalogenase, which removes halides (Cl, Br, I) from hydrocarbons by nucleophilic displacement mechanism resulting in the formation of a covalent ester bond. Halo tag binds chloroalkanes rapidly and under physiological conditions has been used for such applications as fluorescent labelling and modification of nanomaterial surfaces.

4.5 Covalent Biofunctionalisation Strategies

Covalent biofunctionalisation strategies are based on water-friendly chemical reactions, using either natural building blocks or non-native functional groups introduced to the biomolecule of interest. The preferred covalent biofunctionalisation strategies involve either use of covalently binding protein tags (see Section 4.4.3), amide coupling (see Figure 4.9a) or **click chemistry** routes. The term click chemistry refers to reactions done under mild conditions (pH, T, solvents), with minimal use of catalysts and in the absence of side products (Back to Basics 4.6).

| Back to Basics 4.6 | Click Chemistry |

Click chemistry, as first introduced by Barry Sharpless' group in 1999 at the 217th American Chemical Society annual meeting, describes a group of reactions that

... must be modular, wide in scope, give very high yields, generate only inoffensive by-products that can be removed by non-chromatographic methods, and be stereospecific (but not necessarily enantioselective). The required process characteristics include simple reaction conditions (ideally the process should be insensitive to oxygen and water, readily available starting materials and reagents, the use of no solvent or the solvent that is benign (such as water) or easily removed, and simple product isolation.

(Sharpless and Kolb, 1999)

There are few classes of chemical transformations that meet these requirements:

Cycloadditions such as copper(I)-catalyzed Huisgen cycloadditon between azide (N≡N–N) and alkyne (–C≡C–) (CuAAC) and its copper-free strain-promoted version (SPAAC), as well as Diels–Alder transformations and light-triggered nitrile-imine mediated tetrazole-ene cycloaddition (named NITEC).

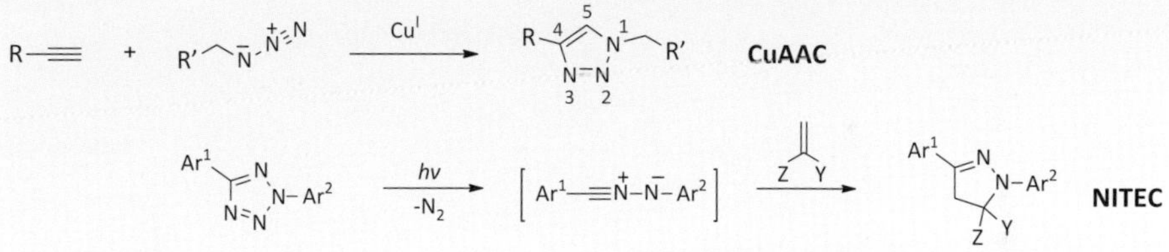

(Ar stands for aromatic group)

Nucleophilic substitution reactions, such as the ring-opening reactions of strained heterocyclic electrophiles (electron-loving species), for example epoxides (contain oxygen), aziridines (contain nitrogen, NR), aziridinium ions ($^+NR_2$), and episulfonium (^+SR) ions (R is a general representation of a functional group).

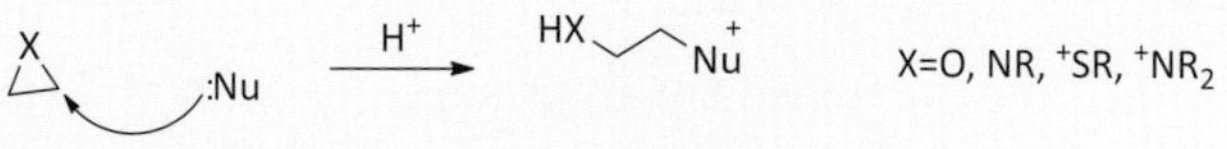

Carbonyl reactions of the 'non-aldol' type such as formation of oxime ethers and hydrazones (a), ureas/thioureas (b) aromatic heterocycles and amides. Carbonyl reactions of the 'aldol' type generally have low thermo-dynamic driving forces resulting in longer reaction times, formation of side products, and therefore cannot be considered click reactions.

(a) Hydrazone/oxime ether formation

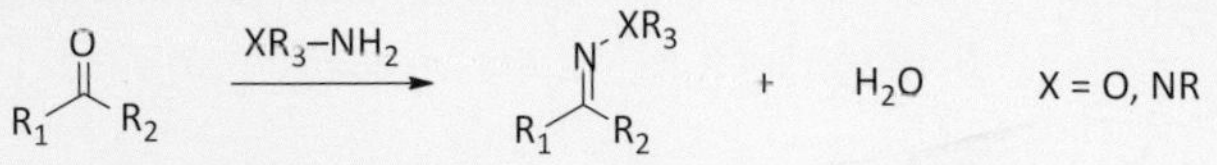

(b) Amide/isourea formation

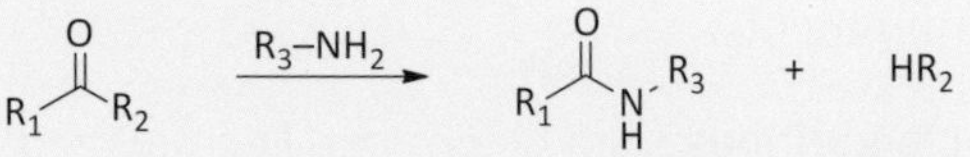

Additions to carbon–carbon multiple bonds, such as including epoxidation (a), dihydroxylation, aziridination and sulfenyl-halide addition, but also Michael additions (b).

(a) Formation of three-member rings

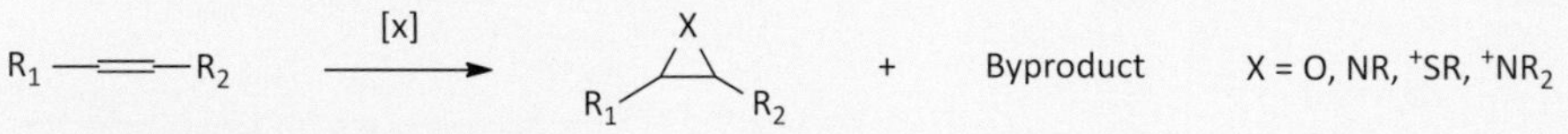

(b) Certain Michael additions

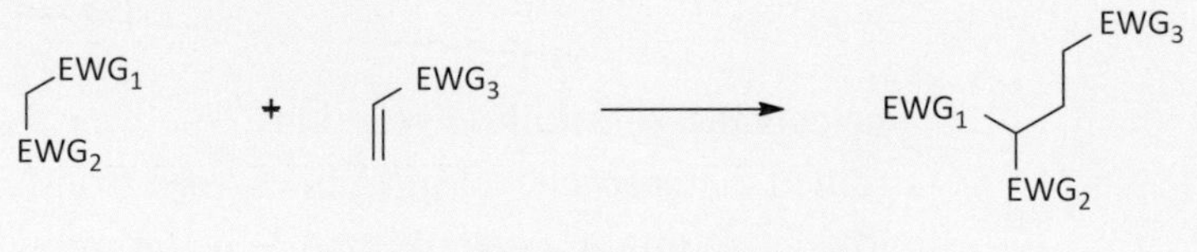

(EWG stands for electron-withdrawing group)

An extensively used click reaction is Michael addition, which results in thioether formation between a thiol and a maleimide group (see Figure 4.9b). Other click chemistry procedures employed for nanomaterial bi-functionalisation are Huisgen cycloadditions based on the interaction of alkynes with azides in presence or absence of catalytic amounts of copper(I) catalyst (Figure 4.16a), and Diels–Alder cycloaddition (Figure 4.16b).

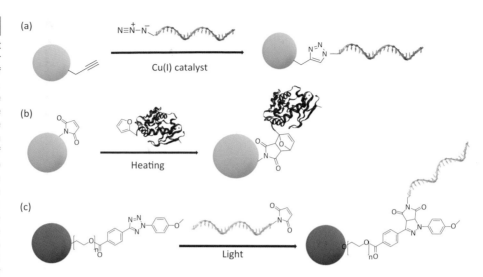

Figure 4.16

Examples of covalent click strategies used for biofunctionalisation of nanomaterials. Biomolecules can be attached to the surface using (a) alkyne–azide click chemistry in presence or absence of copper(I) catalyst; (b) Diels–Alder cycloaddition between maleimide furan under application of heat; and (c) nitril-imine mediated tetrazole-ene cycloaddition (NITEC) between tetrazole and maleimide under irradiation.

Particularly interesting are coupling strategies that can be triggered on demand, as they allow for a spatio-temporal control over surface functionalisation. Such reactions require use of external stimulus such as light. Photo-click reaction between tetrazole and -ene groups such as maleimide (nitrile-imine mediated tetrazole-ene cycloaddition or NITEC; Figure 4.16c) can not only be triggered by light, but it also results in a fluorescent product. Such easily detected product reports on a reaction status and allows for the quantification of molecules on the surface (Stolzer et al., 2015).

Although they have many advantages, click strategies require an additional modification of biomolecules with non-native groups. Such functional groups are easily introduced to DNA or small peptides during synthesis, but modification of proteins is more complex. Addition of groups such as maleimide is usually achieved with the help of **bifunctional coupling agents** that contain maleimide and a group that can bind to specific amino acids. Coupling agents that can bind to lysine, cysteine, tryptophan or tyrosine amino acids and introduce a non-native functional group to proteins have been developed and some are commercially available (Figure 4.17). It is important that these groups are **bioorthogonal**, meaning that they do not react with any functional group present within a native protein.

When the use of chemical strategies is not an option due to protein sensitivity, desired functional groups can be introduced to proteins through unnatural amino acids incorporated during protein synthesis. Such a strategy is both expensive and complex, and it requires the design of specific molecular tools, and is not straightforward to use. Although unnatural amino acids are used in molecular biology to introduce novel functions to native proteins, and

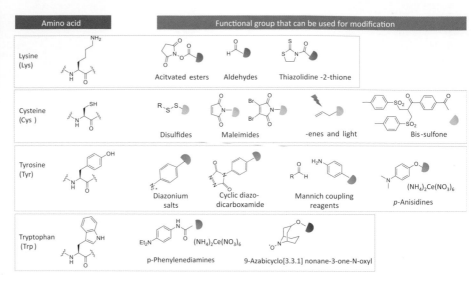

Figure 4.17

Coupling agents employed for modification of proteins through some amino acids.

are explored for design of therapeutic proteins (Wals and Ovoa, 2014), they have limited application in biofunctionalisation of nanomaterials.

Introduction of non-native functional groups is not required for a strategy known as **native chemical ligation** (NCL). Native chemical ligation is a chemo-selective coupling that results in the formation of peptide bond between a peptide fragment containing cysteine residue, and another peptide fragment bearing a thioester group (Figure 4.18). Peptide bond formation is followed by an irreversible S–N acyl shift under physiological conditions, at pH 7 and temperature from 20 to 37 °C. Native chemical ligation is usually catalysed by the thiol-containing compounds such as 4-mercaptophenylacetic acid (MPAA) and 2-mercaptoethanesulfonate sodium (MESNa). A semisynthetic version of the native chemical ligation is expressed protein ligation (EPL) in which synthetic or recombinant polypeptides are joined together through NCL in the final step.

Expressed protein ligation has been successfully used to assemble proteins from smaller polypeptides, and has been employed for the preparation of protein–DNA conjugates (more on their importance in Chapter 6), but less often for modification of nanomaterials. Despite few advantages such as simplicity and high yield, both NCL and EPL usually require higher concentrations of either one or both chemical reagents. Thiols needed for the reaction are also prone to formation of disulfides (S–S bridges), which can result in undesired agglomerates and poor protein solubility.

Choice of the biofunctionalisation strategy depends on both the nature of the starting materials and the ultimate fate of bionano conjugates.

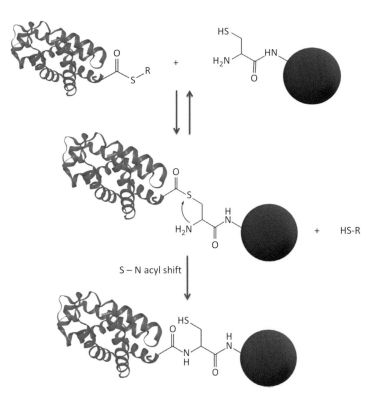

Figure 4.18

Native chemical ligation (NCL) for surface attachment of the protein to the nanoparticle. NCL is a chemo-selective coupling reaction between the terminal cysteine group (shown on nanoparticle) and thioester group (protein).

Biofunctionalisation is usually a critical step for application of nanomaterials in biosensing and medicine, and requires careful design and an interdisciplinary approach.

Key Concepts

Antibody–antigen interaction: specific interaction between antibody and its antigen, and a major regulative processes of our immune response. One of the most common strategies for modification of nanomaterials.

Click chemistry: chemistry of reactions that result in the formation of covalent bonds but under mild conditions, using readily available starting materials and reagents, with little or no side products which can be easily removed.

DNA aptamers: DNA-based antibodies with high affinity and specificity towards particular target (bio)molecules.

DNA-directed immobilisation: use of DNA hybridisation to immobilise (bio)molecules onto various surfaces including those of nanomaterials.

His, SNAP, CLIP and HALO tags: peptide or small protein tags genetically fused to the proteins and employed for protein purification and immobilisation.

Opsonisation: binding of opsonin proteins to the surface of nanomaterials (or organic materials) that guide the macrophage uptake and removal of foreign substances from blood.

PEGylation: attachment of polyethylene glycol groups to the surface of (nano)materials to increase their blood circulation time and minimise the uptake by immune system cleaner cells.

Self-assembly: spontaneous organisation of small elements into larger structures.

Surface binding linkers: molecules used for stabilisation and modification of nanomaterial surface, usually composed of surface binding group, spacers and a functional group.

Problems

4.1   Group the following events as static or dynamic self-assembly and explain what is the difference between the two. In the case of dynamic self-assembly, what could you use to keep each event you have chosen in a steady state?

Nanoparticle growth	Formation of SAMs of thiols on gold surface
Formation of single-walled carbon nanotubes	Magnetosome formation within magnetotactic bacteria
Viral shell formation	Assembly of metal-organic frameworks (MOFs)
Formation of a bacterial colony	Concentric rings of charged polymer nanoparticles in electric field
Assembly of a ribosome structure	

4.2   How could you modify the surface of CdSe nanorods to induce a self-assembly into chains of nanorods?

4.3   Which functional groups could be introduced to the surface of Au nanoparticles to enable interaction with a phospholipid cell membrane?

4.4 Which surface binding groups are most suitable for modification of
  (a) 15 nm carbon nanodiamonds
  (b) 30 nm porous SiO_2
  (c) 10 nm Au nanorods
  (d) 5 nm Pt nanocubes

4.5 Explain the steps needed to prepare antibody-coated graphene.

4.6 Oxidation of a methyl group produces a carboxylate group. How will the wetting properties of an alkanethiol SAM on Au NP change if the methyl group is oxidised?

4.7 Commercial iron oxide nanoparticles you bought are nicely dispersed in organic solvents such as toluene, but precipitate upon addition of water.
  (a) How would you make your nanoparticles stable in aqueous solution?
  (b) Which strategy could you use to attach an enzyme to the surface taking into account that the resulting conjugate will be used for catalysis in a large-scale industrial reactor?
  (c) What do you need to take into account when you are preparing the same nanoparticles for applications in imaging of cancer cells?

4.8 Design a linker which would enable modification of mesoporous silica nanoparticle with a cysteine-containing antibody specific for breast cancer cells.

4.9 Describe two methods by which DNA can be attached to Au nanoparticles using relevant chemical structures.

4.10 Surface of a silver nanorod was coated with 20 streptavidin molecules. What is the maximum number of biotinylated-DNA strands that can be attached to the nanorod?

Further Reading

Best, M. D. (2009). Click chemistry and bioorthogonal reactions: unprecedented selectivity in the labelling of biological molecules. *Biochemistry*, **48**(28), 6571–6584.

Conde, J., Dias, J. T., Grazu, V., et al. (2014). Revisiting 30 years of biofunctionalisation and surface chemistry of inorganic nanoparticles for nanomedicine. *Frontiers in Chemistry*, **2**, 48.

Kumar, C. (ed.) (2006). *Biofunctionalisation of Nanomaterials*. John Wiley and Sons.

Mendes, A. C., Baran, E. T., Reis, R. L. and Azevedo, H. S. (2013). Self-assembly in nature: using the principles of nature to create complex nano-biomaterials. *Wiley Interdisciplinary Reviews: Nanomedicine and Nanobio-technology*, **5**, 517– 661.

Nagamune, T. (2017). Biomolecular engineering for nanobio/biotechnology. *Nano Convergence*, **4**(1), 9.

Spicer, D. C. and Davis, B. G. (2014). Selective chemical protein modifica-tion. *Nature Communications*, **5**, 4740.

References

Bai, Y., Mara-Sero, I., De Angelis, F., Bisquert, J. and Wang, P. (2014). Titanium dioxide nanomaterials for photovoltaic applications. *Chemical Reviews*, **114**, 10095–10130.

Boyer, C., Whittaker, M. R., Bulmus, V., Liu, J. and Davis, T. P. (2010). The design and utility of polymer-stabilised iron-oxide nanoparticles for nano-medicine applications. *NPG Asia Materials*, **2**, 23–30.

Chen, Y. Z., Yang, C. T., Ching, C. B. and Xu, R. (2008). Immobilisation of lipases on hydrophobilised zirconia nanoparticles: highly enantioselective and reusable biocatalysts. *Langmuir*, **24**(16), 8877–8884.

Feng, Z., Wang, H., Cheng, X. and Xu, B. (2017). Self-assembling ability determines the activity of enzyme-instructed self-assembly for inhibiting cancer cells. *Journal of American Chemical Society* **139**, 15377–15384.

Fialkowski, M., Bishop, K. J. M., Klajn, R., et al., (2006). Principles and implementation of dissipative (dynamic) self-assembly. *Journal of Physical Chemistry B*, **110**, 2482–2496.

Geiseler, B., and Fruk, L. (2012). Bifunctional catechol based linkers for modification of TiO_2 surfaces. *Journal of Materials Chemistry*, **22**, 735–741.

Jonerst, J. V., Lobovkina, T., Zare R. N. and Gambhir, S. S. (2011). Nanoparticle PEGylation for imaging and therapy. *Nanomedicine*, **6**(4), 715–728.

Lerner, M. B., Dailey, J., Goldsmith, B. R., Brisson, D. and Johnson, A. T. (2013). Detecting Lyme disease using antibody-functionalised single-walled carbon nanotube transistors. *Biosensors and Bioelectronics*, **45**, 163–167.

Lin, C. J., Sperling, R. A., Li, J. K., et al. (2008). Design of an amphiphilic polymer for nanoparticle coating and functionalisation. *Small*, **4**, 334–341.

Lodahl, P., Mahmoodian, S., Stobbe, S., et al. (2017). Chiral quantum optics. *Nature*, **541**, 473–480.

Mastroianni, A. J., Claridge, S. A. and Alivisatos, A. P. (2009). Pyramidal and chiral groupings of gold nanocrystals assembled using DNA scaffolds. *Journal of the American Chemical Society*, **131**(24), 8455–8459.

Menger, F. M. (2002). Supramolecular chemistry and self-assembly. *Proceedings of the National Academy of Sciences of the USA*, **99**, 4818–4822.

Murata, Y., Hari, H., Taga, A. and Toda, H. (2015). Surface charge-transfer complex formation of catechol on titanium(IV) oxide and the application to bio-sensing. *Journal of Colloid and Interface Science*, **458**, 305–309.

Niemeyer, C. M., Sano, T., Smith, C. L. and Cantor, C. R. (1994). Oligonucleotide-directed self-assembly of proteins: semisynthetic DNA-streptavidin hybrid molecules as connectors for the generation of macroscopic arrays and the construction of supramolecular bioconjugates. *Nucleic Acids Research*, **22**, 5530–5539.

Nuzzo, R. G. and Allara. D. L. (1983). Adsorption of bifunctional organic disulfides on gold surfaces. *Journal of the American Chemical Society*, **105**, 4481–4483.

Peckys, D. B., Baudoin, J-P., Eder, M., Wener, U. and de Jonge, N. (2013). Epidermal growth factor receptor subunit locations determined in hydrated cells with environmental scanning electron microscopy. *Scientific Reports*, **3**(2626), 1–6.

Proske, D., Blank, M., Buhmann, R. and Resch, A. (2005). Aptamers-basic research, drug development, and clinical applications. *Applied Microbiology and Biotechnology*, **69**, 367–374.

Ramachandran, G. K., Hopson, T. J., Rawlett, A. M., et al. (2003). A bond-fluctuation mechanism for stochastic switching in wired molecules, *Science*, **300**, 1413–1416.

Sharpless, K. B. and Kolb, H. C. (1999). *Book of Abstracts*, 217th ACS National Meeting, Anaheim, CA, 21–25 March, American Chemical Society, p. 145538.

Stolzer, L., Vigovskaya, A., Barner-Kowollik, C. and Fruk, L. (2015). A self-reporting tetrazole-based linker for the biofunctionalization of gold nanorods. *Chemistry: A European Journal*, **21**(41), 14309–14313.

Termonia, Y. (2014). Entropy-driven self-assembly of nanoparticles into strings. *Colloids and Surfaces A: Physiochemical and Engineering Aspects*, **447**, 23–27.

Volker, K. W., Reinitz, C. A. and Knull, H. R. (1995). Glycolytic enzymes and assembly of microtubule networks. *Comparative Biochemistry and Physiology. Part B, Biochemistry & Molecular Biology*, **112**(3), 503–514.

Wals, K. and Ovoa, H. (2014). Unnatural amino acid incorporation in *E. coli*: current and future applications in the design of therapeutic proteins. *Frontiers in Chemistry*, **2**, 15.

Whitesides, G. M. and Grzybowski, B. (2002). Self-assembly at all scales. *Science* **295**, 2418–2421.

Zhou, J. and Rossi, J. J. (2014). Cell-type-specific, aptamer-functionalised agents for targeted disease therapy. *Molecular Therapy Nucleic Acids*, **3**(6), e169, 1–17.

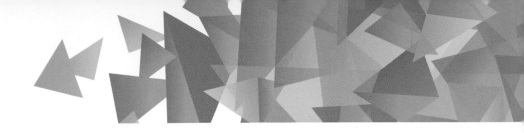

5 Analytical Methods in Bionanotechnology

Characterisation of nanomaterials, whether this refers to their physicochemical properties or their interactions with biomolecules and cells, requires a combination of analytical strategies. Before we explore some of the main instrumental methodologies for analysis of bionano constructs and devices, it is important to define the main questions we are trying to answer using analytical techniques (Figure 5.1).

Figure 5.1

Analytical techniques in bionanotechnology help us in characterisation of (bio)nano hybrids. They are used to decipher the physiochemical properties of materials and improve the understanding of their interactions with the environment.

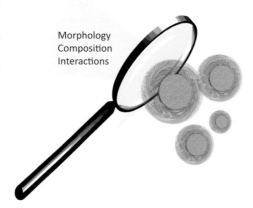

Morphology
Composition
Interactions

First, we would usually like to know – *what does the nanomaterial or nano hybrid look like?* What is its shape, size, crystallinity and stability? Are there any defects or signs of undesired aggregation? In short, we want to understand their morphology. We would also like to know – *what is the material made out of?* The reagents we use to make a particular material will be known to us, so we can make a prediction as to what we are producing, but for further applications we need to know the purity, composition of the core material and the functional groups or layers present on its surface. Finally, we need to know – *what are the properties of our material and how does it behave in different environments*? Are there any changes in hydration and aggregation? Are properties different when our hybrid nanomaterial is exposed to a range of temperature or pH? And, particularly important for design of nanotherapeutics explored in Chapter 9, what happens when our material is introduced to complex biological fluids such as blood or saliva? Materials used in nanomedicine need to fulfil stringent requirements, and they need to be well-characterised before they can be used to diagnose diseases or deliver drugs.

Describing bionano hybrids means putting together a puzzle using pieces of information obtained from different analytical techniques, some of which might be destructive to the sample, and others that are not but require advanced equipment and expert knowledge. As we will see throughout this chapter, whichever technique we use, it comes with its own set of advantages and disadvantages, and these need to be taken into account to prevent misinterpretation of data. We did not include nuclear magnetic resonance (NMR) or mass spectrometry in this description, which are standard techniques used to study of chemical structures and extensively covered elsewhere. Although these two strategies can be employed to assess the bionano hybrid structures, like other techniques described here, they cannot be used as standalone techniques, but always in combination with other strategies.

Characterisation of nanomaterials and nanostructures as well as biomolecules has been, to a large extent, based on existing characterisation strategies used to explore bulk materials. However, development of some analytical strategies such as high-resolution fluorescence microscopy or surface-enhanced Raman was directly driven by the need to explore nanosized features and surface properties of nanomaterials.

In this chapter we have grouped characterisation techniques broadly into those that can be used to explore the morphology of nanomaterials, those to assess the composition and surface properties, and those explored to study physiochemical properties and interactions.

5.1   Assessing the Morphology of Nanostructures

Broadly speaking morphology describes the shape, size and texture of the material. As we have seen already in earlier chapters, these properties are directly related to the unique features we find within different classes of nanomaterials. In quantum dots, size will determine fluorescent properties, in noble metals the specific wavelength of the surface plasmons depends on the size and the shape of the particle, and magnetic and catalytic properties of metal oxide nanomaterials very much depend on the presence of particular crystalline phases. Assessing the size and shape of material is usually a first step in **nanomaterial characterisation**. In fact, nanotechnology as a field advanced due to the developments in design of transmission and scanning electron microscopes (Back to Basics 5.1) and novel X-ray techniques such as small angle X-ray scattering (SAXS).

Back to Basics 5.1   A Short History of Electron Microscopy

When Robert Hooke (1635–1703) designed and described the first optical microscope in 1665, he noted that 'by the help of microscopes, there is nothing so small as to escape our inquiry; hence there is a new visible World discovered to the understanding' (Hooke, 1665). He was fascinated by the beauty of previously unseen things such as the intricate structure of plant (cork) cell walls.

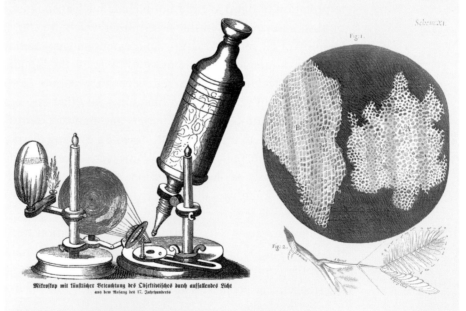

Hooke's microscope (left), and his illustration of the cork structure (right).
Source: Bettmann/Contributor/Getty Images (left); Robert Hooke, *Micrographia*, cork.
Published: 1665. Wellcome Library, London (right).

The structures Hooke observed reminded him of *cellulae*, the structures in honeycomb and *cella*, 'small chamber', the rooms inhabited by monks. Although Hooke described the cork as 'much like a Honey-comb ... these pores, or cells, were not deep but consisted of a great many little boxes', strictly speaking, what he observed were not cells, but rather dead cell walls. Robert Hooke went on to become one of the most important figures of modern science leaving his mark in the fields of mathematics and physics (Hooke's law), astronomy, science of time keeping, meteorology, palaeontology and biology.

Despite the huge advances enabled by optical microscopes, their resolution was limited to 200 nm due to the physics of light, and the best optical microscopes today can still only reach a magnification of $1500\times$.

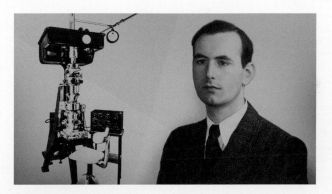

The first commercial electron microscopy and its designer Ernst Ruska.
Source: Wellcome Library, London.

This limitation of optical microscopy, together with the discovery and understanding of electrons, led to the development of electron microscopes. The theoretical groundwork for **electron microscopy** was laid by German scientists Ernst Ruska (1906–1988) and Max Knoll (1897–1969) in 1931. Ernst Ruska went on to build the first model in 1933, and the first commercial instrument was put on the market by Siemens in 1939.

The first scanning electron microscope debuted in 1942, but due to the complexity of the electronics needed to move the electron beam across the sample, it took more than 20 years to develop a commercial model, which was finally available in 1965.

5.1.1   Electron Beam

When a beam of high-energy electrons hits a sample, the electrons can get transmitted, scattered or used for production of X-rays (Figure 5.2). The interactions that lead to the transmission electrons are useful for thin samples (transmission electron microscopy), while bulk or thick samples would usually be probed using backscattered electrons (scanning electron microscopy). X-rays provide information on the chemical composition (see Section 5.2.1), while Auger electrons, which are applied within Auger electron spectroscopy, enable layer-by-layer profiling and qualitative analysis of solid surfaces (see Section 5.2.3).

Figure 5.2

What happens when an electron beam hits a sample? If the sample is thin enough, electrons can be transmitted through the sample. When bulk and thick samples are employed, electrons can get scattered, or transformed into Auger electrons or X-ray events. Only the most basic events are illustrated here.

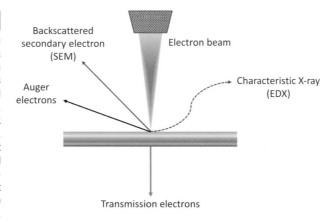

5.1.2 Transmission Electron Microscopy

Figure 5.3

Transmission electron microscope. Electrons are produced by an electron gun and condensed into a beam by a condenser, while the objective lens focuses the electrons after passing the sample. The projector lenses project the electrons onto a fluorescent screen, from which the image recording system produces the TEM micrograph (a). (b) Modern electron microscope (courtesy of Kobi Felton, Cambridge University) and (c) transmission electron micrograph of gold nanorods (courtesy of Lukas Stolzer, Karlsruhe Institute of Technology; Stolzer et al., 2014).

In **transmission electron microscopy** (TEM; Figure 5.3), electrons are produced by electron guns. In conventional electron guns, a positive electrical potential is applied to the anode, and the cathode, made of tungsten filament, is heated until a stream of electrons is produced. These electrons are then accelerated to 100 keV or higher (see In Numbers 5.1), and focused onto the thin specimen (less than 200 nm) by use of the electromagnetic condenser lens.

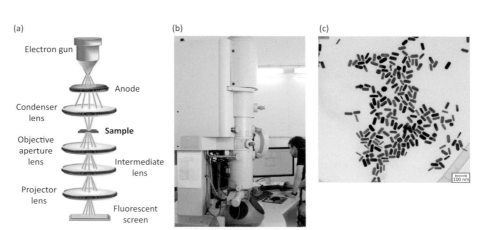

The condenser lens allows only electrons with a certain energy to pass through, so that all of the electrons hit the sample as a beam with a well-defined energy. The biggest advantage of TEM is the high magnification (up to 1 000 000 times), which is the result of the small electron wavelengths as given by the **de Broglie relationship**:

$$\lambda = \frac{h}{\sqrt{2mE}} = \frac{1.22}{\sqrt{E}}.$$ (5.1)

In Numbers 5.1 Electronvolts

Photon energy is commonly expressed in electronvolts, a unit corresponding to the energy acquired by a charge of a single electron that has been accelerated through a potential of one volt, and 1 electronvolt is equal to 1.602×10^{-19} J.

Calculate the energy of a 5.3 Å (1 Å = 0.1 nm) X-ray photon and express it in electronvolts (eV).

Solution

The photon energy equation is used:

$$E = h\nu = \frac{hc}{\lambda},$$

where h is Planck's constant, ν is the photon's frequency and c is the speed of light in a vacuum. So the energy is:

$$E = \frac{(6.63 \times 10^{-34}\,\text{Js})(3.00 \times 10^8\,\text{ms}^{-1})}{5.30 \times 10^{-10}\,\text{m}} = 3.75 \times 10^{-16}\,\text{J}$$

$$= 2340\,\text{eV}.$$

Particles originating from the 'solar wind', the burst of particles released from the Sun, can have energies up to 10^6 eV, while a typical red light emitting diode (LED) has energy of 1.7 eV.

In a transmission electron microscope, transmitted electrons are refocused using an objective lens system, and enlarged and projected onto the screen using projector lenses (Figure 5.3a). The higher the operating voltage of a TEM instrument (shown in Figure 5.3b), the greater is its resolution. High voltage TEM also produce electrons with greater sample penetration ability. In general, high-energy electrons interact less strongly with matter than lower energy electrons, allowing thicker samples to be explored, although ideally, the sample thickness should not exceed 100 nm. Samples are generally drop casted onto a hollow grid, usually made of copper, nickel or gold, which act as a support, while holes allow the electrons to pass through.

Usually, TEM is the first choice of analytical method to determine the shape, crystal structure and surface defects of various nanomaterials (Figure 5.3c). However, it is limited by the in-depth resolution and small analysed area, which might not be representative of the whole sample. In addition, the use of high-energy electrons is not suitable for the study of soft biomolecules and cells. This has been partially overcome by the use of **cryogenic electron microscopy** (cryo-EM), in which thin layers of frozen samples are used as substrates (Back to Basics 5.2).

Back to Basics 5.2 Cryogenic Electron Microscopy

Biomolecules are not compatible with the high energy electrons or vacuum conditions used to obtain TEM images, which cause the water that surrounds the biomolecules to evaporate and molecules themselves burn and get destroyed. To overcome these issues cryo-EM uses frozen samples, lower energy electrons and extensive data processing to obtain high resolutions of biomolecules. The technique has been particularly useful to decipher structures of proteins, which could not be crystallised (and those are many) or explore the interactions between different bioelements or even within the whole cell and tissues (cryo-EM tomography).

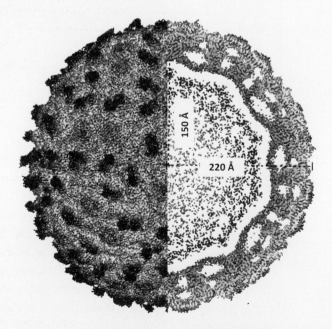

Source: Reprinted from Sevvana et al. (2018), with permission from Elsevier.

The first image of a protein using cryo-EM was obtained by Richard Henderson from the MRC Laboratory for Molecular Biology in Cambridge, UK in 1990. It was an image of a membrane protein bacteriorhodopsin and the resolution was as good as that achieved by X-ray analysis (0.3 nm). Image processing developed by Joachim Frank enabled reconstruction of 3D images from 2D projection, and James Dubochet introduced the water freezing strategy that minimised the interference from regular ice crystals. All three scientists were awarded the Nobel Prize in 2017 for their contributions for development of cryo-EM.

Meanwhile, a large number of proteins, cell organelles and even tissues were explored using this strategy, changing our understanding of cell biochemistry. Cryo-EM was particularly useful to study dynamic protein interactions as well as to provide 3D images of various pathogens in atomic resolution. For example, during the recent outbreak of Zika virus infections, scientists were able to obtain a 3D structure within a few months (shown here, Sevvana et al., 2018), enabling the search for a potential treatment, which was considered not possible only a few decades ago.

5.1.3 Scanning Electron Microscopy

Like TEM, **scanning electron microscopy** (SEM) uses a focused beam of electrons to probe the sample. However, SEM electrons have a much lower energy, usually a few hundred to 50 000 eV, and are rastered over the surface of the specimen using scanning coils. SEM images are produced by collecting **backscattered electrons** by a detector placed above the sample (Figure 5.4a and b), and as a result, scanning electron micrographs are particularly useful to assess the topology of the samples. The areas with different chemical composition will scatter differently providing distinct contrast information about the sample surface. In a mix of atoms, atoms of heavier elements generally scatter more electrons and will appear brighter. Using the differences in scattering but also a unique X-ray photon produced by each element, large areas of the sample can be imaged, providing information on morphology, topography, and composition (more on that in Section 5.2).

Unlike for TEM, the preparation of an SEM sample requires the deposition of the conductive layer, usually gold, on top of the specimen. The conductive layer aids the removal of the charges within the sample, which can affect the generation of backscattered electrons and result in blurred images. Due to the lower energy of the electron beams used, SEM has been extensively employed to study biological samples ranging from microorganisms (Figure 5.4c) to

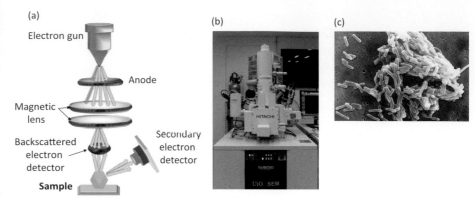

larger insects and plant samples. However, the use of the conductive coating also means that the samples cannot be reconstituted or reused after the measurement.

Electron microscopy has in many ways impacted material science and in particular, nanotechnology. Although it is irreplaceable for the study of shapes, sizes and elemental composition, TEM and SEM micrographs (Table 5.1) need to be complemented by other techniques, especially in the case of biological samples, which can be damaged by high-energy electrons. In particular, in the case of TEM, a careful analysis of larger areas of the samples is needed to obtain a statistic distribution of nanoparticle sizes over

Table 5.1 Comparison of TE and SE microscopy

TEM	SEM
• Transmitted electrons recorded • Determination of morphology, topology and composition • Thin samples needed (up to 100 nm) • Samples are drop cast onto a meshed grid • Energy of used electrons is 100 keV and higher • Information is obtained from a small area • Destructive to soft samples, but cryo-TEM can be used for exploration of biomaterials	• Backscattered and secondary electrons recorded • Determination of the shape, size and composition • Thick samples can be used • Samples need to be coated with a conductive layer, usually gold • Large areas of the sample can be explored

a larger area and in such a way, provide a more realistic image of size and shape distribution.

5.1.4 X-ray Diffraction

X-ray diffraction (XRD) – developed by father and son William (1862–1942) and Lawrence (1890–1971) Bragg in Cambridge in 1912 – is used to study crystallinity of nanomaterials and provide the crystal lattice parameters, and provide data on the presence of different crystalline phases.

In XRD, X-rays with wavelengths typically ranging from 0.7 to 2 Å generated by cathode ray tube are filtered and focused onto a crystalline sample, and then diffracted by its crystalline phases (Figure 5.5a). Diffraction follows the **Bragg law**, which states that:

$$n\lambda = 2d (\sin \theta), \tag{5.2}$$

where $n\lambda$ is the wavelength of the characteristic X-rays, d is the lattice interplanar spacing of the crystal and θ is the X-ray incidence angle or Bragg angle (Figure 5.5b).

Figure 5.5

Principle of X-ray diffraction. (a) The X-ray beam is focused onto a crystalline sample and diffracted by a crystal. (b) Diffraction follows Bragg's law which relates the wavelength of X-rays (λ) to interplanar distance d and X-ray incidence angle θ.

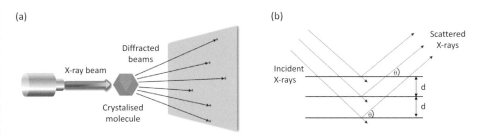

The intensity of diffracted X-rays is measured as a function of the diffraction angle 2θ and the orientation of the sample. A shift in the diffraction peak is used to calculate the change in d-spacing, which is the result of the change in the lattice constants used for crystal identification. Typically, the crystal is identified by comparison of d-spacings with standard reference patterns.

We have already seen that different crystal lattices might lead to different properties of nanomaterial, in particular in terms of surface ligand binding or photocatalytic activity (Chapter 1). X-ray technique provides information about the crystal phase, orientation and even dynamics of crystal changes under different conditions (see Section 5.1.5 and Table 5.2), and what is very important, it is non-destructive and does not require elaborate sample preparation.

However, one of the disadvantages of XRD, compared to, for example, electron diffraction (described in Section 5.1.2) is the low intensity of diffracted X-rays. This means that XRD usually requires a significant amount of sample, which is not always readily available when working with nanomaterials and their hybrids.

5.1.5 Small Angle X-ray Scattering

Strong diffraction peaks result from the constructive interference of scattered X-rays from an ordered array of atoms and molecules, but a lot of information can also be obtained from the angular distribution of scattered X-rays at small angles ($2\theta < 5°$, Figure 5.6a).

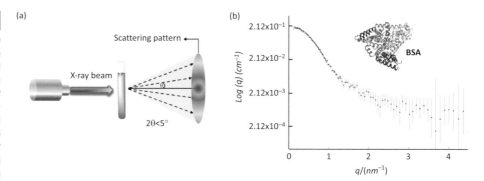

Figure 5.6

Principle of small angle X-ray scattering. (a) Sample of nanosized particle or molecule in solution can be directly studied by exploring X-rays scattered at small angles. (b) Typical SAXS curve is a plot of intensity (log scale) vs scattering angle represented as a scattering vector q. Shown here is a plot of bovine serum albumin protein adapted from SAXS Biological Data Bank (SASBDB) and Bucciarelli et al. (2018).

Small angle X-ray scattering (SAXS) occurs when X-rays hit samples with diameters ranging from 1 to 100 nm, which is ideal for nanomaterials and biomolecules. The principle was first explained by Andre Guinier (1911–2000) in 1939 although it was not until 1955 that the true potential of SAXS was demonstrated by studying metal alloys (Guinier, 1939 and Guinier and Fournet, 1955). In 1960, SAXS became a tool to study biological macromolecules, but the significant advancement was enabled by use of X-ray photon beams generated by particle accelerators known as **synchrotrons** in the 1970s. More than 60 synchrotrons are currently in use globally to study various physicochemical phenomena and act as radiation sources for methods such as SAXS and X-ray diffraction.

SAXS provides information on the size and shape of nanostructures, but also on their internal structure, density and porosity. Such information can be obtained regardless of whether the sample is crystalline or amorphous, which is particularly useful in the study of soft biomolecules such as proteins (Figure 5.6b) and DNA nanostructures. Unlike some other methods, SAXS provides information on the entire sample and complements the information obtained by, for example, electron microscopy. In addition, it also requires little sample preparation, and it can be used for study of biomolecules and nanoparticles in solution, for example, under physiological conditions.

A summary of the main properties that can be deciphered using X-ray strategies can be found in Table 5.2.

Table 5.2 Comparison of XRD and SAXS techniques

XRD	SAXS
• Phase identification and quantification	• Shape, size and crystallinity
• Crystal lattice parameters	• Internal structure
• Crystallinity	• Porosity
• Orientation	• Orientation
• Dynamic changes in crystallinity under different temperature or solvents	• Density
	• In-solution measurements

5.2 Composition and Surface Properties of Nanostructures

With the advancement of nanotechnology, it became important to obtain detailed information on the composition and the structure over larger areas but with an atomic resolution. Such a resolution enables the detection of small differences in elemental composition or presence of defects, both of which can dramatically impact the properties of nanomaterials. The crucial development which marked the beginning of nanotechnology as a research field was the design of the **scanning probe microscope (STM)** by Gerd Binning and his colleagues in 1982, and its use to obtain a topographic map of platinum metal (Binning et al., 1982). Four years later, the **first atomic force microscope (AFM)** was designed using the principles of STM (Binning et al., 1986). Both techniques made an immense impact on nanotechnology as a field, with AFM becoming an invaluable technique to study not only topology but also interactions of soft materials such as biomaterials and various bionano hybrids. Whereas **scanning probe microscopy** was a powerful strategy to obtain detailed information on topology, the elemental analysis of the nanomaterial core and surfaces can be done using either **electron spectroscopy**, which provides specific X-ray signatures with the help of an electron beam or with the help of **time of flight secondary ion mass spectrometry (TOF-SIMS)**, which has lately been applied to design 3D maps of biological and engineered tissues.

5.2.1   Energy Dispersive X-ray Analysis

Energy dispersive X-ray analysis (EDX) is an X-ray technique used to identify the elemental composition of samples and it is usually coupled with scanning or transmission electron microscopy (more on electron microscopy in Section 5.1). The impact of the electron beam on the sample produces X-rays specific to the elements present within that sample. All elements except hydrogen and helium produce characteristic X-rays, and their presence can be determined simultaneously. EDX can be used for quantitative analysis as the amount of X-rays emitted by each element present in a sample directly relates to the amount of that element.

EDX analysis can be used to determine the elemental composition of individual points and line scans (Figure 5.7) along the nanosized area, but also allows for the mapping of the lateral distribution of elements from the imaged area. It is a versatile, inexpensive and quantitative method for analysis of nanomaterials, but usually requires flat, polished and homogeneous samples, which is not always easily achieved.

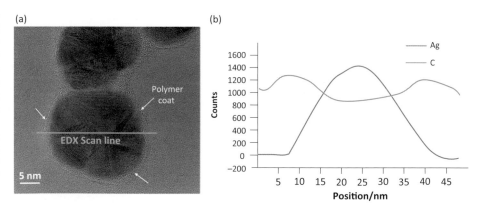

Figure 5.7

EDX analysis of polymer coated 30 nm silver nanoparticles. The elemental analysis across the line (marked orange in (a)) shows the distribution of silver (Ag) over 30 nm, and carbon distribution corresponding to the surrounding polymer carbons (b) (Stolzer et al., 2014).

5.2.2   X-ray Photoelectron Spectroscopy

X-ray photoelectron spectroscopy (XPS), also known as **electron spectroscopy for chemical analysis (ESCA)**, is based on recording the kinetic energy of photoelectrons (e^-) emitted when an incident beam of X-ray photons hits the sample S (Figure 5.8):

$$S + h\nu \rightarrow S^{+*} + e.$$

Figure 5.8

X-ray photoelectron spectroscopy. (a) Incident beam of X-ray photons results in ejection of a photoelectron, which is collected using a hemispheric electron acceptor connected to a detector. (b) Modern X-ray photoelectron spectrometer (Escalab Xi$^+$ XPS used with permission of Thermo Fischer Scientific).

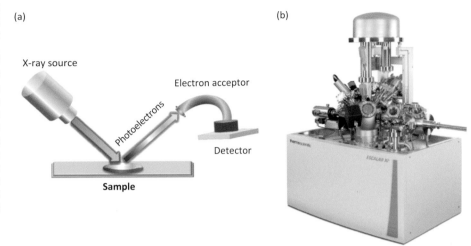

The kinetic energy of emitted photoelectron E_k is measured in an electron spectrometer and used to determine the binding energy of the electron E_b:

$$E_b = E_{hv} - E_k - w, \qquad (5.3)$$

where w is a factor related to a spectrometer, that corrects for the environment in which the electron is formed and measured.

The binding energy of the electron, E_b, is characteristic of the atom and the orbital from which the photoelectron is emitted. As a consequence, the elemental composition of the sample surface can be obtained, including the information on the oxidation states of a particular element. The depth of XPS analysis is limited to 10 nm. Although X-rays can penetrate deeper, photoelectrons generated in lower layers usually collide with the electrons in the upper layers without providing any useful data about the composition. In addition, XPS needs to be performed in an ultra-high vacuum environment and with pressures as low as 1.3×10^{-8} Pa to prevent the collision of high speed photoelectrons with gas molecules. For comparison, the atmospheric pressure is usually 1.0×10^5 Pa – reaching such low pressure requires specialised equipment.

A typical X-ray source of modern XPS spectrometers has a bandwidth of about 0.3 eV, and XPS is considered a non-destructive method due to the non-destructive nature of X-rays. Pioneered by the Swedish physicist Kai Siegbahn (1918–2007) in the late 1950s to early 1960s, XPS has been continuously improved (Siegbahn et al., 1967). Today it is used to extract quantitative information about organic, biological and inorganic coatings as well as contamination on nanoparticles, and to determine the oxidation states of various nanomaterials.

5.2.3   Auger Electron Spectroscopy

Auger electrons may be emitted when an electron from the outer energy level fills the inner vacancy produced by electron beam bombardment (Raman et al., 2011). These electrons were named after a French physicist Pierre Auger (1899–1993) who explained their origin in 1923, whereas the principle of **Auger electron spectroscopy (AES)** and its use to study chemical composition of surfaces was postulated by J. J. Lander in 1953 (Lander, 1953).

The kinetic energy of an Auger electron is equal to the difference between the energy released in relaxation of an excited ion ($E_b - E_b'$) and the energy required to remove the second electron from its orbital (E_b'):

$$E_k = (E_b - E_b') - E_b' = E_b - 2E_b', \qquad (5.4)$$

where E_b is the binding energy of non-excited electron, and E_b' is the energy of the excited electron pushed out of outer shell.

The intensity of Auger transition is characteristic of a particular element and all but light elements, hydrogen and helium can be detected by Auger electron spectroscopy. Auger peaks are independent of the input energy, which means that, unlike the photoelectrons generated in XPS, Auger spectroscopy does not require a single wavelength (monochromatic) source. The instrumental design is based on the same principles as XPS and the measurements require high-vacuum conditions. A summary comparison of XPS and AES techniques can be found in Table 5.3.

Table 5.3 Comparison of XPS and AES techniques

XPS	AES
• High vacuum	• High vacuum
• Dependent on the monochromatic X-ray beam	• Independent of the incident wavelength (no need for monochromatic source)
• Produced when X-ray hits the sample	• Produced when an electron beam hits the sample
• Depth of up to 10 nm	• High-resolution chemical composition and content
• Used for surface exploration	• Line scanning over large lengths
• Provides information on chemical composition and oxidation states	• Low–energy electrons penetrate to max 3 nm in depth
• Non-destructive	

Auger signals can be quantified to provide information on the surface composition in a surface resolution often lower than 10 nm and a depth of a few nanometres. This is particularly useful to obtain the chemical composition profile of very small nanostructures (Figure 5.9) and expose any defects not easily seen by other strategies. The incident beam can also move across the surface in a straight line of 100 mm and more, to provide information on oxidation states or elemental composition as a function of distance along a line.

Figure 5.9

Chemical composition maps obtained by Auger electron spectroscopy. (a) SEM micrography of nanocone. Map of nitrogen (b) and (c) iron distribution. Overlay of both maps shows the tip composed of Fe (red in d). Adapted from Raman et al. (2011). © Microscopy Society of America 2011/ Cambridge University Press.

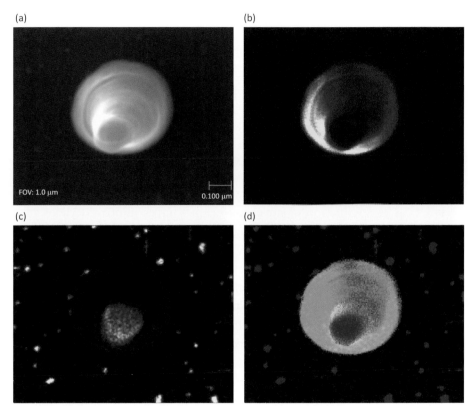

5.2.4   Time of Flight Secondary Ion Mass Spectrometry

Although we are not going into the details of mass spectrometry, the commonly used strategy for chemical analysis, we will briefly mention a subgroup of mass spectroscopy based on the generation and detection of secondary ions from the target surface. Secondary ions can be produced by the bombardment of the target surface with a primary ion source (Figure 5.10), usually a bismuth ion source. Extracted secondary ions provide distinct signature of the material, and can be used to make maps of the surface, or obtain an in-depth profile of a particular structure. Elemental composition can be achieved with 1 nm depth resolution within 3D samples. In-depth studies are possible due to the layer peeling induced by the primary ion beam, so that layer-by-layer maps can be obtained.

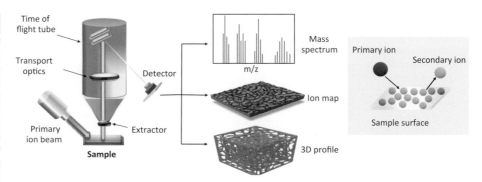

Figure 5.10

Components of time of flight secondary ion mass spectrometry (TOF-SIMS). TOF-SIMS provides either mass spectra, ion maps of the surfaces or full 3D profile of the sample. It uses the generation of secondary ions after the sample surface is bombarded with the primary ion beam.

Initially developed in the 1960s (Benninghoven, 1969), TOF-SIMS was quickly adopted by polymer science and continuously improved. The introduction of novel ion beam sources improved yields of generated secondary ions resulting in significantly enhanced resolution and less sample damage. Today, TOF-SIMS is used to obtain 3D profile of biological samples such as tissues and cells, but also elemental profile of nanocomposites (see Chapter 9) and bionano hybrids.

Unlike electron microscopy or EDX, TOF-SIMS can detect both heavy and light ions and it can distinguish between different isotopes. It can also be used to measure specimens of several tens of millimetres in size with nanoscale resolution, and it does not require particular sample preparation. Due to the resolution and ease of use, it is particularly interesting to study materials used for tissue engineering (see Chapter 9), providing nanoscale information on composition and elemental distribution over larger areas.

5.2.5   Scanning Tunnelling Microscopy

Scanning tunnelling microscopy (STM) exploits the principle of **electron tunnelling**. When two surfaces (metal or semiconductor) are separated by an insulator, electrons cannot transfer from one surface to another since there is an energy barrier between them. However, if there is a voltage applied between two surfaces, the shape of the barrier changes. As a consequence, the electrons can move across the barrier by tunnelling, producing a low tunnelling current.

In STM a conductive tip moves back and forth over a planar surface in very small intervals (Figure 5.11a). The height of the tip is continuously adjusted to keep the tunnelling current constant. The position of the tip at the given interval is then used to construct a topographic map of the surface. One of the first STM images was the topographic map of the silicon surface showing the arrangement of the individual atoms (Figure 5.11b).

In the case of STM, the tip tunnelling current I_t can be given as

$$I_t = Ve^{-Cd}, \tag{5.5}$$

where V is the voltage between the conductors, C is a constant that is characteristic for the composition of the conductors and d is the spacing between the lowest atom of the tip and the highest atom on the sample.

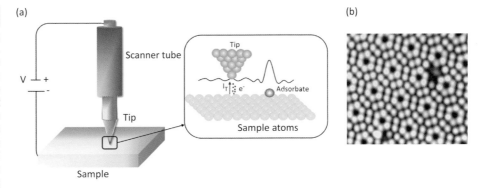

Figure 5.11

Scanning tunnelling microscopy.
(a) A conductive tip moves back and forth over a surface. The tunnelling current between two conductive surfaces is produced as a consequence of the applied voltage and small distances between surfaces. (b) By keeping the current constant, atomic resolution of the surfaces can be obtained such as shown for silicon surface.
Courtesy of Unisoku Co, Ltd.

As can be seen from Equation 5.5, tunnelling current decreases exponentially with the distance between the tip and the sample, and STM images can be obtained only for very small, nanometre, distances. Typically, when the distance between the tip and the surface is 0.2–0.6 nm, tunnelling current of 0.1–10 nA will be generated. The best images are obtained when the tip contains a single atom at the top, which can be relatively easily achieved by cutting platinum/iridium wires or by etching of tungsten metal. Blunt tips reduce STM resolution by inducing electron tunnelling to occur across a wider spatial range. Typical scanning resolution is around 0.01 nm along the x-axis and 0.002 nm in the z-direction, which amounts to a true atomic resolution.

Initially developed and used as an imaging technique, STM has been employed to study electronic properties of the surface, measure lifetime of surface electrons and even assemble atoms on demand (Eigler and Schweizer, 1990).

Although it provides high-resolution images, STM requires electrically conductive surfaces since it depends on the tunnelling current directly related to the bias voltage between conductive surface and tip. It is also very sensitive to the surface properties and environmental conditions. To address these challenges, **atomic force microscopy (AFM)** was developed in 1986 using the principle of STM, but allowing for the measurements on both the conducting and insulating surfaces.

5.2.6 Atomic Force Microscopy

In AFM, a **force sensitive cantilever** probe with an nanoscale tip is scanned over a surface (Figure 5.12). The force between the probe and the surface causes very small upward and downward deflections of the tip. These deflections are recorded as deflections of the laser beam pointed towards the cantilever (Figure 5.12). Unlike STM, which is based on a continuous readjustment of the tip to maintain a constant tunnelling current, AFM measures very small upward and downward deflections of the tip while maintaining the constant force of the contact. AFM can probe the sample in xy and z directions, allowing for the measurements of the height (for example, of the particles) or depth (if there are indentations or holes on the surface). Although initially AFM was used to image hard surfaces in air or vacuum, it works also in liquids, which is particularly well-suited to image biological samples.

Figure 5.12

Atomic force microscopy. A cantilever with a nanosized tip is moved over the sample keeping the constant force between the sample and the tip. Cantilever movements are recorded as deflections of the laser beam projected onto the cantilever. This work is licensed under a CC-BY-SA-3.0 licence.

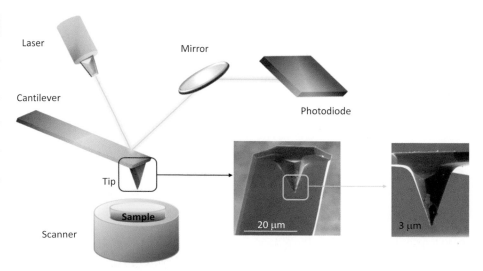

The cantilever and the tips are usually made of silicon, or silicon nitride which is more flexible. Combination of both materials results in excellent cantilevers and superior resolution. The shape and size of the tip influences the resolution of the image, and high-resolution cantilevers are available that have tips with 1 nm radius.

The preparation of an AFM sample is very simple: there is no cutting, no coating, no drying, no fixation needed. The only requirement is the use of a regular and reproducibly flat surface onto which the samples are deposited. Most commonly used AFM surfaces are made of the silica-based mineral **mica** with general formula $X_2Y_{4-6}Z_8O_{20}(OH, F)_4$, in which X are K, Na, Ca, Y are Al, Mg, Fe and Z is Si.

There are also several modes of measurements, which can be used depending on the nature of the sample. A **contact mode**, in which a physical contact between the surface and the tip occurs, allows for high resolution but it can cause damage to the soft tissue and result in image artefacts. A **non-contact mode** is slower, but it does not cause damage, although resolution usually suffers. As a compromise, a **tapping mode** can also be employed based on the intermittent and short contact between the sample and the tip, resulting in high resolution and minimal damage to the sample.

Besides being useful for imaging, AFM can be used to study the force of intramolecular interactions (Burnham et al., 1990), adhesive forces and even the strength and nature of chemical bonds (Research Report 5.1), and it could easily be grouped into a family of techniques used to explore physiochemical properties of nanostructures.

Research Report 5.1   Chemical Bond Formation Explored by AFM

AFM has extensively been used in bionanotechnology to study DNA nanostructures (see Chapter 6), conformational changes of proteins and to determine interactive force between various molecular species or surface-binding force.

To study the interactive force, the cantilever generally needs to be modified with the species of interest. For example a cantilever modified with the protein fibrinogen was used to probe the health of red blood cells. Interaction of this protein with healthy red blood cells differs from its interaction with the diseased or damaged cells. By measuring the interactive force, detection of early signs of cardiovascular diseases can be achieved (Guedes et al., 2016).

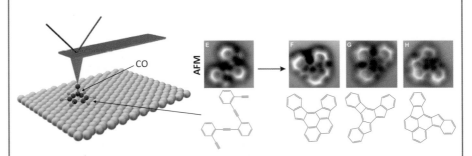

Source: de Oyteza et al. (2013). Reprinted with permission from AAAS.

One of the most exciting applications of the AFM technique is the study of chemical bonds. One such study performed in 2013 resulted in the 'photographs' of the bond formation (de Oteyza et al., 2013). This has been achieved by designing an atomic needle by depositing a single carbon monoxide molecule onto the tip of a cantilever. Such an atomic tip can be deflected when moving over the molecule, much as the ordinary AFM tip deflects when it encounters different topographic features on the surface. This requires a very smooth surface, and a planar silver surface was prepared onto which a molecule from a family of enediyne was deposited. Enediynes can undergo cyclisation when heated, which results in several products. An image of each of these products was obtained by heating the reagent molecule and moving the AFM tip over the structures, resulting in real-time image of newly formed products, which is an incredible feat of the modern microscopy.

In the past decade AFM has extensively been applied to study protein interaction or adhesion, DNA and protein imaging (Figure 5.13) and conductive and thermal analysis of surfaces. For example, in conductive AFM (C-AFM) a bias voltage of the tip is discharged on the sample generating a tunnelling current. Measurement of this current provides the conductivity profile of the surface (Avila and Bushan, 2010), resulting in conductivity maps with resolution down to 1 nm. A summary comparison of STM and AFM techniques can be found in Table 5.4.

Table 5.4 Comparison of scanning probe techniques

STM	AFM
• Conductive surface and tip needed • Tunnelling current measured, which depends on distance between the surface and the tip • Size of the tip determines resolution • Atomic resolution achieved • Information on topology and electronic properties • Can be employed to move around atoms	• Can be used for non-conductive surfaces • Based on force between the tip and the sample • Can be used for soft samples and measured in liquid • Atomic resolution can be achieved • The resolution depends on the size of the tip • Can be used to obtain conductive and thermal profile, adhesive force and strength of molecular interaction

Figure 5.13

AFM images of protein DNA complex. DNA (long string) is wrapped around 12 histone proteins (white spheres). Prepared by Dr Joyce Ratti, University of Cambridge. Image courtesy of Dr Ioanna Mela, University of Cambridge.

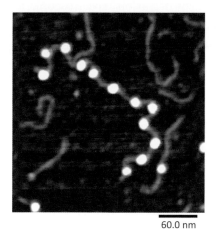 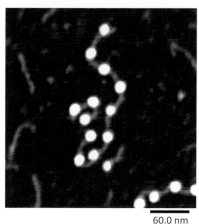

60.0 nm   60.0 nm

2.5 nm

Height indicator

5.3   Exploring Physiochemical Properties on the Nanoscale

Physicochemical properties might be defined as physical properties, solvation properties related to interactions with different media, and molecular attributes that define the reactivity or unique character of nanomaterials and hybrids. **Atomic force microscopy**, initially developed to study topology of surfaces, has quickly become a useful tool also to explore the forces and interactions between different species deposited on the surface. **Molecular and vibrational spectroscopy** provide information on reactive groups present within the nanostructure, explore the interaction with light, changes in fluorescence properties and the behaviour of surface plasmons. All of these changes are closely linked to the changes in the structure and surface of nanomaterials, and very important for exploration of interactions with various species in their environment, in particular those used in medicine (see Chapter 9). Interactions of nanomaterials with biomolecules largely depend on the hydrophilicity, hydrodynamic radius and surface charges of the interacting species, which can be determined by **dynamic light scattering** and **zeta potential measurements**.

Techniques for characterisation of physiochemical properties of materials are many, but they need to be used in combination with other strategies to provide a fuller profile of the studied material.

5.3.1   Molecular Spectroscopy

When light interacts with matter, it can get reflected, scattered, transmitted or absorbed. All of these events can provide useful information and have been exploited for the development of various spectroscopic analytical techniques. Although, in general terms, **spectroscopy** is a field that deals with the interaction of various types of irradiation with matter, within this section we will explore techniques concerned with electromagnetic spectrum covering the UV (~100–380 nm), visible (~380–740 nm) and IR (~740 nm to 1 mm) range, which have been most widely used in bionanotechnology. We will not explore atomic spectroscopy, which deals with the interaction of photons and electrons within an isolated atom, but rather **molecular spectroscopy** that results in more complex spectra and provides information on the molecular structure and bond strength.

To explain different interactions of an incoming photon of a particular wavelength with molecular species, spectroscopist constructed energy diagrams often referred to as **Jablonski diagrams** which illustrate electronic (energy) states of a molecule and transitions between them (Back to Basics 5.3). Jablonski diagrams are a useful tool for describing the processes of light absorption and emission in terms of transitions between the energy and vibrational levels within a molecule. The diagrams were named after Polish physicist Alexander Jablonski (1898–1980), who is regarded as a father of fluorescence spectroscopy. However, the diagrams should more precisely be referred as **Perrin–Jablonski** diagrams, due to the large contributions to the theory of fluorescence made by French physicists, father and son Jaen Baptiste (1870–1942) and Francis (1901–1992) Perrin. Jean Perrin is considered to be the first person to use a molecular energy level diagram to illustrate the absorption and emission of light.

Back to Basics 5.3   The Jablonski Diagram Explained

In a Jablonski diagram, energy levels are shown as bold black lines. Thin lines in between energy levels represent vibrational levels of each electronic state and are often denoted as v_n (n representing any number from 0 onwards). The ground energy level is known as S_0 (S stemming from singlet state referring to a total spin angular momentum equal to zero). S_1 is the first excited singlet state and there are S_n of these. T_1 denotes first excited triplet state (triplet means that the total angular momentum is equal to one).

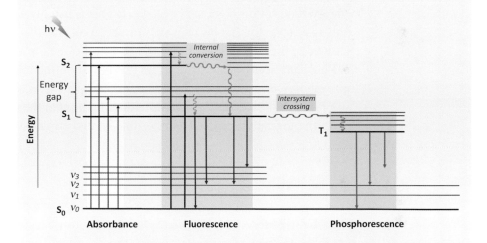

Absorbance (black arrows): At room temperature, the majority of molecules are in the lowest vibrational level (v_0) of the ground energy level (S_0). When light is absorbed the energy of the photon is converted into internal energy of the molecule. Absorption spectrum will depend on the type of molecule. For example, DNA strands absorb strongly in the UV region (260 nm), haem proteins in both the UV and visible region (~405 nm), and 15 nm spheric gold nanoparticles in the visible (~520 nm).

Vibrational relaxation (wiggly yellow arrows): After absorption, the molecule is promoted to an excited state, but it will eventually return to the lowest vibrational level within the state. This is achieved by the dissipation of energy through a process of vibrational relaxation within the same energy level.

Internal conversion (wiggly yellow arrows): Vibrational relaxation happens from higher to lower vibrational level from one to another energy level of the same spin ($S_2 \rightarrow S_1$, $S_3 \rightarrow S_2$, the energy gap between S_1 and S_0 is usually too big so that the process is too slow and competes with other processes).

Fluorescence (red arrows): After light is absorbed, rapid vibrational relaxation and internal conversion in some molecules might lead to fluorescence. Fluorescence emission usually occurs from the lowest vibrational level of the excited state (i.e. v_0 of S_1 to vibrational levels of the ground state S_0). Fluorescence has lower energy than the absorbed light, and this will result in an emitted light of longer wavelengths. For example, green fluorescent protein absorbs 395 nm light and emits green fluorescence at 509 nm.

Intersystem crossing (wiggly blue arrow): A non-radiative transition can occur between the vibration levels of the same energy but belonging to the energy states of different spin ($S_1 \rightarrow T_1$). This is usually a forbidden process and it is too slow to be relevant for the majority of organic molecules. However, it can be enhanced by the addition of heavy atoms.

Phosphorescence (blue arrow): As it is based on the intersystem crossing, phosphorescence is usually very slow and happens over longer periods. It is similar to fluorescence, the only difference being that the transition happens from the lowest vibrational level of the excited triplet state, instead of the singlet.

5.3.2   Ultraviolet–Visible Spectroscopy

When light is absorbed, the energy of the photon can be used to excite the absorbing molecular species from ground S_0 into a higher energy states S_n (Back to Basics 5.3). Almost instantaneously the excited species releases its absorbed energy and relaxes to the ground state by transferring the excess energy to other molecules in the form of thermal energy, which is so small that it is virtually undetectable. The process of absorption and relaxation occurs continuously as long as the species is irradiated by light.

Absorbance (A) is given by:

$$A = - \log_{10} \left(\frac{I_s - I_b}{I_r - I_b} \right), \tag{5.6}$$

where I_s is the intensity of light irradiated from a sample, I_b is the background intensity and I_r is the reference intensity.

Absorbance depends on the molecular structure of the species as well as its concentration and this relationship is defined by **Lambert–Beer's law**:

$$A = \varepsilon b c, \tag{5.7}$$

where ε is an extinction coefficient constant for a particular species, b is the length of the path through which the light is passing, and c is the concentration of the species within the sample.

In ultraviolet–visible (UV–Vis)spectroscopy, a continuous light source is used such that the power does not change sharply over a range of wavelengths. This can be achieved by employing deuterium or tungsten halogen lamps. Absorbance spectra are obtained by placing the sample into a sample holder known as a **cuvette** (Figure 5.14a). Quartz and fused silica cuvettes are required when working in the UV region as the glass absorbs strongly at wavelengths less than 350 nm. Silicate glass and disposable plastic cuvettes can be employed for the 350 to 1000 nm range. The most common length for the cuvette is 1 cm, corresponding to the path length b equal to 1. The quality of absorbance data depends a lot on the quality of the used cuvettes; any impurities will impact the measurements and should be avoided. UV–Vis spectroscopy is a quick method for identification of molecular family and determination of the concentration is easily performed using an affordable UV–Vis spectrometer (Figure 5.14b).

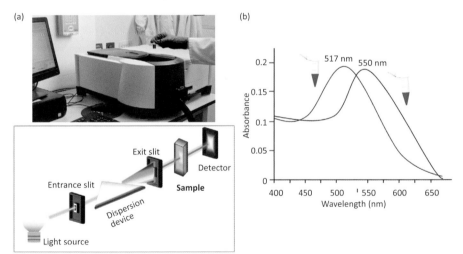

Figure 5.14

UV–Vis spectroscopy. A continuum source is used to irradiate the sample placed in a cuvette. Absorbed light is recorded with the help of a spectrometer. Shown here is a single-beam instrument. Modern UV–Vis spectrometers (a) are often used to determine the concentration of plasmonic nanoparticles (b) and other absorbing nanospecies.

The study of plasmonic nanoparticles such as gold has benefitted largely from UV–Vis spectroscopy (Haiss et al., 2007). In the case of plasmonic nanoparticles, the collective vibrations of an electron cloud (Back to Basics 1.2, Chapter 1) can strongly interact with electromagnetic radiation resulting in unique optical properties such as absorbance in the visible region. Moreover, the position of the peak maximum depends strongly on the size and the shape of the nanoparticles (Figure 5.14b), making UV–Vis spectroscopy a valuable tool for determination of their shape, size and concentration (In Numbers 5.2).

In Numbers 5.2 Determining the Concentration of Functionalised Silver Nanoparticles

Calculate the concentration of the streptavidin-coated silver nanoparticles (15 nm) using the absorbance at 450 nm $A_{450} = 2.0$ and the extinction coefficient, $\varepsilon(\text{Ag NPs}) = 4.5 \times 10^8\,\text{M}^{-1}\,\text{cm}^{-1}$.

Solution

Using Lambert–Beer's law and the path length of 1 cm:

$$c = \frac{A}{b\varepsilon} = \frac{2.0}{4.5 \times 10^8\,\text{M}^{-1}} = 4.4 \times 10^{-9}\,\text{M} = 4.4\,\text{nM}.$$

Due to their extensive use, the extinction coefficients for spherical gold and silver nanoparticles of different sizes have been determined and can be found in reference tables. This eases the determination of the concentration, which is particularly important for any biomedical applications of such materials as well as for biofunctionalisation.

5.3.3 Fluorescence: Spectroscopy and Microscopy

When light is absorbed, the energy of the photon is transferred to the molecule (Back to Basics 5.3). If the absorbed photon's energy is greater than the energy gap, transition between S_0 and S_n (usually S_1 or S_2) level will occur resulting in an excited state, which ultimately relaxes back into an equilibrium ground state. The time needed to excite the molecule from the ground to the excited state is very short and measured in femtoseconds (10^{-15} s), whereas fluorescence emission usually takes 10^{-10} to 10^{-7} s. Due to the relaxation processes taking place before the fluorescence emission, the energy of emission is lower than absorption leading to longer wavelengths of emitted light (Figure 5.15a). It is also possible for two photons with half the energy to act jointly and match the energy required for the transition of electron to an excited energy level. Such is the principle of the **two-photon excitation** and **two-photon fluorescence** (Figure 5.15b). Since the absorption process is very fast (10^{-15} s), only high-intensity light such as produced by **lasers** (Back to Basics 5.4) provides sufficient probability for multiple low-energy photons to be in the same place at nearly the same time to provide enough energy for the two-photon process.

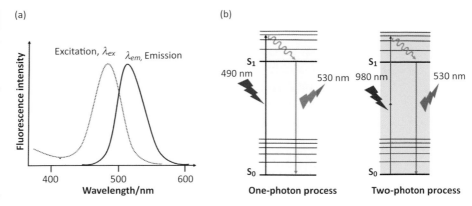

The probability that a fluorophore (a fluorescent compound) will absorb a
photon is contained within its molar **extinction coefficient** ε. The higher the
value of ε, the more efficient will be the absorption of light. Small organic
fluorophores have ε values from around $25\,000$ to $200\,000\,\mathrm{M}^{-1}\,\mathrm{cm}^{-1}$
(Figure 5.16a). For comparison, enhanced GFP (EGFP; Chapter 3) often
used for protein labelling has a value of approximately $60\,000\,\mathrm{M}^{-1}\,\mathrm{cm}^{-1}$.
Organic fluorophores such as fluorescein or AlexaFluor^{TM} dyes are characterised by aromatic and heterocyclic structural elements (Figure 5.16a). Other
fluorophores developed and successfully used for fluorescence imaging belong
to the classes of fluorescent proteins (Figure 5.16b; Chapter 3) or fluorescent
nanoparticles such as quantum dots (Figure 5.16c) or carbon nanodiamonds
(Chapter 2).

(a)

AlexaFluor^{TM} 555
$\lambda_{ex} = 555\ \mathrm{nm}$
$\lambda_{em} = 580\ \mathrm{nm}$

Fluorescein
$\lambda_{ex} = 490\ \mathrm{nm}$
$\lambda_{em} = 520\ \mathrm{nm}$

(b)

Green fluorescent protein (GFP)
$\lambda_{ex} = 490\ \mathrm{nm}$
$\lambda_{em} = 520\ \mathrm{nm}$

(c)

$\lambda_{ex} = 535\ \mathrm{nm}$

$\lambda_{ex} = 560\ \mathrm{nm}$

$\lambda_{ex} = 585\ \mathrm{nm}$

$\lambda_{ex} = 640\ \mathrm{nm}$

Quantum dots
$\lambda_{ex} = 360\ \mathrm{nm}$

The quality of fluorophore is usually assessed by its **quantum yield (QY)**, which is a measure of the total light emission over the entire fluorescence spectral range. When very intense light sources such as lasers are used, quantum yield provides an accurate measure of the maximum intensity that can be obtained from a fluorophore. Fluorophores with QY closer to 1 will be more suitable for fluorescence imaging. For example, the widely used fluorescein dye has a QY of 0.9, while GFP has 0.8.

In bionanotechnology, fluorescence is widely used to characterise different materials, decipher biochemical events with the help of biosensors (see Chapter 8) and aid cell imaging.

Fluorescence imaging is typically done using **fluorescence microscopy**, which can measure the distribution of fluorophores within a particular volume by imaging their emission. Such an ability is particularly useful for studying intracellular components and interactions between biomolecules. The only requirement is that the studied biomolecules are fluorescent, which, with notable exceptions of fluorescent proteins, is often not the case. As a consequence, to enable imaging, biostructures have to be labelled with fluorescent species (Figure 5.16) either through a genetic fusion, i.e. with fluorescent proteins (Chapter 3), or by covalent bond formation.

The first fluorescence microscope was constructed by Oscar Heimstädt (1879–1944) in 1911 and used for imaging of bacteria employing a UV light source and autofluorescence. Heimstädt was not sure about the potential of the fluorescent microscopy and wrote: 'If and to what degree, fluorescence microscopy will widen the possibilities of microscopic imaging only future will show' (Rusk, 2009).

Significant advances in terms of the resolution were made after the introduction of fluorescence compounds, named fluorochromes by Max Haitinger (1868–1946). Using fluorescent dyes he stained biological samples, significantly improving the resolution. Incident light similar to that found in modern fluorescent microscopes was first employed in 1929 by Philip Ellinger (1887–1952) and August Hirt (1898–1945) to image kidney and liver tissue in live rodents injected with fluorescein. In early 1940 fluorescent labelling with antibodies was developed, and since the early 1990s fluorescent proteins to prepare fusions with proteins of interest.

A fluorescence microscope is in many ways similar to the traditional optical microscope, differing only in the light source and the complexity of the filter-objective set-up (Figure 5.17a). High-intensity light sources such as lasers, high-power light-emitting diodes (LEDs) or xenon or mercury arc lamps are commonly used. A set of filters is employed to tune the excitation and emission wavelengths, and the dichroic filter directs the excitation light

The term laser is an acronym for light amplification by stimulated emission of radiation.

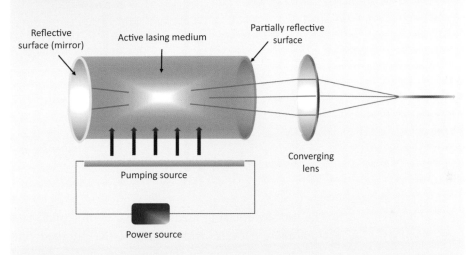

The main components of a laser are an **active lasing medium** with required energy level distribution, a **pumping source** connected to a power supply, and a **resonator** composed of a set of mirrors, which can move the radiation produced by the lasing action back and forth through the medium numerous times. The first laser, described by Theodore Maiman (1927–2007) in 1960, contained ruby as a lasing medium (Maiman, 1960). Since then semiconductors, solutions of organic dyes or gases such as argon or krypton have been used as lasing media. Pumping can be achieved by radiation from an external source, by application of electrical current or by an electrical discharge.

In short, lasers are devices that amplify the photon production of the excited atoms. This is achieved through a sequence of absorption, relaxation and emission processes. In a **four-level laser** shown below, four energy levels are involved in the amplification process. A widely used four-level laser is **Nd:YAG** (neodymium-doped yttrium aluminum garnet crystal), often used in fluorescence microscopy.

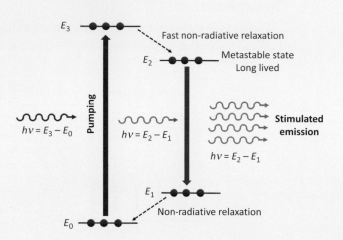

The four-level lasing medium consists of ground energy (E_0) and three excited energy levels. Absorption of the pumped photon results in the excitation of electrons to the higher excited level (E_3). Due to the high instability of this state, fast non-radiative relaxation causes electrons to drop into a long-lived metastable state E_2. Electrons from a metastable state are forced to return to the ground state by the interaction of an incoming photon with the energy corresponding to the energy gap between E_2 and E_1. A photon is produced as the electron relaxes from E_2 to E_1 and eventually to E_0 state, ultimately resulting in the overall production of two photons. Such a process is known as the **stimulated emission**. It is an artificial process in which a photon is used to force an electron to get back to the ground energy level while releasing an additional photon. As a result, two photons are emitted, an incident photon and the photon released when the electron moves to the ground energy level. Multi-level energy systems are used in lasers to achieve **population inversion**. This means that the higher number of electrons is present in the excited energy level (for example, E_2) than the ground energy level (E_0), which is, of course, an equilibrium state and favoured under normal conditions.

Ultimately, the laser light is:

Monochromatic: it contains photons of the same wavelength.
Coherent: the photons are in phase in space and time, unlike those from ordinary light sources such as lamps.

Directional: all photons travel in the
   same direction.
Collimated: it has a narrow beam width.

Laser beams can travel over
long distances without
significant change in their width.

High power: lasers with power up to 10^{12} W have been produced (Fujioka,
   2012). A laser pointer has the power of approximately 1 mW.

towards the sample and the emission towards the detector. The majority of
the fluorescence microscopes (Figure 5.17b) used to study biological samples
are **epi-microscopes** in which both the excitation and the observation of the
fluorescence occur above the sample. The most common microscope found in
imaging laboratories is a **confocal fluorescence microscope**, which contains a
pinhole in front of the detector to block any out-of-focus light, resulting in
improved 3D resolution (Combs, 2010).

Figure 5.17

Fluorescence
microscope. (a) High-
intensity light source is
passed through an
excitation filter to achieve
wavelengths suitable for
the excitation of a
fluorescent sample. The
emitted light is passed
through a dichroic mirror
and emission filter and
collected in the detector.
(b) Commercial confocal
fluorescence
microscope, in which a
pinhole in front of the
detector blocks out any
out-of-focus light
(photo by Kobi Felton,
University of Cambridge).

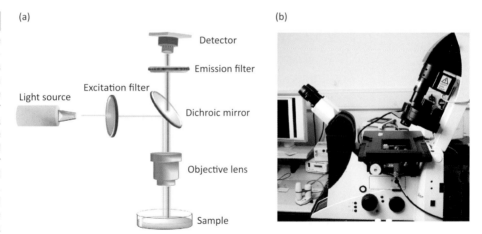

(a)

(b)

Detector

Emission filter

Excitation filter

Light source

Dichroic mirror

Objective lens

Sample

Compared to other imaging techniques such as electron microscopy, conventional fluorescence microscopy is limited by relatively low spatial resolution due to the diffraction of light. The diffraction limit of 200–300 nm in a
lateral direction and 500–700 nm in the axial direction is much larger than
some of the cellular components and biomolecules. This limitation was for
long thought to be insurmountable and directed by the basic properties of
light. However, in 1994 the diffraction limit was overcome and the first **super-
resolution fluorescence microscope** (Hell and Wichmann, 1994) known as

stimulated-emission depletion (STED) fluorescence microscopy was developed (Back to Basics 5.5). Different types of super-resolution microscopies followed and these developments allowed for the imaging of the intricate cellular structure in unprecedented detail (Figure 5.18).

Figure 5.18

Liver cell imaged by super-resolution fluorescent microscopy. Structured illumination microscopy (SIM) image of a live liver cell THLE-2 stained with the dye tetramethylrhodamine methyl ester (TMRM, red) specific to mitochondria and lysosome vesicles (SiR-lysosome, green). Courtesy of Meng Lu (Kaminski group), University of Cambridge.

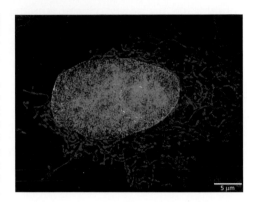

5 μm

Back to Basics 5.5   Types of Fluorescence Microscopy

Two classes of fluorescence microscopy can be distinguished based on the resolution they can achieve: diffraction-limited microscopy and super-resolution microscopy.

Diffraction-limited microscopy provides images which are within the diffraction limit of 200–300 nm in a lateral direction, and 500–700 nm in the axial direction.

Confocal microscopy	The first type of fluorescence microscopy that was developed and is still in use today. A typical setup is shown in Figure 5.17b.
Spinning disk microscopy	Spread laser beam is passed through a rotating disc holding an array of micro lenses so that many spots in the biological specimen can be illuminated.
4 pi microscopy	A spherical focal point can be achieved using a combination of lenses resulting in improved resolution.

Two-photon excitation microscopy

Photons of lower energy (longer wavelengths, Figure 5.16b) are used for excitation resulting in less photobleaching and deeper tissue penetration.

Total internal reflection fluorescence (TIRF) microscopy

Based on total internal reflection of light as it moves from a transparent medium of high refractivity (glass) to low refractivity (water). It can be used only to excite fluorophores in about 150 nm distance from the surface.

Selective plane illumination (SPIM) microscopy

Cylindrical lens is used to focus an incoming exciting light only on the focal plane, resulting in less photobleaching and phototoxicity.

Super-resolution microscopy was developed in the 1990s and enables imaging of subcellular compartments with high resolution and even the visualisation of single molecule events.

Stimulated emission depletion (STED) microscopy

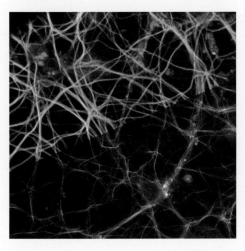

Two laser beams are employed, one to excite the fluorophores and the other to create a doughnut shape pattern, in which illuminated fluorophores are activated but the core of the doughnut remains unaffected. In such a way, fluorescence detection is reduced to an area smaller than the diffraction-limited spot, which results in dramatically improved resolution. STED can provide images in thick samples, and lateral resolution of 60 nm was achieved for brain slices at depth up to 120 μm. The image shown here is of

	neurons with stained Tau proteins (courtesy of Oliver Vanderporten and Colin Hockings, University of Cambridge).
Stochastic optical reconstruction microscopy (STORM)	Image is constructed from highly localised fluorophores that are switched on and off. Resolution of 10–50 nm can be achieved enabling single molecule localisation.
Photoactivated localisation microscopy (PALM)	Similar in principle to STORM, it uses fluorescent photoactivable proteins, which are first activated by a laser pulse, and then bleached in cycles. This enables high precision localisation of studied events, allowing a single molecule to be tracked within a cell.

The disadvantage of both STORM and PALM is the difficulty to obtain temporally resolved images, meaning that imaging of dynamic processes in live cells is difficult.

Structured illumination microscopy (SIM)	SIM provides high-resolution images over many time points and it is a method of choice when live-cell imaging is needed. SIM uses patterned illumination, usually stripes to excite the sample. Pattern position and orientation are changed several times and the emitted fluorescence is measured for each one of these positions. Striped fluorescence excitation and emission from a sample will result in interference patterns known as Moire patterns, from which detailed spatial information can be extracted using image processing.

A combination of super-resolution fluorescent microscopy with other techniques can also be used to improve the resolution and image heterogeneous biological tissue. The main limitations of super-resolution microscopy are the availability of suitable fluorophores, expensive equipment and low acquisition time for images.

Although very sensitive, fluorescence microscopy is often faced with the problem of **photobleaching**. The process of photobleaching or fading occurs when a fluorophore permanently loses the ability to fluoresce due to the photon-induced structural damage or covalent bonding. In principle, fluorophores can cycle between ground and excited states, but the number of such cycles, in particular for organic fluorophores, is limited and depends largely on the environment of the fluorophores. The typical organic fluorophore can go through around 10 000 to 40 000 cycles before it is permanently bleached. This might seem like a big number, but in real-life application to cell studies this is not much, and a permanent fading of fluorescence might lead to false results and unwanted intracellular effects. Although bleaching is still not fully understood, it is clear that it occurs readily in the presence of molecular oxygen, which can be converted into highly reactive singlet oxygen by interaction with an excited state of fluorophores. Such a reactive species can alter the structure of fluorophores and also interact with other biomolecules within the cell. As opposed to organic fluorophores, fluorescent nanomaterials such as quantum dots and noble metal clusters are much more resistant to fluorescence bleaching and are particularly used for cell labelling and design of stable biosensors.

5.3.4   Vibrational Spectroscopy: Infrared Spectroscopy

Molecules are not static entities. Their bonds are in a continuous state of vibration. For simple molecules containing two or three atoms, these vibrations can be defined and described, but as the molecule gets more complex, so does the number of possible vibrations. To make everything simpler, we distinguish between two basic categories of vibrations; stretching and bending (Figure 5.19a), each of which comes with their own subtypes. Stretching refers to continuous changes in interatomic distances along the axis of the bond, whereas bending is characterised by a change in the angle between two bonds. Furthermore, a coupling of vibrations usually occurs, making the systems even more complex. Vibrational spectroscopy uses these vibrations to characterise and quantify molecular species and the type of bonds they contain.

IR spectroscopy provides information on the vibration of molecules. Molecular vibrations can be grouped into stretching and bending vibrations (a), and when incoming IR light is matched to a particular vibration, the light will be absorbed corresponding to the dip in transmittance (b).

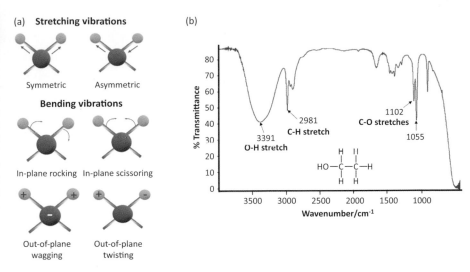

In vibrational infrared spectroscopy, infrared (IR) light, typically in the mid-IR range with wavelengths between 2.5 and 25 μm (which can also be expressed in wavenumbers, 4000–400 cm^{-1}, the number of waves per unit distance), is used as the excitation light. The energy of IR light is not enough to induce transitions between energy levels such as seen in UV–Vis and fluorescence spectroscopy. Rather, if the energy of IR light matches one of the vibrational energy levels (Back to Basics 5.3), a net transfer of energy will take place that results in the amplitude change of the molecular vibration and absorption of light.

To absorb IR radiation, a molecule must undergo a net change in a dipole moment as a consequence of its vibrational and rotational motion. Most of the molecules absorb IR radiation, the only exception being homonuclear species such as O_2, N_2 or Cl_2, and IR has been one of the most widely used techniques for the characterisation and quantification of molecules. The principles of IR interaction with molecules were described as early as 1800 by William Herschel (1738–1822), although commercial instruments became available in the 1960s. Infrared spectrometers became widely used after an introduction of Fourier transform infrared (FTIR) instruments (Back to Basics 5.6) in the 1980s, which improved resolution and allowed for rapid scanning by allowing for the simultaneous collection of information from multiple frequencies. Despite many advantages, the major disadvantage of IR spectroscopy is the high absorbance of water in the mid-infrared region, limiting the application of FTIR for biological samples.

Infrared spectroscopy can achieve resolutions of about 5 to 10 μm, which is not suitable for chemical analysis of submicrometre or nanoscale material features. The resolution limitation was overcome by combining AFM and IR into nanoscale IR spectroscopy (Figure 5.20).

Back to Basics 5.6   Fourier Transform IR

Advancement in IR spectroscopy came with the introduction of Fourier transform spectrophotometers, which increased the signal-to-noise ratio, enabled faster measurements and multiplexing.

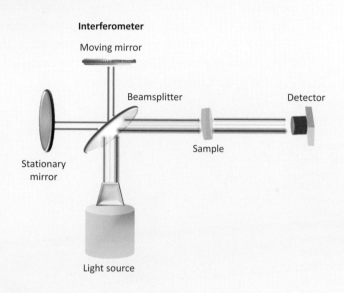

The main component of the Fourier transform spectrometer is the Michelson interferometer composed of two mirrors and a beam splitter. The principle behind the interferometer is simple: a beam of incoming light is split into two beams with different paths. These beams are then reflected off the stationary and moving mirror resulting in their interference. Such beams meet at the beam splitter and pass through the sample. Some of the energy will be absorbed, some transmitted. Transmitted light will be detected and recorded as an interferogram, in which the signal is a function of time. Using a mathematical method known as Fourier transform named after the physicist Jean-Baptiste Joseph Fourier (1768–1830), the interferogram is converted from function of time to a function of frequency:

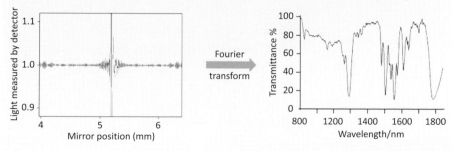

In nanoscale IR, high speed, tunable IR laser light is focused onto the sample at the AFM tip location. If the light is matching the absorbance bands of the material, rapid thermal expansion occurs, which causes the change of the height within the sample, and in turn, the oscillation of the AFM cantilever. Spectra obtained by measuring cantilever oscillation amplitude as a function of IR wavelength contain unique chemical information about the surface. Using nanoscale IR, a chemical composition map of a particular surface at the chosen wavelength can be obtained with less than 10 nm resolution. Spectral data can also be extracted to provide information on topology and mechanical properties.

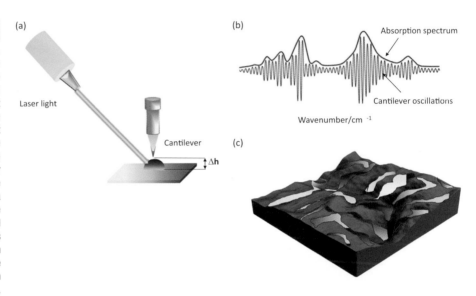

Figure 5.20

Nanoscale IR. (a) Tunable IR laser beam is focused onto the sample, causing thermal expansion when it matches the absorbance band of the material. Heat expansion leads to the change of the height (ΔH) resulting in AFM cantilever oscillation. (b) Nanoscale IR spectrum is a combination of the absorption spectrum and cantilever oscillations which are then transformed into the chemical composition map of the surface (c).

5.3.5 Raman Spectroscopy and Surface-Enhanced Raman Scattering

Raman spectroscopy is based on the phenomenon of Raman scattering, which is a result of the same type of vibrational changes that are associated with infrared spectroscopy. However, whereas in IR the absorbed light that corresponds to a particular vibration is measured, Raman scattering reports on the difference between the incident and scattered visible radiation. This difference was first observed by Indian physicist Sir Chandrashekhara V. Raman (1888–1970) in 1928, he also noticed that the value of the difference can be attributed to a particular molecule and depends on its chemical structure.

When the light of a wavelength which is different from absorption peaks of the molecule is used for excitation, 1 out of 10 million photons will interact with the molecule in such a way to cause the excitation into a higher vibrational level. The increase of energy will be equal to the energy of the photon (Figure 5.21), and the molecule can assume any of an infinite number of values or virtual states between the ground and first excited energy level.

Raman spectroscopy. (a) Absorption of light promotes an electron to a virtual vibration level from which it can relax to one of the ground level vibrations without the change in energy (Rayleigh), or with changed energy (Stokes and anti-Stokes). (b) Raman spectrum is composed of regions corresponding to vibrational relaxation of particular bonds and the fingerprint region useful for fast characterisation of molecules.

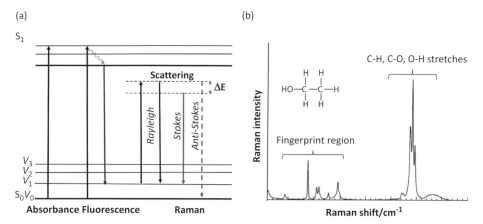

Three different scattering events can occur following the photon impact: **Rayleigh**, **Stokes** and **anti-Stokes scattering** (Figure 5.21a). The energy of Rayleigh scattering will be the same as the energy of the incident photon. Although this is the most probable and most intense scattering event, it is not useful for molecular fingerprinting. Of two events that result in the difference in scattering, anti-Stokes is the least probable, and as a consequence, only the Stokes part of the spectrum is used for analytical purposes. Due to the rarity of the scattering events, Raman signals are very weak, often 0.001% of the intensity of the source. For this reason, Raman scattering was not considered as particularly useful until the powerful laser light sources were introduced in the 1960s.

Raman and IR spectrum for a given molecule often resemble one another, but there are enough differences between Raman and IR active groups within the molecule to make both methods complementary to each other.

Due to the weak signals, Raman spectroscopy was not considered as particularly sensitive even after the introduction of the laser light sources. However, in 1974, researchers at the University of Southampton, UK, observed that Raman signals can be enhanced 10^4 to 10^5 times when a target molecule is placed in the proximity to a roughened noble metal surface (Fleischmann, 1974).

A few years later **surface-enhanced Raman spectroscopy (SERS)** or **Raman scattering** was coined and the technique soon became an invaluable tool in bionanotechnology and biosensor design (Figure 5.22a).

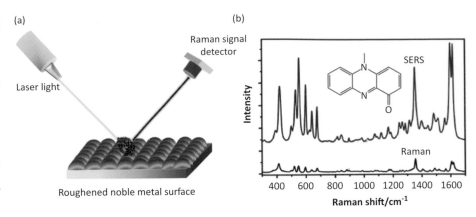

The main contributor to the enhancement of the Raman signal is an electromagnetic effect, which is a consequence of the excitement of the localised surface plasmon when the incident laser light hits the roughened noble metal surface. Such plasmon excitement enhances an electric field E, impacting both the incident and scattered light, and resulting in Raman signal enhancement proportional to E^4 (McQuillan, 2009). Smaller contribution to SERS comes from chemical enhancement due to the charge transfer between the studied molecules interacting with metal nanoparticles. Depending on the type of interaction with the surface and the chemical structure of the molecule and the incident wavelength, the enhancement up to 10^{12} can be achieved allowing for the detection of an analyte in concentrations as low as an attomolar ($1\,aM = 10^{-18}\,M$) (Figure 5.22b). For example, using hydrophobic gold surfaces to concentrate the dilute solution, $75\,aM$ concentration of rhodamine dye could be detected (Yang et al., 2016).

Noble metal nanoparticles are commonly used as surfaces for SERS enhancement as their plasmons are observed in a visible region, and can be excited with visible light lasers, resulting in a large localised plasmon enhancement. The effect is even more enhanced at the hotspots present on an irregular, roughened surface, which is preferred to the smooth surfaces as it leads to larger signal. Unlike for other nanoparticle applications, the formation of irregular aggregates is desirable in SERS as it results in hot spots of strong plasmon leading to significant signal enhancement.

SERS has also largely benefitted from the developments in nanoparticle preparation and surface nanostructuring strategies, which led to the design of roughened surfaces suitable for imaging of different biomolecules such as proteins, DNA and lipids (Bruzos, 2018), detection of small molecules in complex mixtures as well as the DNA sequence analysis (Graham and Faulds,

2008). In recent years, SERS has also been used for live-cell imaging and single-molecule detection (Sharma et al., 2012).

As in Raman, the vibrational spectra obtained by SERS contain fingerprint areas specific to a particular molecule enabling identification of various species in a solution. Particular chromophores such as aromatic ring containing compounds will have particularly strong Raman bands, and these are additionally enhanced if the molecule is chemisorbed onto the noble metal substrates. Many common fluorophores have been used as SERS labels since they absorb strongly in a visible region giving the characteristic Raman signal, while their fluorescence is quenched by the presence of the noble metal.

SERS can be used not only for the measurements in research facilities but also in real-life settings due to a relatively simple set-up and potential for quantitative measurements. Portable SERS instruments were already successfully used in forensic science, in particular in the detection of explosives or drugs, for detection of environmental pollutants and non-invasive biomedical screening (Sharma, 2012).

Being a relatively young technique, its potential has still not been fully exploited. Recent years have seen the development of new SERS strategies such as UV–SERS, although a challenge has been to find a plasmonic surface capable of enhancing the incoming UV light. The advantage of UV–SERS is in its ability to be used to study biomolecules, many of which absorb in the UV region (many proteins have absorption bands around 280 nm, while DNA has a strong band at 260 nm). But one of the most promising SERS-based techniques is a **tip-enhanced Raman spectroscopy** or **TERS**, which combines the principles of scanning probe microscope and SERS (Back to Basics 5.7). TERS has been used to obtain chemical composition data of area with a nanometre resolution.

Back to Basics 5.7	Tip-Enhanced Raman Spectroscopy

In TERS, the electromagnetic field enhancement is achieved around the metallic tip that is irradiated with laser light. When the tip is moved to the proximity of the sample, it provides localised SERS enhancement and information on the structural and chemical properties with a resolution of a few nanometres. Practically this is achieved by combining STM or AFM instruments with Raman spectrometry optics. Tips are either made of metal using electrochemical etching methods, by depositing a layer of gold or silver plasmonic nanoparticles onto an AFM cantilever tip made of silicon nitride. Although silver is preferred in SERS as it results in a high enhancement within a visible light region, it is also easily oxidised, and has often been replaced by gold.

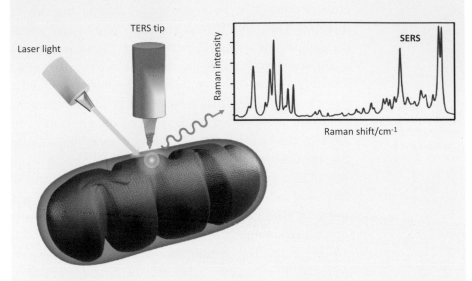

Depending on the sample, illumination in TERS can be achieved from the bottom, top or from the side, and the technique has been particularly useful for investigation of biological systems (Gao et al., 2018). Individual DNA and RNA bases were identified by moving a silver-coated AFM tip along a nucleic acid strand (Bailo and Deckert, 2008). Topography and chemical composition of complex proteins such as amyloid fibrils involved in Alzheimer's disease (Paulite et al., 2013) was obtained, receptors were identified on cancer cells (Xiao and Schulty, 2016), and molecular maps of whole cells produced.

Two of the challenges of TERS are the difficulty in calculating the enhancement area around the tip and the production of reproducible and reliable TERS tips.

5.3.6 Dynamic Light Scattering

Dynamic light scattering (DLS), sometimes referred to as quasi-elastic light scattering (QELS), is a non-invasive, well-established technique to determine the size and size distribution of molecules and particles typically in the submicrometre region, and with the latest technology, down to 1 nm. As opposed to reflection, in which the angle of the incident light will be equal to the angle of reflection, scattering results in light being scattered at all angles from the original path.

In a typical DLS experiment, the sample is exposed to a monochromatic wave of light and scattering from the sample is detected as a signal. When a monochromatic light hits a dispersion containing macromolecular species or spherical nanoparticles, the light scatters in all directions as a function of the size of in-solution species (Figure 5.23).

Figure 5.23

Dynamic light scattering. Scattering of the light depends on the size of the particles in solution. Brownian motion is monitored over time (a) and converted into particle size distribution (b).

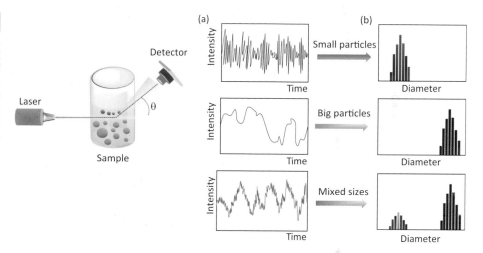

In dynamic light scattering, the intensity of fluctuations of scattered light can be used to determine a diffusion coefficient D which is related to the hydrodynamic radius R_h through the **Stokes–Einstein equation**:

$$D = \frac{kT}{6\pi\eta R_h},\qquad(5.8)$$

where η is the viscosity of the solvent, T is the temperature and k is the Boltzmann constant.

DLS primarily measures Brownian motion, the random motion of particles in the solution, which is a consequence of collisions with the solvent molecules, and relates this motion to the size of particles. When the movement of particles over time is monitored, particle size can be determined since the larger particles diffuse more slowly than the smaller ones.

According to the Rayleigh approximation, the scattering intensity monitored by DLS is approximately proportional to the sixth power of the particle size, and as a consequence, the technique is very sensitive to the presence of small aggregates. This means that it can be used for fast determination of the stability of the nanoparticles or biomolecules in solution.

DLS is a non-invasive method that requires low amounts of the sample, enables fast assessment of particle sizes and the measurements are straightforward. However, the range of the studied concentrations, in particular for nanoparticle solutions, is highly dependent on the type of material and its size. If a sample is very dilute, there might not be enough scattering events to make a proper assessment. On the other hand, if it is too concentrated, multiple scattering events might occur, which together with the inter-particle interactions, and the randomness of the motion within the solution might skew the data. Moreover, although some types of rod-shaped nanoparticles can be analysed by readjusting the DLS equations, use of DLS for assessment of other shapes is less reliable than for spherical particles. Careful interpretation of DLS data is needed as several other factors can impact the data such as the presence of absorbing and fluorescing species and the rotational diffusion often present in dispersions of colloidal nanoparticles.

In short, DLS needs to be used in combination with other techniques and the interpretation of data has to be done carefully.

5.3.7   Zeta Potential

Often DLS measurements are done in combination with zeta potential determination, and modern DLS instruments often contain a zeta potential add-on. **Zeta potential, ζ**, or **electrokinetic potential** is a measure of the potential at the slipping boundary when the charged particle moves under an external electric field (Back to Basic 5.8) and it is expressed in millivolts (mV).

If all the particles in suspension have a large negative or a large positive zeta potential they are considered to be stable due to the repulsion forces between them and consequently have a low tendency to agglomerate. Low zeta potential (> 5 mV) leads to agglomeration. As a general rule, the particles with zeta potentials more positive or negative than 30 mV are considered stable (-30 mV $> \zeta < +30$ mV).

Zeta potential cannot be measured directly, but it can be calculated from the measurements of electrophoretic mobility. When the electric field is applied across the colloid sample the charged particle moves towards the electrode with the opposite charge. The velocity of the particle depends on the strength of the electric field, the dielectric constant and viscosity of the medium and the zeta potential. Zeta potential can be derived from the Henry equation:

$$U_{\mathrm{E}} = \frac{2\varepsilon f(\kappa a)}{3\eta},\tag{5.9}$$

where U_E is electrophoretic mobility, ζ is zeta potential, ε dielectric constant, η viscosity and $f(\kappa a)$ is Henry's function. The κ, termed the Debye length, is reciprocal to length and κ^{-1} refers to the 'thickness' of the electrical double layer.

A zeta potential measurement system commonly comprises six main elements (Figure 5.24). A laser beam from a **laser source** is split to provide an incident and a reference beam. An **attenuator** adjusts the intensity of light reaching the sample and hence the intensity of scattering. The incident beam passes through the centre of the sample cell which contains a positive and negative electrode to generate an electrical field, and the scattered light is **detected** at an angle of 13°. **Compensation optics** are installed to correct the cell wall thickness and the dispersant refraction. The particles moving through the measured volume at applied electric field induce the fluctuation of light intensity with a frequency proportional to the particle speed. This information is processed to obtain the zeta potential value for a particular system. Zeta potential depends not only on the surface properties of the nanoparticle (nanoparticle surface charge, nature of attached ions/ligands) but also the nature of the solvent such as its ionic strength and pH. For example, a curve of zeta potential versus pH will be positive at low pH values and negative for high pH values. The point with a zero zeta potential is called the isoelectric point, which is a point at which the colloidal system is least stable and will agglomerate.

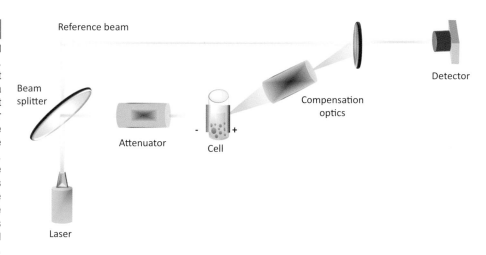

Figure 5.24

Zeta potential measurement set-up. The laser beam is split into an incident and a reference beam. Incident beam is scattered after passing through the sample within the electrode-containing cell. The fluctuation of the light intensity, which is proportional to the particle speed within the electrical field is recorded and processed to obtain zeta potential.

Considering the complex nature of nanomaterial surfaces, DLS and zeta potential measurements need to be taken with caution. Even the smallest changes in the surface properties might lead to misleading results. This is particularly the case when measurements are attempted for nanoparticles dispersed in a complex biological solution such as blood. However, they can be used for quick assessment of the size, stability, and charge of nanoparticles and bionano hybrids, and are particularly useful for quick and cost-effective assessment of nanoparticle functionalisation, prior the use of other more complex analytical methods.

Back to Basics 5.8   Zeta Potential ζ

When a charged particle is suspended in liquid, an electric double layer (EDL) is formed around its surface. EDL consists of two layers: a region closest to the surface that is considered immobile and may include adsorbed ions known as the **Stern layer**, and an outer region or the **diffuse layer**. The diffuse layer allows for the diffusion of ions under the influence of the electrical forces and thermal motion. Within the diffuse layer, there is a boundary called the surface of hydrodynamic shear or the **slipping plane**, where the particles and ions form a stable entity. When the particle moves, ions within this boundary move with it, whereas the ions beyond the boundary do not. The difference in potential between the EDL and the slipping boundary of a particle moving under an electric field is the **electrokinetic potential** or **zeta potential** ζ.

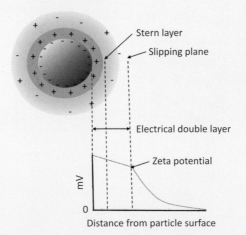

For a negatively charged particle, the Stern layer will contain negative charges, whereas a diffuse layer consists of both negative and positive charges. The diffuse layer is a dynamic entity and it will depend on pH, ionic strength and concentration. When placed in an electric field, the particle moves towards the positive electrode, and the velocity of such movement can be used to determine zeta potential. This is the principle behind the widely used electrophoretic light scattering instruments. Another type of measurement is based on the electroacoustic phenomenon, which uses high frequencies to induce particle oscillations. These oscillations depend on the particle size and zeta potential, allowing for the fast characterisation.

5.4 Exploring (Bio)Molecular Interactions on the Nanoscale

Biological systems are dynamic. Ultimately bionanotechnology is trying to design probes to explore them and the materials that can change them. In order to design suitable nanocomposites for tissue engineering or nano hybrids to deliver drugs or detect the presence of a particular pathogen, we need to characterise the interactions of engineered materials with (bio)molecules. We also need to characterise and monitor the biomolecular folding and binding in the absence and presence of nanomaterials, but also time-dependent changes on the nanoscale. Such dynamic processes require not only imaging of the explored materials but also the strategies that can provide kinetic data and binding constants.

5.4.1 Fluorescence (Förster) Resonance Energy Transfer

Fluorescence resonance energy transfer known simply as FRET is a physical phenomenon of radiation-less transfer of energy between two fluorophores positioned at a particular distance to each other. Fluorescence and Föster resonance energy transfer are often used interchangeably in honour of Theodor Förster (1910–1974) and his contribution to the understanding of FRET theory.

FRET depends on the distance between the fluorophores, but also their excitation and emission profiles, which need to show significant spectral overlap (Figure 5.25a). FRET theory is based on the concept of treating an excited fluorophore as an oscillating dipole that can undergo an energy exchange with a second dipole having a similar resonance frequency. One can imagine these fluorophores behaving like a pair of tuning forks, which vibrate at the same frequency when coupled to each other. When two fluorophores are close together, the dipole moment of one interacts with the other, and the dipole energy at the overlap of the excitation and emission energies is delocalised between them (Figure 5.25b). Thus, if a donor dye is optically excited, it will transfer the energy directly to the acceptor and then relax into a ground state. One of the key factors for successful FRET is the choice of the right donor–acceptor pair, and this choice was made easier with the introduction of fluorescent proteins and quantum dots.

Fluorescence resonance energy transfer (FRET). Donor and acceptor fluorophore need to have matched excitation profiles and be in proximity to allow for energy transfer between them. As a consequence, excitation at the donor $\lambda_{ex}(D)$, will result in the emission of acceptors λ_{em} (A).

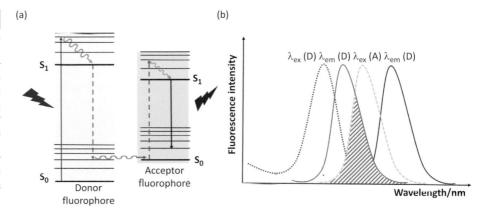

Since the energy transfer efficiency is distance-dependent, FRET can only occur over distances d smaller than the Förster radius R_0:

$$E_{FRET} = \frac{1}{1 + \left(\dfrac{d}{R_0}\right)^6},$$ (5.10)

where the Förster radius is given by

$$R_0 = 9.78 \times 10^3 (\kappa^2 n^{-4} Q_D J(\lambda))^{1/6},$$

where κ factor is dependent on the relative orientation of the donor and acceptor ($0 \leq \kappa^2 \leq 4$), n is the refractive index of the medium, Q_D is the quantum yield of the donor, and $J(\lambda)$ is an overlap integral between the appropriate states of the donor and acceptor (Weiss, 1999). Factor κ tells us if the orientation of dipoles are ideal for energy transfer. When κ^2 is 4, the dipoles are aligned to each other well and energy transfer will happen, but the value of 0 would mean that they are positioned perpendicular to each other. No matter how close the donor and acceptor are, in that case, the energy transfer will not occur.

As can be seen from Equation 5.10, FRET interaction gets weaker with the sixth power of the distance between the two fluorophores, and FRET intensity can be essentially used as a molecular ruler to determine the distance between molecules or different parts of the same molecule. The maximum distance requirement for FRET to occur is 8 to 10 nm, which means that FRET is well within the range of sizes of many proteins and nucleic acids. Consequently, FRET is particularly useful to explore conformational changes such as folding (Research Report 5.2) and cleavage.

| Research Report 5.2 | Protein Folding Studied by FRET |

One of the most powerful applications available is the use of FRET to study protein folding, which cannot be easily studied by other methods. Before measurements, the protein of interest needs to be labelled by donor and acceptor dyes at different sites. As the protein folds, the two dyes will come close to each other which will result in fluorescence resonance energy transfer. Such a principle is not only useful to explore the folding of a single protein but has been extensively employed to study interactions of different domains within the multi-domain proteins such as streptavidin composed of four domains (see Chapter 3).

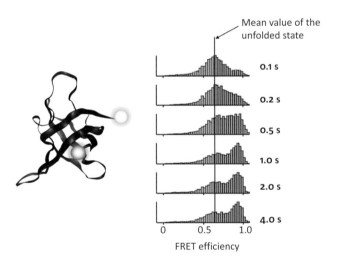

Source: Lipman et al. (2003). Reprinted with permission from AAAS.

FRET is particularly useful to obtain data on the kinetics of folding as demonstrated in 2003 in work by Lipman and colleagues (2003). Cold shock protein (CSP) from *Thermotoga maritima* (Kramer, 2001) was first labelled with a green fluorescent donor (Alexa Fluor 488 dye) and red fluorescent acceptor (Alexa 594) via cysteine positioned at the amino (N) and carboxylic acid C terminal end of the protein. Denaturing agent guanidium chloride is then added to the solution of the protein to keep it in the unfolded state. To explore the kinetics of folding, the denaturing agent is continuously diluted allowing for the protein to fold. In an unfolded state, when the average distance between the dyes is the greatest (this happens 0.1 seconds into the measurement), the FRET efficiency is low and most of the fluorescence comes from the donor dye. After 4 s, an increase in the acceptor fluorescence indicates that dyes have come together into the folded structure.

With the introduction of fluorescent proteins and super-resolution micro-scopy, FRET has been extensively used to probe the interaction of biomo-lecules in cells and in real time, significantly advancing our understanding of biomolecular processes and aiding the design of therapeutic strategies. Add-itional improvement of the FRET strategy came with the introduction of fluorescent quantum dots as both the donor and to a lesser extent, acceptor fluorophores. As inorganic nanoparticles, quantum dots are characterised by remarkable photostability and are often 10 to 100 times brighter than organic fluorophores, which makes them particularly suitable for long-term and live imaging. However, unlike fluorescent protein they cannot be genet-ically fused to a protein of interest, they are larger than organic fluorophores (2–10 nm) making them often unsuitable for intramolecular measurements and are often composed of toxic elements not always suitable for live-cell imaging.

Like other analytical techniques in bionanotechnology, FRET suffers from several practical pitfalls such as fluorescence quenching upon fluorophore labelling, non-ideal fluorophore behaviour or non-specific FRET when the density of donor and acceptor molecules are not well-matched, and it should be complemented with other strategies. Nevertheless, with such a diverse toolbox of fluorophores ranging from small organic molecules to inorganic nanoparticles, there are many available options for the design of suitable FRET systems.

5.4.2 Surface Plasmon Resonance

When an incident beam of polarised light strikes an electrically conducting thin gold layer at the interface of high refractive index material n_h (glass prism) and a material with low refractive index n_l (i.e. water) total internal reflection will occur. The thin gold layer is characterised by the presence of a surface plasmon, an oscillating wave propagating along the surface of gold, which interacts with the incident light resulting in an **evanescent wave**. The amplitude of the evanescent wave decreases exponentially with the distance to the gold surface and decreases significantly at approximately 300 nm from the surface.

At a given angle, the incident light will be in resonance with the surface plasmon oscillations resulting in a sharp decrease in the intensity of the reflected light. **Surface plasmon resonance (SPR)** technique provides information on the change in **resonance angle** as the composition of the medium on the gold layer surface changes. The reason for this is a dependence of the resonance angle on the refractive index of the media surrounding the gold surface as shown in Equation 5.11:

$$\theta_{SPR} = \sin^{-1}\left(\frac{1}{n_h}\sqrt{\frac{n_l^2 n_{Au}^2}{n_l^2 + n_{Au}^2}}\right), \tag{5.11}$$

where θ_{SPR} is the resonance angle, n_h is the high refractive index, n_l is the low refractive index and n_{Au} refractive index of the gold film.

Equation 5.11 tells us that if n_h and n_{Au} are kept constant, the resonance angle will depend on the refractive index n_l. In an SPR instrument n_h corresponds to the index of the glass prism, which does not change (Figure 5.26). However, small changes in the refractive index of the medium on the surface of the gold film (n_l) will have a significant impact on the resonance angle.

Figure 5.26

Surface plasmon resonance (SPR). (a) In SPR, the angle of the incident polarised light is changed until it reaches the value at which the frequency of the incident light corresponds to that of the surface plasmon (resonance angle) within the gold film. (b) When this happens, a dip in reflection intensity will occur and it will depend on the species present on the film surface. Resonance angle of an antibody alone will differ significantly from a protein-bound antibody. (c) The change in the resonance angle can be monitored over time proving a time-resolved (kinetic) data on the interacting event on the film surface.

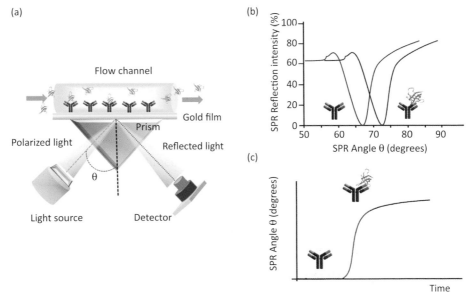

Let us imagine we have a sample from a patient previously diagnosed with cancer, but successfully treated and free of symptoms. The patient is undergoing regular check-ups to screen for the presence of a known cancer biomarker. The antibody that binds the protein biomarker is known and readily available, and we have an SPR set up to perform the screening. The first step in our SPR sensing strategy is the immobilisation of the antibody on the gold surface, which can be performed using one of the surface biofunctionalisation strategies explored in Chapter 4. Once this is achieved, the SPR resonant angle is measured showing a strong dip in reflectance (Figure 5.26b, blue curve). The next step is to check if any of the proteins in the patient's sample binds to the antibody. This is achieved by passing the sample over the antibody-functionalised surface through a flow channel. If the binding occurs, the antibody–protein complex will cause the change in refractive index shifting the resonance angle (Figure 5.26b, red curve). The change in the angle can be plotted as a function of time (Figure 5.26c) providing information on the kinetics of the binding event.

Surface plasmon resonance is a versatile method that can be used to study binding events between a diverse range of species. The only requirements are that the binding occurs within 300 nm, after which the amplitude of the evanescent wave decreases significantly, and that the conditions that might affect the change of refractive index, such as temperature or solvent, are kept constant.

Besides high sensitivity and kinetic constant determination, the major advantage of the SPR method is a label-free detection. Since SPR is widely used to study biomolecular interactions, commercial gold chips are available which can also be coated with binding molecules required for a particular application. Numerous SPR sensors have been designed to explore inter-actions between proteins, lipids, carbohydrates and nucleic acids (more on sensor design in Chapter 8).

5.4.3 Quartz Crystal Microbalance

When a piezoelectric material (from *piezin*, a Greek word for 'squeeze'; Back to Basics 5.9) such as crystal quartz is placed in an alternating electric field of the right frequency, it will oscillate in a mechanically resonant mode. Due to the **piezoelectricity**, the resonant mode of a crystal can be affected by external physical loading. This loading can either be gravimetric (referring to a mass change) or viscoelastic (acoustic fluid damping interaction when the quartz crystal microbalance (QCM) is in a liquid medium).

Back to Basics 5.9   Piezoelectric Materials

Piezoelectricity was first observed by French physicist, and husband of Marie Skłodowska Curie, Pierre Curie (1859–1906) and his brother Jacques (1855–1941) in 1880. Based on earlier experiments showing that a change in temperature in a crystalline material generates electricity, the Curie brothers set out to check if the same is true for a mechanical strain. They tested various crystals such as quartz, topaz and cane sugar, and found that the strain indeed results in electrical potential. The strongest effect was observed in quartz. The following year the Curie brothers also showed that the reverse is true; the application of the electric field to a crystal causes the material to deform. After a few rather research-quiet decades, the first practical application was devised by Pierre Langevin (1872–1946) in 1917. He developed an ultrasonic transducer based on quartz for use in submarines.

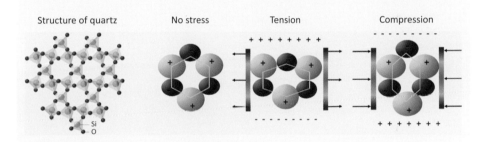

The basis of piezoelectric materials lies in their asymmetric crystal lattice. Despite the asymmetric arrangement of ions, the charges are balanced when there is no stress applied, and a piezoelectric material has a zero net charge. However, when mechanical stress is exerted onto the crystal, the force causes the charges to get displaced, resulting in separation of a negative and positive charge on the opposite crystal faces.

Piezoelectric materials are important components of many devices such as microphones, speakers, sonar, ultrasound imaging systems, inkjet printers just to name some. For example, in a microphone the sound energy is converted into an electrical signal with the help of a piezoelectric element; the pressure of the voice excites the piezoelectric crystal generating a measurable electrical signal.

The relationship between the change in frequency, Δf, of the crystal and the change of mass is given by the Sauerbrey equation (Equation 5.12) named after the German physicist Günther Sauerbrey (1933–2003):

$$\Delta f = \frac{Cf^2 \Delta m}{A}, \tag{5.12}$$

where f is the oscillation frequency of the crystal, C is a proportionality constant, A is the surface area and m is the mass of the crystal.

QCM measures mass per unit area by recording the change in frequency of a quartz crystal resonator (Figure 5.27), and it can be used both in the gas phase and liquid environments.

Figure 5.27

Quartz crystal microbalance (QCM). The resonant frequency of a piezoelectric quartz crystal changes with mass. When an antibody is attached to the quartz crystal surface containing top and bottom electrode elements, a sharp decrease in frequency is recorded, which additionally changes when an antigen binds to the antibody surface.

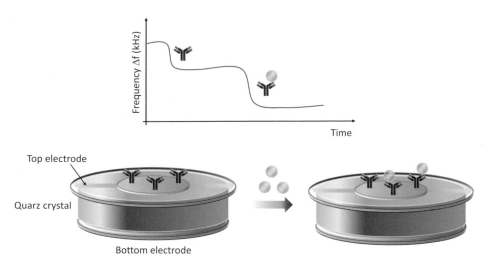

Depending on the resonance of QCM, it can be used to detect masses down to $20 \, \text{ng cm}^{-2}$ for 5 MHz QCM. A higher frequency will lead to higher sensitivity, although this would require the quartz crystal to be thin, which is difficult to achieve.

The current limit of detection is around $2 \, \text{ng cm}^{-2}$ with the response time of 1 sec. In many ways, QCM can be considered similar to SPR, although, for some applications such as kinetic and multiplex studies, SPR is more useful as it requires lower sample volumes and has a lower limit of detection. However, QCM can be used for fast determination of mass changes on the NP surface.

QCM has been used to study nanoparticle interactions with cells, binding of drugs to the cell receptors, studies of novel nanocomposite materials (Heydari and Haghayegh, 2014), and detection of protein biomarkers in blood serum (Research Report 5.3).

Research Report 5.3 | Detection of Cancer Biomarker Using SPR and QCM

One of the biggest challenges in the design of biosensors (see Chapter 8) is the use of complex clinical samples to detect a particular analyte. Often other (bio)molecules present in serum, saliva or urine interfere with detection. For example, injection of serum onto SPR or QCM causes a bulk shift response due to the higher refractive index and viscosity of the serum medium. This can often mask the signal corresponding to binding of an analyte to the immobilised capture species such as an antibody.

To address this issue, a sandwich assay can be used in which a bound analyte is additionally labelled with a gold nanoparticle carrying secondary antibody specific to the analyte. This strategy was used by Uludag and Tothill (2012) to develop SPR and QCM-based sensors for detection of the prostate cancer biomarker, total prostate-specific antigen, tPSA.

Serum containing PSA was passed over the sensors containing capture anti-PSA antibody. Once PSA is bound and the sensor washed, gold nanoparticles modified with anti-PSA antibody are added, resulting in a sandwich assay and increased sensor response.

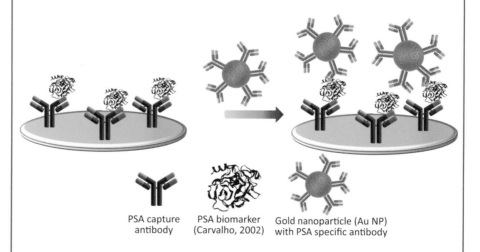

PSA capture antibody   PSA biomarker (Carvalho, 2002)   Gold nanoparticle (Au NP) with PSA specific antibody

When two different sizes of Au nanoparticles were compared (20 and 40 nm), significant improvement in both SPR and QCM response was recorded with 40 nm Au NP. The PSA in serum that could be detected was 2.3 ng ml^{-1} with 20 nm Au NP, and 0.23 ng ml^{-1} with 40 nm

Au NP. Not only could a significant increase in detection limit be achieved by the use of larger plasmonic Au NPs, but this limit was way beyond the required clinical detection threshold of $2.5\,\mathrm{ng\,ml^{-1}}$. Moreover, in both methods data were acquired within minutes (Uludag and Tothill, 2012).

Key Concepts

Electron microscopy: a microscopy technique based on the measurements of electron transmitted through or scattered from the sample and widely used to explore the shape and the size of nanomaterials, but also the morphology of larger structures in nanometre resolution.

Electron spectroscopy: an analytical technique that exploits the kinetic energy of electrons emitted when an incident X-ray beam hits the sample. Each atom is characterised by a unique binding energy of the electron, which can be used to provide the information on the composition of the studied material.

Fluorescence microscopy: an optical microscopy technique based on recording the fluorescence emission within a sample, and a powerful tool to study nanomaterial–cell interactions. Advanced fluorescence microscopy (super-resolution fluorescence microcopy) is capable of studying a single molecule interaction and also dyanimc processes within cells.

Fluorescence resonance energy transfer (FRET): a physical phenomenon of energy transfer between two fluorophores positioned close to each other. It is extensively used to explore the dynamic processes within a single molecule such as protein folding, or interactions between different classes of materials and molecules. Used extensively for design of biosensors, it has also been widely used as a helper tool in super-resolution fluorescence microscopy.

Jablonski diagram: a representation of different processes within a molecule as it interacts with light. It illustrates the possible transitions between various energy and vibrational levels within the molecule, and it is an important tool in spectroscopy.

Nanomaterial characterisation: requires analytical methods that explore morphology, physiochemical properties and their interaction with biomolecules and dynamic biological systems.

Piezoelectricity: is the property of a certain class of materials to generate electrical current after they are exposed to mechanical stress or pressure. Piezoelectricity of quartz crystal is exploited in the design of very sensitive **quartz crystal microbalance (QCM),** which can measure very small mass changes.

Scanning probe microscopy: a microscopy technique based on the scanning of the surface of material to provide morphological maps with nanosized resolution. **Scanning tunnelling microscopy (STM)** exploits the principle of electron tunnelling between the electrically conductive tip and the surface. **Atomic force microscopy (AFM)** records small movements of the cantilever as it scans the surface, from which the surface morphology can be inferred.

Surface-enhanced Raman scattering (SERS): a vibrational spectroscopy technique based on the enhancement of Raman scattering in the presence of rough plasmonic metal nanosurfaces. It provides fingerprint signals useful for identification of molecules on the surface of nanomaterials and has been extensively explored for design of sensitive bionanosensors.

Surface plasmon resonance (SPR): an analytical technique used to study interactions between different molecular classes and molecules and engineered materials by exploring the changes in the surface plasmon of a thin gold film. Unlike FRET or SERS, it does not require the use of any labels.

TOF-SIMS: a mass spectrometry technique used for 3D elemental mapping of nanocomposites based on the measurements of specific secondary ions produced by the bombardment with ions produced from a primary ion source.

X-ray diffraction: exploits the diffraction of X-rays from a crystal to determine the crystal lattice parameters and decipher crystalline phases of the materials. **Small angle X-ray scattering (SAXS)** can be used to study biomolecules and soft nanomaterials, and **energy dispersive X-ray (EDX)** analysis can be used to identify the elemental composition of samples.

Problems

5.1 Calculate the energy of:
   (a) a 9 Å X-ray photon
   (b) a 530 nm photon of visible radiation.
5.2 Calculate the wavelength of electrons with energy of 100 keV. Explain why these electrons can be effectively transmitted through a 0.6 μm silicon wafer.
5.3 How would you determine that iron oxide nanoparticle contains a magnetite or maghemite iron oxide form?

5.4　Explain the difference between the X-ray used for X-ray diffraction and for SAXS?

5.5　Name the two types of scanning probe microscope.
(a) How do they differ?
(b) What are the advantages and disadvantages of each?

5.6　Why is it important to control the size of a cantilever in AFM?

5.7　Besides being used for surface imaging, AFM can be used to study forces between interacting molecules, for example interaction between two complementary DNA strands. How would you attach a 24 base long DNA molecule on the surface of an AFM cantilever?

5.8　What is the difference between spontaneous and stimulated light emission?

5.9　What is the advantage of a Fourier transform infrared spectrometer?

5.10　What is the structure of fluorophore within the fluorescent protein and how is that fluorophore formed?

5.11　The extinction coefficient of GFP protein is relatively small (around 60 000) in comparison to some organic fluorophores (200 000). How could the extinction coefficient of GFP be increased?

5.12　In a single molecule FRET, the green channel (direct fluorescence) counts 1000 units, and the red channel (FRET signal) counts 200 units in a given interval. The dye used has $R_0 = 6$ nm. What is the separation of the donor and the acceptor dyes, assuming that their alignment remains fixed during the experiment? ($d = 4.7$ nm)

5.13　You need to prepare gold nanorods coated with a bacteria-binding antibody for a collaborator who is designing a bacterial biosensor. Explain which methods you would employ to characterise the nanorods, prove that you have a bound peptide on the surface and that the bionano hybrids bind to the bacteria.

5.14　Citrate-coated gold nanoparticles aggregate in the presence of a high concentration of sodium chloride. Which method could you employ to study the aggregation and determine the concentration of the salt needed?

5.15　In which analytical method is the aggregation of plasmonic nanoparticles desirable?

5.16　Compare and contrast IR and Raman spectroscopy.

5.17　Which method can be used to determine the hydrodynamic radius of DNA-coated silver nanoparticle in aqueous solution?

5.18   Describe methods that can be used to obtain time-sensitive (kinetic) data on binding of biotin-modified quantum dot and streptavidin?

5.19   Specify which analytical method(s) would you use to:
   (a) determine the size of Ag NPs;
   (b) determine that QDs are modified with STV;
   (c) check that the surface of the cell is coated with Au NPs;
   (d) determine the crystallinity of TiO_2 NPs;
   (e) investigate the folding of the protein biomarker under various conditions;
   (f) prove that a short DNA sequence is attached to the surface of the protein;
   (g) map the elemental composition of a nanomaterial's surface.

Further Reading

AFM

Dufrene, Y., Ando, T., Garcia, R., et al. (2017). Imaging modes of atomic force microscopy for application in molecular and cell biology. *Nature Nanotechnology*, **12**, 295–307.

Müller, D. and Anderson, K. (2002). Biomolecular imaging using atomic force microscopy. *Trends in Biotechnology*, **20**(8), S45–S49.

DLS and Zeta Potential

Bhattacharjee, S. (2016). DLS and zeta potential: what are they and what they are not? *Journal of Controlled Release*, **235**, 337–351.

Stetefeld, J., McKenna, S. A. and Patel, T. R. (2016). Dynamic light scattering: a practical guide and applications in biomedical sciences. *Biophysical Reviews*, **8**, 409–427.

Fluorescence Microscopy

Huang, B., Bates, M. and Zhuang, X. (1999). Super-resolution fluorescence microscopy. *Annual Reviews in Biochemistry*, **78**, 993–1016.

Lichtman, J. W. and Conchello, J. A. (2005). Fluorescence microscopy. *Nature Methods*, **2**(12), 910–919.

SERS

Bruzas, I., Lum, W., Gorunmez, Z. and Sagle, L. (2018). Advances in surface-enhanced Raman spectroscopy (SERS) substrates for lipid and protein characterisation: sensing and beyond. *Analyst*, **143**, 3990–4008.

Jamieson, L. E., Asiala, S. M., Gracie, K., Faulds, K. and Graham, D. (2017). Bioanalytical measurements enabled by surface-enhanced Raman scattering (SERS) probes. *Annual Reviews in Analytical Chemistry*, **10**, 415–437.

SPR

Nguyen, H. H., Park, J., Kang, S. and Kim, M. (2015). Surface plasmon resonance: a versatile technique for biosensor applications. *Sensors*, **15**(5), 10481–10510.

TEM and Cryo-TEM

Kourkoutis, L. F., Plitzko, J. M. and Baumeister, W. (2012). Electron microscopy of biological materials at the nanometer scale. *Annual Review of Materials Research*, **42**, 33–58.

TERS

Verma, P. (2017). Tip-enhanced Raman spectroscopy: technique and recent advances. *Chemical Reviews*, **117**, 6447–6466.

TOF-SIMS

Fearn, S. (2014). Characterisation of biological material with TOF-SIMS: a review. *Materials Science and Technology*, **31**(2), 148–161.

Malmberg, P., Jennische, E., Nilsson, D. and Nygren, H. (2011). High-resolution, imaging TOF-SIMS: novel applications in medical research. *Analytical and Bioanalytical Chemistry*, **399**(8), 2711–2719.

References

Avila, A. and Bhushan, B. (2010). Electrical measurement techniques in atomic force microscopy. *Critical Reviews in Solid State and Materials Science*, **35**, 38–51.

Bailo, E. and Deckert, V. (2008). Tip-enhanced Raman spectroscopy of single RNA strands: towards a novel direct-sequencing method. *Angewandte chemie*, **47**, 1658–1661.

Benninghoven, A. (1969). Analysis of submonolayers on silver by negative secondary ion emission. *Physica Status Solidi B*, **34**(2), K169–K171.

Binning, G., Rohrer, H., Gerber, C. and Weibel, E. (1982). Surface studies by scanning tunnelling microscopy. *Physical Review Letters*, **49**, 57–61.

Binning, G., Quate, C. F. and Gerber, C. (1986). Atomic force microscope. *Physical Review Letters*, **56**, 930–933.

Bucciarelli, S., Midtgaard, S., Nors Pedersen, M., et al. (2018). Size-exclusion chromatography small-angle X-ray scattering of water-soluble proteins on a laboratory instrument. *Journal of Applied Crystallography*, **51**, 1623–1632.

Burnham, N. A., Dominguez, D. D., Mowery, R. L. and Colton, R. J. (1990). Probing the surface forces of monolayer films with an atomic-force microscope. *Physical Review Letters*, **64**, 1931–1934.

Combs, C. A. (2010). Fluorescence microscopy: a concise guide to current imaging methods. *Current Protocols in Neuroscience*, **50**(1), 1–14.

De Oteyza, D. G., Gorman, P., Chen, Y-C., et al. (2013). Direct imaging of covalent bond structure in single-molecule chemical reactions. *Science*, **340**, 1434–1437.

Eigler, D. M. and Schweizer, E. K. (1990). Positioning single atoms with a scanning tunnelling microscope. *Nature*, **334**, 524–526.

Fleischmann, M., Hendra, P. J. and McQuillan, A. J. (1974). Raman spectra of pyridine adsorbed at a silver electrode. *Chemical Physics Letters*, **26**, 163–166.

Fujioka, S., Zhang, Z., Yamamoto, N., et al. (2012). High-energy-density plasmas generation on GEKKO-LFEX laser facility for fast-ignition laser fusion studies and laboratory astrophysics. *Plasma Physics and Controlled Fusion*, **54**, 124042.

Gao, L., Zhao, H., Li, T., et al. (2018). Atomic force microscopy-based tip-enhanced Raman spectroscopy in biology. *International Journal of Molecular Science*, **19**(4), 1193.

Graham, D. and Faulds, K. (2008). Quantitative SERRS for DNA sequence analysis. *Chemical Society Reviews*, **37**, 1042–1051.

Guedes, A. F., Cavalho, F. and Santos, N. M. C. (2016). Atomic force microscopy as a tool to evaluate the risk of cardiovascular diseases in patients. *Nature Nanotechnology*, **11**, 687–692.

Guinier, A. (1939). Diffraction of X-rays of very small angles: application of an ultramicroscopic phenomenon. *Annales de Physiques*, **12**, 161–237.

Guinier, A. and Fournet, G. (1955). *Small-Angle Scattering of X-rays*, Wiley.

Haiss, W., Thahn, N. T., Aveyard, J. and Fernig, D. G. (2007). Determination of size and concentration of gold nanoparticles from UV–Vis spectra. *Analytical Chemistry*, **79**(11), 4215–4221.

Hell, S. W. and Wichmann, J. (1994). Breaking the diffraction resolution limit by stimulated emission: stimulated-emission-depletion fluorescence microscopy. *Optics Letters*, **19**(11), 780–782.

Heydari, S. and Haghayegh, G. H. (2014). Application of nanoparticles in quartz crystal microbalance biosensors. *Journal of Sensor Technology*, **4**, 81–100.

Hooke, R. (1665). *Micrographia: Or Some Physiological Descriptions of Minute Bodies Made By Magnifying Glases with Observations and Inquiries Thereupon*, Royal Society.

Kremer, W., Schuler, B., Harrieder, S., et al. (2001). Solution NMR structure of the cold-shock protein from the hyperthermophilic bacterium *Thermaotoga maritima*. *European Journal of Biochemistry*, **268**, 2527–2539.

Lander, J. J. (1953). Auger peaks in the energy spectra of secondary electrons from various materials. *Physical Review*, **91**, 1382–1387.

Lipman, E. A., Schuler, B., Bakajin, O. and Eaton, W. A. (2003). Single-molecule measurement of protein folding kinetics. *Science*, **301**, 1233–1235.

Maiman, T. H. (1960). Stimulated optical radiation in ruby. *Nature*, **187**, 493–499.

McQuillan, A. J. (2009). The discovery of surface-enhanced Raman scattering. *Notes and Records of the Royal Society*, **63**, 105–109.

Paulite, M., Blum, C., Schmid, T., et al. (2013). Full spectroscopic tip-enhanced Raman imaging of single nanotapes formed from β-amyloid (1–40) peptide fragments. *ACS Nano*, **7**, 1911–1920.

Raman, S. N., Paul, D. F., Hammond, J. S. and Bomben, K. D. (2011). Auger electron spectroscopy and its application to nanotechnology. *Microscopy Today*, **19**, 12–15.

Rusk, N. (2009). The fluorescence microscope. *Nature Cell Biology*, 11, S8–S9.

Sevvana, M., Long, F., Miller, A. S., et al. (2018). Refinement, and analysis of the mature Zika virus cryo-EM structure at 3.1 Å resolution. *Structure*, **26**, 1169–1177.

Sharma, B., Frontiera, R. R. Henry, A-I., Ringe, E. and van Duyne, R. P. (2012). SERS: materials, applications, and the future. *Materials Today*, **15**(1-2), 16–25.

Siegbahn, K., Nordling, C., Fahlman, A., et al. (1967). *ESCA: Atomic, Molecular and Solid-State Structure Studied by Means of Electron Spectroscopy. Nova acta regiae societatis scientiarum upsaliensis*, series 4, vol. **20**, Almqvist & Wiksells.

Stolzer, L., Ahmed, I., Rodriguez-Emmenegger, C., et al. (2014). Light-induced modification of silver nanoparticles with functional polymers. *Chemical Communications*, **34**, 4430–4433.

Uludag, Y. and Tothill, I. E. (2012). Cancer biomarker detection in serum samples using surface plasmon resonance and quartz crystal microbalance sensors with nanoparticle signal amplification. *Analytical Chemistry*, **84**, 5898–5904.

Weiss, S. (1999). Fluorescence spectroscopy of single biomolecules. *Science*, **283**, 1676–1683.

Xiao, L. and Schulty, Z. D. (2016). Targeted-TERS detection of integrin receptors on human cancer cells. *Cancer Cell Microenvironment*, **3**(4), e1419.

Yang, S., Dai, X., Stogin, B. B. and Wong, T-S. (2016). Ultrasensitive surface-enhanced Raman scattering detection in common fluids. *Proceedings of the National Academy of Sciences of the USA*, **113**(2), 268–273.

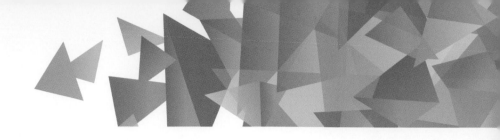

6 DNA Nanotechnology

The understanding of double helix structure has brought revolution to the fields of molecular biology and genetics. The structural properties of DNA such as specific base pairing, a combination of stiffness and flexibility as well as remarkable stability (see Chapter 3) have made a huge impact in fields ranging from drug delivery to sensor design. With increased availability of chemically synthesised DNA strands and developments of super-resolution microscopy, DNA nanotechnology established itself as an independent area of research within bionanotechnology. DNA nanotechnology uses DNA as a versatile building block rather than a genetic code carrier. Although the genetic information of DNA was recognised soon after the discovery of the double helix in the 1950s, the potential of DNA assembly for the design of programmable structures was for the first time hinted in a theoretical paper written by Ned Seeman in 1982 (Seeman, 1982). His early theoretical work was followed by experimental studies that demonstrated the programmability of short DNA strands and their use for self-assembly of larger ordered structures.

The field of DNA nanotechnology was further advanced by the introduction of DNA-directed immobilisation, the conjugation strategies by which DNA can be added to various molecular species, and DNA origami – the programmable folding of long DNA strands. However, all of these advances were facilitated by chemical synthesis of short DNA strands known as oligonucleotides and the design of an automated synthesiser, which enabled fast and affordable production of short DNA strands.

6.1   Chemical Synthesis of DNA

Oligonucleotides can be prepared by solid phase chemical synthesis using several different strategies with **phosphoramidite** being the most common one (Back to Basics 6.1).

Phosphoramidites are modified nucleosides used for the sequential addition of new bases to the growing DNA chain during a simple and efficient cyclic

| Back to Basics 6.1 | A Short History of the Chemical Synthesis of DNA |

The foundation of the chemical synthesis of oligonucleotides was laid in 1955 when a di-thymidine dinucleotide was synthesised for the first time using organic coupling (Michelson and Todd, 1955). A further significant contribution was made by Har Gobind Khorana (1922–2011) and his team, who introduced a **phosphodiester method** for the preparation of dinucleotide segments in 1958 (Smith et al., 1958). Following this success, almost two decades later, small segments were combined into 77 units of double-stranded DNA corresponding to the gene for alanine transfer ribonucleic acid (tRNA) from yeast (Agarwal, 1970). Khorana and his colleagues also developed the orthogonal protection/deprotection strategy, a variation of

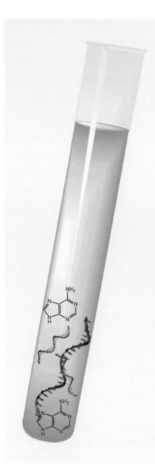

which is still used today (Back to Basics 6.2) (Schaller et al., 1963). The next important step in oligonucleotide synthesis was adapting the solid phase synthesis, initially developed for peptide preparation, and so improving the yields and easing the purification of oligonucleotides (Letsinger and Kornet, 1963; Merrifield, 1963).

Chemical synthesis of oligonucleotides was continuously optimised, finally resulting in the **nucleoside phosphoramidite strategy** by Marvin H. Caruthers (1940–) and colleagues in 1981 (Beaucage and Caruthers, 1981) which is still commonly used today. Their work was an extension of the research that demonstrated the advantages of 2-cyanoethyl phosphoramiditie reagents for solid phase synthesis, and the work done by American biochemist Robert Letsinger (1921–2014) and his team in the late 1970s, which showed that phosphorus (III) is considerably more reactive than the corresponding phosphorus (V) acylating agent (Letsinger and Lunsford, 1976).

reaction (Figure 6.1). Phosphoramidite chemistry exploits higher reactivity of phosphorus (III) compared to phosphorus (V) present in nucleic acids (Letsinger and Lunsford, 1976). In order to prevent side reactions and ensure the stability of the growing oligonucleotide chain, reactive nucleoside hydroxyl (–OH) and amine (NH_2) groups are masked using different protecting groups. In synthetic chemistry, protecting groups are commonly employed to control the reaction sequence and achieve the desired molecular structure while minimising side reactions and therefore, increasing the efficiency of the reaction. Dimethoxytrityl (DMT, green in Figure 6.1) group protects the 5′ hydroxyl group (5′–OH) on the deoxyribose and it can be cleaved easily under acidic conditions. The resulting cleavage product is coloured, which makes it suitable for monitoring the growth of the synthesised strand.

Removal of a diisopropylamino group (yellow in Figure 6.1), with the help of a catalyst, enables binding of the phosphoramidite group to the growing oligonucleotide. A 2-cyanoethyl (orange in Figure 6.1) protects the second hydroxyl group on the phosphite moiety and it is usually removed after the completion of the synthesis using bases such as ammonia. A similar strategy is also used to remove protecting groups for reactive amino groups ($-NH_2$) present in the nitrogenous bases (shown in pink in Figure 6.1 is benzoyl Bz protecting group).

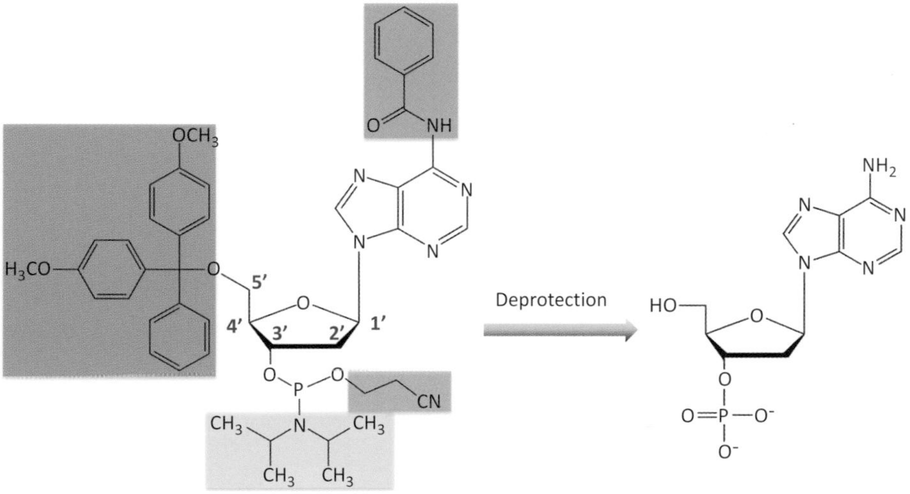

Figure 6.1

Adenosine phosphoramidite with protecting groups used to afford efficient chemical synthesis and prevent cross-reactions; dimethoxytrityl (DMT, green), benzoyl (Bz, pink), diisopropylamino group (yellow) and 2-cyanoethyl (orange).

Before the synthesis, a first base in the growing chain is immobilised onto a solid support in the form of nucleoside phosphoramidite (Back to Basics 6.2). Widely used solid supports are **controlled pore glass (CPG)** and **porous polystyrene beads**, which are easy to modify and cleave, and inert to reagents used for oligonucleotide synthesis.

Depending on the scale of the synthesis, solid carriers can be packed into columns of different dimensions, which can range from 0.05 ml to several litres. By varying the pore size of CPG from 50 to 300 nm, different lengths of oligonucleotides (50–200 bases) can be prepared. However, the yields are significantly decreased on 50 nm CPG when oligonucleotides with more than 40 bases are prepared. The reason for this is limited diffusion of the reagents due to the blockage of the pores caused by growing oligonucleotide. Larger pore CPGs are more fragile but also more suitable for preparation of longer oligonucleotides. For example, 100 nm CPGs can be used for the synthesis of oligonucleotides up to 100 bases, and 200 nm for even larger chains. Porous polystyrene beads are often employed in a small-scale synthesis due to high ligand loading and good moisture exclusion, both of which improve the efficiency of coupling reactions of water-sensitive phosphoramidites.

Back to Basics 6.2   A Single Cycle of the Phosphoramidite Coupling

The phosphoramidite reaction cycle for the synthesis of single-stranded DNA strands involves several steps described below:

deblocking of the 5′-hydroxyl group by treatment with dichloroacetic acid (usually 3% in dichloromethane)

activation with a tetrazole solution

coupling of the nucleoside phosphoramidite to a 3′-end of support-bound growing oligonucleotide. The chain elongation occurs in 3′ → 5′ direction; the phosphoramidites are usually used in excess and due to their

> high reactivity should be handled exclusively under inert reaction
> conditions
>
> **masking** of the non-reacted 5'-OH groups (**capping**) by treatment with
> acetic anhydride and *N*-methylimidazole in order to avoid the forma-
> tion of undesired sequences
>
> **oxidation** of the tri-coordinated phosphite triester linkage to tetra-
> coordinated phosphate triester by treatment with iodine and water in
> the presence of bases such as pyridine.
>
> Further growth is achieved by the addition of the next nucleoside phos-
> phoramidite after the **detritylation** step. When the desired length is
> obtained, the oligonucleotide is cleaved from the solid support by treatment
> with 25% ammonia hydroxide solution (or alternative methods that can
> achieve alkaline conditions) at increased temperature (usually within
> 5 hours at 55 °C).

After attachment to a solid support of choice, protected nucleoside
phosphoramidite goes through a sequence of deprotection and coupling
reactions that result in oligonucleotide growth. Since the reaction between
two nucleotides does not proceed in quantitative yield (the yield per chain
elongation step is mostly around 99%), short chain oligonucleotides are
present in the system alongside desired longer sequences. As a consequence, synthesised oligonucleotides need to be purified, usually by gel
electrophoresis or reversed-phase high-performance liquid chromatography
(HPLC).

Today, short DNA strands (up to 150 bases) can be synthesised in a
relatively straightforward manner using commercially available DNA synthesisers (Figure 6.2). Using the phosphoramidite strategy numerous modifications can be introduced to oligonucleotides either on 5' and 3' end or
internally through direct modification of a base.

As a consequence, a large number of modified oligonucleotides that differ
in length, sequence and functional groups is available. Custom synthesised
DNA oligos cost approximately 0.35 euro per base at a 25 nmol synthesis
scale, and have become a useful tool for functionalisation of materials (Chapter 4) as well as for design of DNA-based biosensors and complex DNA
shapes (more on this in Sections 6.5 and 6.6).

Figure 6.2

A row of DNA synthesisers for continuous DNA production. Courtesy of Integrated DNA Technologies (idtdna.com).

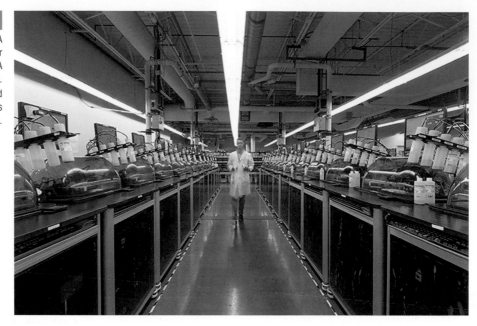

6.2   DNA As an Immobilisation Tool

We have already explored the use of DNA-directed immobilisation for functionalisation of nanomaterials in Chapter 4 (see Figure 4.13). In order to use DNA as an immobilisation tool, a DNA strand needs to be attached to the desired surface (magnetic bead, planar surface, nanoparticle) allowing for the binding of the complementary strand and formation of a double helix, a process referred to as **DNA hybridisation**. DNA hybridisation is enabled by hydrogen bonding between specific pairs of bases (A will bind to T and G to C), base stacking and hydrophobic interaction. The thermodynamic stability of a double helix is determined by the length and the sequence of complementary single DNA strands as well as the presence and the concentration of the salt in the solution. In the absence or at very low concentration of salts such as magnesium chloride ($MgCl_2$), the negative charges on neighbouring phosphate groups are not shielded, resulting in repulsion and helix destabilisation. Very small double helices are also unstable, and about eight bases must be paired for a double helix to be stable at room temperature.

DNA-directed immobilisation (DDI) employs hybridisation of complementary DNA strands to modify large variety of surfaces. It can be used in applications ranging from protein structuring (Figure 6.3) to immobilisation of living cells to explore cell signalling (Research Report 6.1).

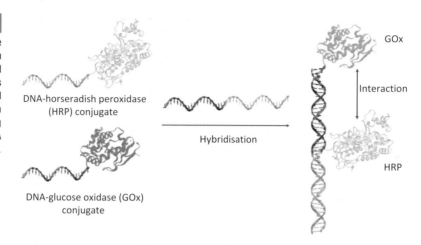

Figure 6.3

Controlling the distance between horseradish peroxide (HRP) and glucose (GOx) proteins using DNA directed immobilisation of both proteins onto a long single-stranded DNA carrier.

The important step for DNA-directed immobilisation is the preparation of modified DNA strands. Small functional groups can often be introduced directly during solid phase synthesis. Amino–, thiol– and biotin–DNAs are readily available from commercial sources and have been used extensively for attachment of various species ranging from small molecules to larger proteins to oligonucleotides.

Research Report 6.1   DNA-Directed Immobilisation to Study Signalling in a Live Cell

Dynamic signalling pathways within cells are not trivial to study, although significant progress has been made with the help of fluorescent protein technology, which enabled real-time exploration of the life and fate of single proteins. Signalling pathways are usually initiated through inter-action with a protein receptor on the surface of the cell. A cell has many of these receptors, which are precisely positioned at defined distances from each other across the cell surface. Activation of a receptor by a protein, peptide or small molecule triggers a signalling cascade that can fork into several pathways. But how can we study this process in real time and in the single cell?

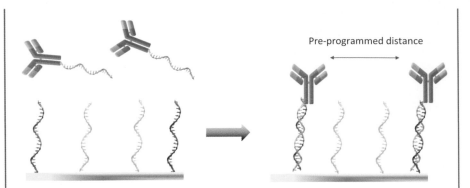

One way is through controlled activation of the receptor such as done by Gandor et al. (2013). They immobilised antibodies that specifically bind to the receptors and activate two signalling pathways. The activation resulted in the attachment of fluorescently labelled proteins to the transmembrane protein's inner membrane domains. DNA-directed immobilisation was used to precisely immobilise antibodies at distances that correspond to the receptor geometry on the surface of the cell, and induce simultaneous activation of the two pathways.

In short, when a cell is added to the surface, each antibody activates a receptor, which in turn activates an intracellular pathway that results in binding of fluorescently labelled protein to the membrane allowing for fluorescence read-out of the activation.

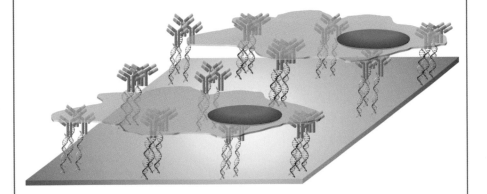

But why use DDI and not attach the antibody directly to the surface? DNA immobilisation has significant advantages over direct chemical immobilisation. The length of DNA can be easily adjusted to control the distance from the surface and prevent any deactivation of the molecules or cells. Antibodies have been shown to bind to antigens more efficiently when immobilised through DNA, most probably due to diminished steric hindrance and more flexibility in terms of orientation. Reproducibility and homogeneity of the surface are also increased, and different antibodies can be attached to the surface without getting damaged, which is often the case when they are directly immobilised through chemical strategies. Finally, DNA-directed immobilisation is a reversible process, and the surface can be easily regenerated for another experiment by heating up or washing with a basic solution.

Preparation of protein–DNA conjugates usually requires DNA strands to be modified with functional groups adjusted to the nature of the specific protein. Such functional groups can either coordinate protein tags, bind covalently to available amino acids on the surface of the protein, or be inserted specifically into the protein through, for example, cofactor reconstitution. Many of the strategies we discussed in Chapter 4, which are employed for attachment of proteins to nanomaterials, can also be used to prepare DNA–protein conjugates (Figure 6.4).

The most common non-covalent methodologies usually employ streptavidin–biotin interaction or protein tags, the requirement being that DNA is modified with the tag binding moiety prior to conjugation. Non-covalent approaches often result in protein–DNA conjugates which are sensitive to temperature or pH and prone to dissociation, making them unsuitable for applications that require the use of complex biological fluids. More robust covalent linkages provide the chemical stability often needed in biosensing applications. A variety of covalent strategies have been used for DNA–protein conjugation and they often rely on the use of oligonucleotides containing amine, thiol or click chemistry groups. Amines and thiols can be used directly with natural amino acids, but other functional groups usually require an additional modification of the protein to introduce a suitable reactive group, most often through lysine, cysteine or tyrosine residues, or through the introduction of artificial amino acids (Lee et al., 2009).

6.3   DNA–Nanoparticle Conjugates

The DNA–gold nanoparticle (DNA–Au) conjugates first prepared in 1996 (Mirkin et al., 1996) laid the foundation for a vast number of DNA–nanomaterial conjugates that followed. Two methods are commonly used to

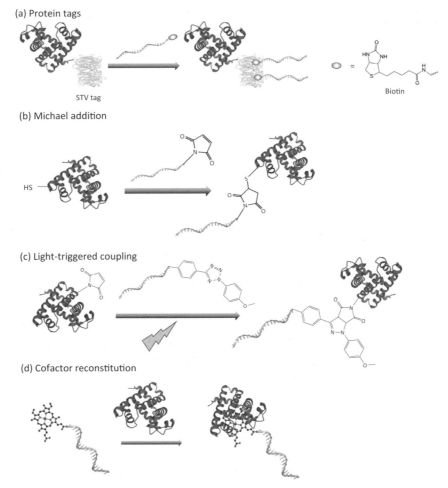

(a) Protein tags

STV tag

Biotin

(b) Michael addition

HS

(c) Light-triggered coupling

(d) Cofactor reconstitution

add DNA onto the nanoparticle surface: either ligand exchange strategy using suitably modified oligonucleotides or direct coupling of oligonucleotides to surface ligands present on nanoparticles. Gold–DNA conjugates are commonly prepared using ligand exchange of the surface stabilising ligand with thiol-modified DNA, whereas metal oxide nanoparticles are usually first coated with a bifunctional linker such as dopamine-maleimide and then allowed to react either with thiol (Michael addition), furan (Diels–Alder cycloaddition) or tetrazole (photo-click reaction) modified DNA.

Once prepared, DNA–nanoparticle conjugates can be used for DNA-directed immobilisation of various molecules, attachment to different surfaces or preparation of larger hierarchical nanoparticle structures through DNA hybridisation with nanoparticles containing complementary strands (Figure 6.5).

Figure 6.5

DNA–nanoparticle conjugates are useful tools in bionanotechnology. They can be used for (a) immobilisation of biomolecules, (b) design of nanoparticle coated surfaces and (c) preparation of larger 3D nanoparticle assemblies.

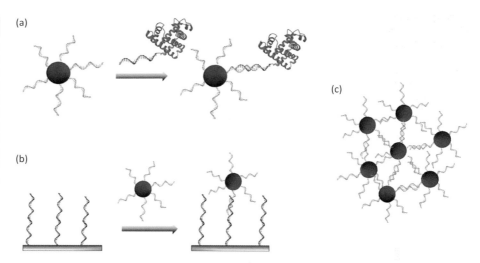

These larger nanoparticle structures can be programmed in such a way to assemble only in the presence of a particular DNA sequence, and such a strategy is used for the design of biosensors for DNA detection in the solution. A simple yet sensitive gold nanoparticle DNA sensor can be made using two batches of nanoparticles modified with short DNA strands with a different base sequence. These strands are not complementary to each other but bind to a larger, target DNA, which can be a whole gene or situated within a gene sequence that needs to be detected. When a target DNA is present in the solution, hybridisation of nanoparticle–DNA conjugates will lead to the assembly of gold nanoparticles, which results in a change of colour (red to violet) due to the interacting plasmons (Figure 6.6).

Figure 6.6

The principle of colorimetric gold nanoparticle-based DNA sensor. DNA hybridisation drives the aggregation of DNA–gold conjugates resulting in the colour change.

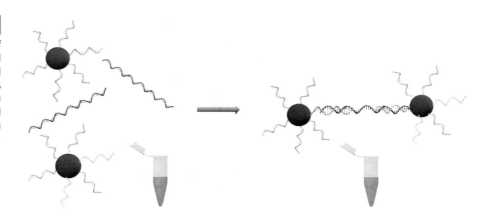

This is the principle of colorimetric gold nanoparticle-based DNA sensor, which can be used for the detection of genes or gene mutations. Different variations of this principle have been used to prepare efficient biosensors employing other classes of plasmonic nanomaterials.

DNA–nanoparticle conjugates are particularly suitable for controlled assembly of nanoparticle elements into different spatial arrangements. Use of nanoparticles modified with complementary strands usually results in large three-dimensional assemblies such as shown in Figure 6.7a. Linear geometry can be achieved using a template-assisted approach in which a template DNA strand is employed for hybridisation of smaller strands containing nanoparticle anchoring groups in a 180° angle to each other (Figure 6.7b). Following nanoparticle binding, template DNA is removed and successively added to the solution to afford a linear assembly of nanoparticles. When flexible geometrical shapes are needed, branched DNA structures obtained by covalent coupling of two DNA strands to a cyclic dithiol can be employed as building blocks (Figure 6.7c). These and similar strategies led to the design of responsive materials useful for biosensing (Peng and Miller, 2011).

An interesting application of DNA–nanoparticle conjugates is DNA barcoding. In zoology, DNA barcoding has been used since 2003 for identification of species through labelling of their short gene regions. Such genetic taxonomy is used to distinguish various species on the basis of their genetic code. DNA barcoding has also been successfully adopted in bionanotechnology, for the design of biosensors and identification of various molecular species in biological samples. Similar to barcodes used to identify products in shops, DNA can be used to identify biomolecules. Whereas traditional barcodes encode data by varying the widths and spacing of parallel lines, DNA encoded information is contained within its unique sequence. Considering the number of possible combinations of DNA bases within a particular oligonucleotide length, a large number of unique DNA barcodes are available for tagging. A successful application of DNA barcoding is the use of barcode DNA-labelled gold nanoparticles to identify unknown biospecies in complex biological samples.

Let us imagine we need to check which one of five protein biomarkers (P1, P2, P3, P4, P5) for cardiac disease is present in a patient's blood sample. We do not know which biomarkers are released into the blood and in which amount, but it is crucial that their presence is detected at the early stage of the disease when the concentration is so small that it evades detection by standard methods such as direct antibody staining. Taking into account such low amounts of a biomarker, as is often the case in biological samples, the first step in our biosensing protocol has to be the separation of the target

Figure 6.7

Controlled assembly of
nanoparticles using (a)
monothiol-modified
nanoparticles, (b)
template-assisted
immobilisation and (c)
branched DNA structures
for flexible assembly of
different geometries.

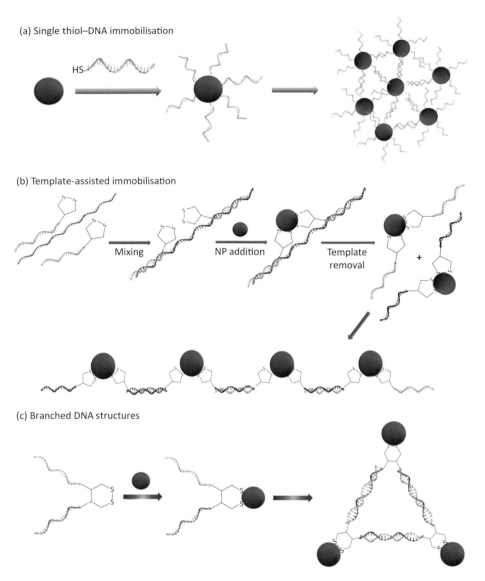

(a) Single thiol–DNA immobilisation

(b) Template-assisted immobilisation

Mixing   NP addition   Template
removal

(c) Branched DNA structures

protein from other proteins in the solution. This is best done using antibody-labelled magnetic particles (MP). As we do not know which biomarker is present in our sample, five antibody-MPs each containing one antibody specific to one of five cardiac biomarkers (Ab1-MP, Ab2-MP, Ab3-MP, Ab4-MP and Ab5-MP) are added to the patient's sample. Antibody-MP binds to protein antigen and can be concentrated using magnetic separation. After this is done, we need to identify which biomarker (if any) is bound to MP. The standard method would employ a secondary antibody labelled with a fluorophore, but fluorescence cannot be detected below a certain limiting concentration. In addition, it would be expensive to label five antibodies with five different fluorophores (remember that we do not know which one of five biomarkers we have in the sample) that do not cross-talk and interfere with the fluorescence read-out.

Enter DNA barcoding. A number of unique DNA barcodes is huge, much larger than the number of available antibodies, and we can easily pick DNA sequences that will code for a secondary antibody. In our particular case, we need only five sequences. The secondary antibody can be labelled with a DNA barcode directly, but antibodies are sensitive proteins and the conjugation of DNA can be both expensive and detrimental to their binding ability. To avoid direct antibody–DNA conjugation, we can use gold nanoparticles as carriers of both the secondary antibodies and DNA barcodes. Each DNA barcode corresponds to one secondary antibody; D^1 to Ab1, D^2 to Ab2, D^3 to Ab3 and so on. Gold nanoparticle-Ab^x-D^x binds to the protein biomarker attached to the magnetic particle. Following another round of magnetic separation, D^x is released from the gold nanoparticle by the destruction of thiol–gold bonds usually by the addition of dithiothreitol (DTT). Hundreds of D^x strands are present on the surface of gold nanoparticles, and all of them are released into solution. Once released, D^x can be identified using commercial DNA-chip technology and correlated to an antibody, ultimately leading to the identification of the protein biomarker (Figure 6.8). Detection of a D^2 barcode would mean that a gold nanoparticle carrying antibody Ab2 was bound to a target antigen identifying protein 2 (P2) as the one present in the patient's sample.

Figure 6.8

Use of DNA barcodes to identify (a) the presence of an antigen or (b) gene or target DNA in a complex biological fluid. MP stands for magnetic particle, which can be nm or µm sized.

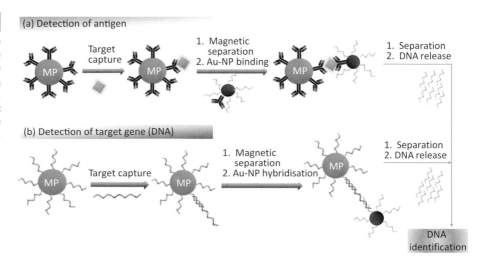

In DNA barcoding, short oligonucleotides are used as labels which store data that enable identification of a particular species or biological interaction in complex samples. Such an approach is particularly useful for detection of pathogens such as viruses and bacteria, or as explained earlier, biomarker proteins related to various diseases in early stages when they are present in low amounts. Nanoparticle-bound DNA barcodes enable fast read-out and improved detection limits, and have found applications beyond biosensing, and also been used in drug screening and investigation of nanoparticle interaction with biological systems (Paunovska et al., 2018).

6.4   DNA for Material Design: DNA Hydrogels

DNA is not only interesting for the structuring of nanomaterials or design of nanostructures, as we will explore later, but could be used for the preparation of various macroscopic materials. As we have already mentioned in Chapter 3, DNA is a biopolymer composed of four repeating elements (bases) and this has been utilised to make polymeric materials such as **DNA hydrogels** either entirely made of DNA strands or combined with other polymers. Hydrogels are cross-linked polymeric networks with a distinct three-dimensional structure, which can absorb large amounts of water and can often adapt to their environment and external stimuli (see Back to Basics 2.5). Such responsiveness is primarily associated with swelling and water release mediated by a change in temperature, pH, ionic strength, solvent and type of photon flux. We usually distinguish between chemical (held together by covalent bonds between individual elements) and physical (held together by weak forces such as hydrogen bonds) hydrogels. Both classes of DNA hydrogels can be prepared using either enzymatic reactions to covalently link DNA strands, or direct hybridisation of complementary regions of employed DNA building blocks. Interestingly, some DNA hydrogels have unusual properties (Research Report 6.2) that depend on the water content and are finding numerous applications, in particular in biomedical areas.

Research Report 6.2	DNA Hydrogels

Using a combination of **rolling circle amplification (RCA**; explained later in Back to Basics 6.3) and another amplification method called **multi-primed chain amplification (MCA)**, Lee et al. (2009) prepared extremely long DNA with regions that can hybridise to each other resulting in a physically linked hydrogel. Prepared hydrogel had unusual macroscale properties stemming from never before observed hierarchical structure consisting of bird's nest-like smaller structures woven together throughout the gel:

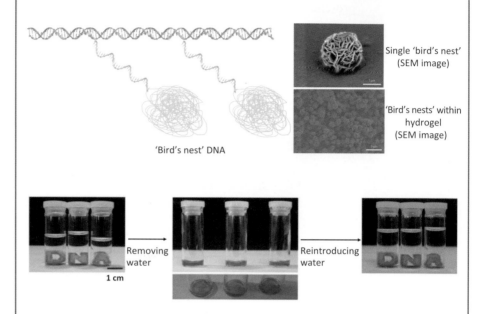

Source: Reprinted by permission from Springer Nature: Lee et al. (2012).

When DNA hydrogel is immersed in water, it exhibits solid-like properties and it can easily be moulded using different shaped templates. After the water is removed, the hydrogel is exposed to air and, as it is extremely soft, collapses under the surface tension and the gravitational force. Addition of water leads again to a reconstitution of the original shape. Switching between two hydrogel shapes happens very quickly (within a few seconds), and can clearly be controlled by the addition and removal of water.

Such materials can be applied as scaffolds for cell seeding and growth, or the cell-free production of proteins (Lee et al., 2012).

DNA hydrogel named P-gel system was prepared that acts as a protein factory, producing functional proteins in absence of the living cell (known as **cell-free protein synthesis**) and with the efficiency about 300 times higher than other solution-based cell-free protocols (Park et al., 2009). Other hydrogels have been shown to enable sustained delivery of drugs over longer periods of time and can be used for triggered drug release using irradiation, pH change or heating (Shahbazi et al., 2018).

In fact, one of the major advantages of hydrogels is the ability to tune their properties by external stimuli, which is particularly desirable for the design of sensors. For example, enzyme-sensitive regions can be incorporated into DNA and the changes in gel properties can be used to detect the presence or absence of a particular enzyme. Or light-sensitive groups can be added that are activated when irradiated, releasing DNA damaging species that can cleave the hydrogel structure and cause a change in mechanical properties.

Slightly less explored, but nevertheless interesting, are hybrid structures made of DNA and other types of polymers such as poly-lysines, PEG or polyacrylamide, and various other polymeric species. Within such hybrids, DNA hybridisation is usually used as a cross-linking strategy to design reversible polymers that can respond to pH or various proteins, and be potentially used for biomedical applications.

6.5   DNA Nanostructuring

Structural properties such as 3.4 nm helical repeats (Chapter 3), base pairing/strand recognition, stability and a unique combination of stiffness and flexibility turned DNA into a versatile building block used to assemble a range of nanostructures. DNA structuring potential was first highlighted in a theoretical paper by Ned Seeman, a pioneer of DNA nanotechnology with a strong background in crystallography, which enabled him to grasp the structural power of the double helix (Seeman, 1982).

Theoretical predictions resulted in DNA assemblies obtained from carefully designed short single-stranded oligonucleotides. One of the first and simplest forms to be made was a quadruplex structure with a stable branching point referred to as a **four-armed junction** (Figure 6.9).

Figure 6.9

Four-armed junction assembled using four different DNA strands (a), and the naturally occurring Holliday junction (b).

(a)   (b)

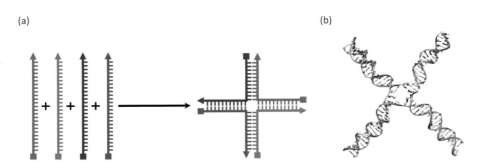

Design of the four-armed junction was inspired by the naturally occurring Holliday junction, a DNA structure formed during the process of genetic recombination in which two double-stranded DNAs exchange their content. Holliday junctions are unstable and short-lived, but Ned Seeman and his team obtained stable four-arm junction by redesigning the sequences and removing the symmetry from the branches. Holliday junctions are not the only multi-strand DNA structures found in nature. There are also three-stranded structures known as replication forks formed, as you can guess, during the process of DNA replication. However, such multi-branched DNA structures are often unstable, they are transition states and designed to have short lifetimes, and therefore not easily reproduced out of living systems. Ned Seeman and his coworkers, many of whom became leaders in the field of DNA nanotechnology, developed the concept of designer DNA structures, which are stable, long-lived and can be assembled from short, chemically synthesised single-stranded DNA. Soon it became clear that a set of rules can be established to select for sequences that result in the most stable structures. Several distinct architectural elements – such as shown in Figure 6.10a–f: **helical regions**, **sticky ends**, **bulge loops**, **loops**, **junctions** and **crossovers** – were also introduced to improve the stability and flexibility of larger DNA nanostructures.

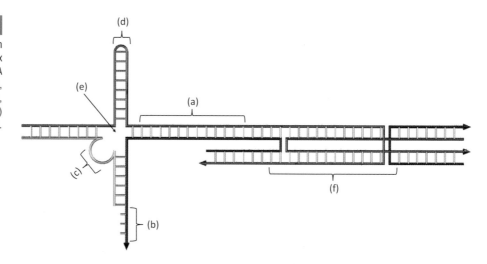

Figure 6.10

Basic structural forms in the design of complex DNA structures. (a) DNA helices, (b) sticky ends, (c) bulge loops, (d) loops, (e) junctions and (f) crossovers.

Assemblies of different levels of complexity can be obtained by varying the length and sequence of oligonucleotides. Smaller assembled structures can further be joined into more complex or larger shapes in a process similar to LEGO assembly. Whereas in LEGO, building blocks are assembled using fitted geometrical shapes on the surface, DNA structures are connected using sticky ends (Figure 6.10b), short single-stranded sequences added to the ends of the DNA structures. Complementary sticky ends enable spontaneous pairing of smaller DNA elements, leading to larger assemblies (Figure 6.11); they are DNA-based molecular glue. Conveniently, this sticky-end hybridisation process can also be reversed by heating or addition of competitive complementary strands, leading to controllable assembly–disassembly processes.

Figure 6.11

Assembly of larger lattice structures from DNA tiles using sticky-end hybridisation.

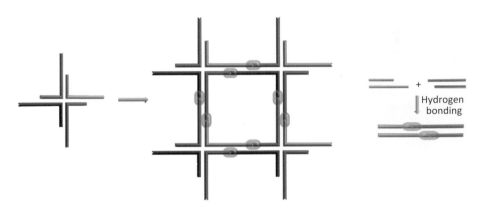

The simplest elements in DNA assembly are often called **DNA tiles** and large assemblies can be obtained by careful design of sticky ends within tiles. Arrays can further be turned into more complex 3D structures with the addition of shaping DNA sequences, which act as pillars for construction of 3D DNA shapes.

The simplest way of adding complexity to planar 2D structures is the introduction of small single-stranded oligonucleotides called **protruding arms** at certain positions within DNA arrays. As the name hints, such oligonucleotides protrude from the planar structure and can serve as anchors for immobilisation of various species such as proteins or nanoparticles through DNA-directed immobilisation (Figure 6.12; Zhang et al., 2006). Using protruding arms a large number of different elements can be attached to the arrays in a programmed way. Providing that the rules of complementarity and base pairing are respected, anything containing a complementary strand can be attached to designer DNA structures.

Figure 6.12

DNA–gold nanoparticles assembled onto 2D arrays using hybridisation through protruding DNA arms. Adapted with permission from Zhang et al. (2006). © 2006 American Chemical Society.

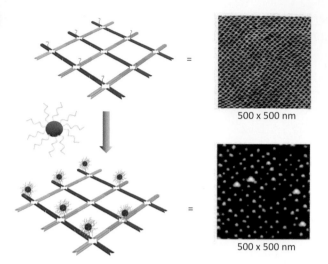

500 x 500 nm

500 x 500 nm

The beauty of this initial DNA nanostructuring strategy lies in its simplicity. Once individual strands are synthesised, they are mixed in a solution containing a small concentration of salt such as magnesium chloride ($MgCl_2$), heated to $90\,°C$ to break any double helices which are spontaneously formed, and then cooled down slowly to allow for the self-assembly. Remarkably, well-designed 2D DNA nanostructures can often be produced in yields close to 100%.

Three-dimensional structures require more careful design of sequences and are usually done in a sequence of several assembly and purification steps. They also require a larger number of individual DNA strands, and structures obtained are often irregular due to the competitive hybridisation and less control over the assembly. In addition, each purification step ultimately results in the loss of DNA, low yields and tedious and time-consuming structuring process.

As we already noted, DNA nanostructuring became a lively research field only after cheap oligonucleotides became available through solid phase synthesis. However, it is worth keeping in mind that chemical synthesis is limited by the yield of each synthetic step, which is never 100%. As a consequence, only short oligonucleotides with sizes up to 150 bases can be made in satisfactory yields. If longer strands are needed, enzymatically driven elongation using DNA polymerases can be employed. However, assembling long DNA strands into programmable 2D and 3D shapes is a challenging task, which requires significant expertise, lots of patience and more than a solid financial background.

To overcome the challenges of complex DNA shape design, a new approach was introduced in 2004 based on the use of 1700-base DNA (Shih

Figure 6.13

Three dimensional DNA structures assembled using 1700 bases long DNA scaffold and a handful of shorter folding strands.
Reprinted by permission from Springer Nature: Shih et al. (2004). https://doi.org/10.1038/nature02307.

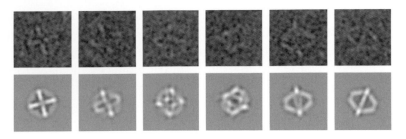

et al., 2004). Such a long DNA scaffold was assembled into defined 3D shapes using five smaller DNA strands (Figure 6.13), and this strategy spearheaded the development of **DNA origami** – named after the ancient Japanese art of paper folding (*ori* standing for folding and *kami* for paper).

6.6   DNA Origami

The term DNA origami was coined by Paul Rothemund in 2006 to describe the method of folding long circular single-stranded DNA (7250 bases) isolated from M13 bacteriophage virus to custom shapes with the help of a number of short oligonucleotide strands (Rothemund, 2006; Figure 6.14). Nanostructures prepared using DNA origami strategy are characterised by higher yields and larger diversity in terms of shape, size and mechanical flexibility than conventional DNA nanostructuring using only smaller DNA strands.

Figure 6.14

Different shapes designed using the DNA folding process known as DNA origami. The top two rows show different designs (a–f), and the bottom two rows AFM images of the folded structures.
Reprinted by permission from Springer Nature: Rothemund, 2006. https://doi.org/10.1038/nature04586.

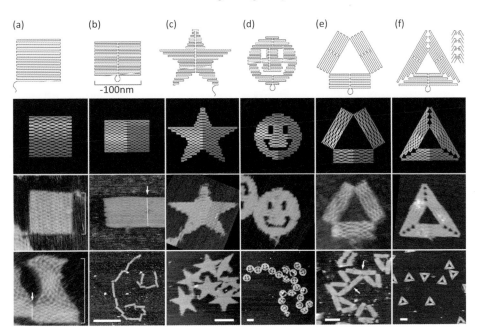

Short single-stranded oligonucleotides which are used to fold the viral DNA scaffold are referred to as **staple strands** and usually contain between 20 to 50 bases. The long scaffold strand has a unique non-repeating sequence, and the power of DNA origami lies in the simplicity of shape formation. Unlike the first complex 3D nanostructures, which are made in a stepwise manner with intermittent washing sequences, DNA origami shapes are formed by mixing staples with the scaffold strand, and allowing for slow, thermally controlled annealing as illustrated in Figure 6.15. Conventional two-dimensional DNA origami structures are comprised of helix rows stabilised by a regular progression of crossovers, which are usually replicated every 1.5 helical turn or 16 bases of B-DNA structure (see Chapter 3). Ultimately, alternating crossovers can be found every 180 degrees, resulting in a folding of the helices into a planar shape. By changing the crossover angles between two helices within the structure, the folding of three-dimensional structures can be achieved (Sacca and Niemeyer, 2012). Approximately 200 short stable strands are required to prepare a simple 100 × 100 nm rectangle such as shown in Figure 6.15.

Figure 6.15

Two-dimensional shape folding using DNA origami strategy starting from a viral circular single-stranded DNA scaffold. Short staple DNA strands are annealed to the scaffold during slow cooling of the solution to afford different shapes. Schematic representation of origami design is shown in the bottom row, as well as AFM images of rectangular DNA origami.

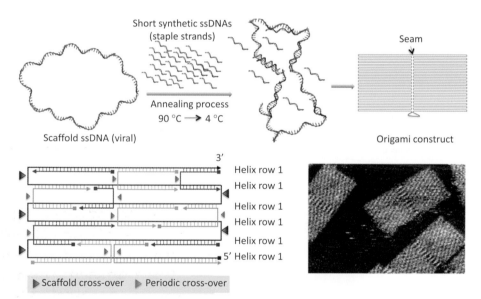

Taking into account the cost of their synthesis (0.30 euro per base for 25 nmol scale), the cost for staple strands needed for origami folding amounts to around 2000 euro. The cost was one of the biggest obstacles to practical applications of origami, but new routes are continuously being developed to reduce the expense. Another challenge is the size of the starting scaffold strand, which ultimately limits the size of the final origami shape to approximately 100 nm. To overcome this limitation, other scaffolds have been introduced such as long circular DNA prepared by rolling circle amplification (RCA, Back to Basics 6.3) or a 51 466 base long single-stranded DNA isolated from a hybrid M13 virus (Marchi et al., 2014). Larger structures can also be assembled from smaller origamis with the help of bridge strands.

Whereas the first publication of the DNA origami principle in 2006 demonstrated that two-dimensional structures such as rectangles, triangles and stars can be assembled from a viral template, more complex geometrical forms and 3D structures quickly followed. Origami tubes, cages and movable structures such as DNA-box with lid (Andersen, 2009) that can open or close by the addition of a 'key' DNA strands (Figure 6.16), were all successfully made. Several software packages such as **CaDNAno** developed in William Shih's group at MIT (Douglas et al., 2009) and **Tiamat** (Williams et al., 2009) are available to aid the design of appropriate staple sequences.

Back to Basics 6.3	Rolling Circle Amplification

Rolling circle amplification (RCA), first introduced by Eric T. Kool in the 1990s, describes a simple and efficient enzymatic process used for the amplification of DNA or RNA from very small amounts of starting material (Mohsen and Kool, 2016). Unlike polymerase chain reaction, which requires thermocycler and thermostable enzyme polymerase, RCA can be performed at a constant temperature (room temperature to 37 °C) in solution, on a solid support or in a complex biological environment (e.g. inside the cell). During RCA, polymerase continuously adds single nucleotides to a primer that is annealed to a circular template resulting in a long nucleic acid strand of tens to hundreds of repetitive sequences complementary to the circular template.

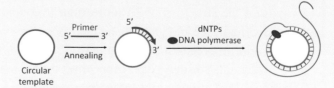

Four components are required for a successful RCA: (1) DNA or RNA polymerase (e.g. Phi29, Bst or Vent exo-DNA polymerases for DNA and

T7 RNA polymerase for RNA) with suitable buffer; (2) a short DNA or RNA primer; (3) a circular DNA template (15–200 nucleotides in length); and (4) deoxyribonucleotides (dNTPs).

Gel electrophoresis is most commonly used to determine the success of RCA. Additionally, fluorescent dyes can be incorporated into RCA product via fluorophore-labelled dNTPs or via hybridisation with fluorophore-tethered complementary strand and analysed by various fluorescence-based techniques.

RCA has been mainly used for the development of sensitive detection methods for various targets including DNA, RNA, proteins, small molecules, and cells. In bionanotechnology, RCA is widely employed in the design of complex DNA nanostructures such as DNA origami and as a template for the controlled periodic assembly of nanosized objects.

Figure 6.16

DNA origami box with a movable lid which can be opened by hybridisation of the 'key' DNA strands with complementary protruding DNA strands within the box.
Adapted by permission from Springer Nature: Andersen et al. (2009).

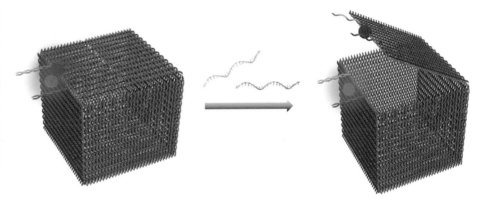

To enable further modification of DNA origami, protruding arms and short staple strands containing various functional groups can be introduced within the structure. With more than 200 unique staple strands, which can individually be modified at defined positions with a resolution up to 6 nm, decoration possibilities are numerous.

Origami strategy has been one of the fastest growing fields within bionanotechnology and, with the continuous development of new scaffold strands and strategies to make reproducible three-dimensional shapes, it is to be expected that the range of applications will be expanded in the near future.

6.7   DNA Origami: Applications

6.7.1   Origami-Guided Assembly

In Chapter 1 we defined plasmons as collective oscillations of conductive band electrons in metal nanoparticles. **Plasmonics** studies the interaction of plasmons with light and the use of this phenomena in biosensing, surface-enhanced Raman and fluorescence spectroscopy (Chapter 5), optics and energy transfer. The plasmonic effect depends on the type, but also on the proximity of metal nanoparticles, and optical behaviour is highly distance dependent. In order to achieve and control plasmon interactions, nanoparticles need to be positioned close to each other in a precisely controlled way, which is not easy to achieve. DNA nanostructuring and in particular DNA origami offer unprecedented structural adaptability, and nanoscale precision, particularly suited for nanoparticle assembly. Origami can enable immobilisation of NPs in a programmed way with <10 nm spacing to allow plasmon coupling. Such small distances between nanoparticles as well as their orientation in space can be employed to generate extremely high field enhancement for construction of nanolenses or conductive nanowires. Preparation of origami-based plasmonic nanostructures relies on modification of nanoparticles with single-stranded DNA (see Section 6.3 for more) and their subsequent hybridisation to carefully positioned protruding arms (Figure 6.17; Schreiber, 2013). Noble metal nanoparticles of different shapes have been immobilised onto various origami structures affording the library of plasmonic materials.

Figure 6.17

Assembly of gold nanoparticles into a plasmonic system using DNA origami. Reprinted by permission from Springer Nature: Schreiber (2013).

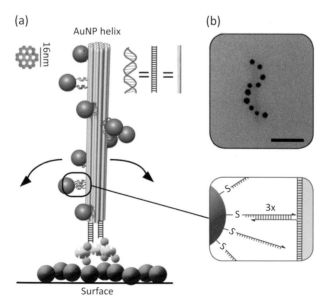

Equally exciting is the use of origami to act as a platform for the precise positioning of proteins. The advantage of origami-guided protein assembly is two-fold: first, various proteins can be brought together to study their interactions and second, sensing or light-harvesting devices can be designed, which benefit from precise positioning of proteins and enzymes. For immobilisation of proteins, protruding DNA strands are employed which either contain protein-binding groups or can be directly hybridised to protein–DNA conjugates. Binding groups depend largely on the type of the protein and the ease of functionalisation and often comprise of either protein tag binders, small interacting molecules (i.e. cofactors) or functional groups that react with surface amino acids, many of which we have already mentioned in Chapter 4. Figure 6.18 illustrates an early example of protein array design using origami strategy. Planar origami with regularly spaced well-like structures was assembled to enable positioning of streptavidin proteins with the help of biotin-containing protruding arms positioned within wells (Kuzuya, 2009).

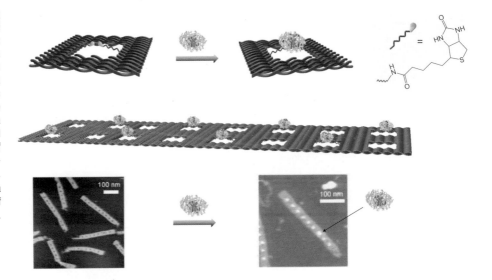

Figure 6.18

Protein nanoarrays designed using DNA origami: biotin incorporated as a DNA protruding arm is used to immobilise streptavidin protein in a regular, pre-designed pattern. AFM images of empty (left) and protein-filled wells (right). Adapted from Kuzuya (2009), by permission of John Wiley and Sons.

Protein–origami arrays can be used for whole cell immobilisation (cell receptors can be precisely positioned to interact with proteins on a cell surface), biosensing, drug screening and, interestingly, also for studying single molecule behaviour (Research Report 6.3).

As well as for immobilisation of nanoparticles and proteins, DNA-guided assembly can be employed for encapsulation of proteins. In general, proteins have a different level of stability but are generally very sensitive to changes in

Research Report 6.3	DNA Origami for Studying Chemical Reactions at the Single Molecule Level

One of the most interesting aspects of (bio)chemistry is to be able to study various events at or close to the single molecule level. This is being enabled by the development of super-resolution fluorescence microscopy and a range of advanced spectroscopies, which often require expensive instrumentation. Origami, on the other hand, can provide information on reaction conditions or protein behaviour with the help of AFM microscopy as demonstrated by Voigt et al. (2010).

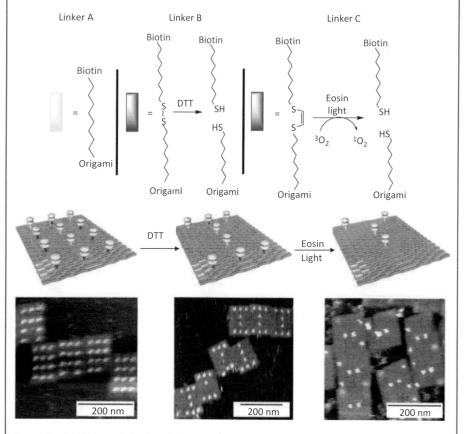

Source: Reprinted by permission from Springer Nature: Voigt et al. (2010).

Removal of the proteins immobilised onto an origami square using three types of linkers was employed to explore reaction conditions. Each linker can be cleaved using different chemical reagents, with protein removal acting as an identifier of a particular reaction. Out of 12 positions, 4 linkers contained a non-cleavable linker type A, and 4 had a linker type B which contains a disulfide moiety that can be cleaved by DTT-mediated reduction. The final four positions contain an electron-rich thiol-ethene moiety, which can be cleaved by singlet oxygen generated with light in the presence of a singlet oxygen photosensitiser Eosin.

Such an approach to studying chemical reactions enables selective monitoring of chemical reactions offering a fundamental insight into the conditions required for reactions to proceed in a biological setting. And all of this is done using relatively straightforward AFM monitoring.

pH, temperature, salt concentrations and solvent combinations. Such sensitivity limits their applications in catalysis (enzymes) or design of biotherapeutics and requires carefully controlled storage conditions if they can be stored at all. Encapsulation of proteins can be achieved using porous materials or polymeric species such as hydrogels, but DNA origami enables encapsulation of a single protein molecule. Most of the early origami-based encapsulation strategies involved the use of protein tags or covalent chemical conjugation, which requires protein modification that can result in deactivation or loss of structural integrity. More recent strategies are utilising principles of supramolecular interactions, and origami capsules have been designed that adapt to the shape of the proteins creating a perfect host–guest complex in which protein encapsulation is guided by non-covalent interactions only (Sprengel et al., 2017).

6.7.2   DNA Origami for Drug Delivery

Among the advantages of DNA structured materials are their biocompatibility and increased stability in biological fluids as densely packed DNA regions prevent binding of any cleaving enzymes. In addition, reproducible shapes and structures can be made, which are chemically adaptable and relatively easy to assemble. All of these properties make origami structures suitable for design of nanocarriers to deliver both small molecules or biomolecular (proteins, nucleic acid, peptides) drug cargoes (more on nanocarriers in Chapter 9).

In one of the early examples, simple DNA origami structures were employed to deliver chemotherapeutic doxorubicin (see Back to Basics 6.4 for more on this potent anti-cancer drug) to breast cancer cells (MCF-7 cells).

Back to Basics 6.4	Battling Cancer: Doxorubicin

Doxorubicin is one of the most commonly used and the most potent chemotherapeutic drugs to date. It is used in the treatment of multiple cancers including breast and ovarian cancer, leukaemia, neuroblastoma, Hodgkin and non-Hodgkin lymphoma.

Doxorubicin combats rapidly dividing cells such as found in tumour tissues by intercalating between base pairs in the DNA helix and preventing DNA replication, ultimately inhibiting protein synthesis. It also inhibits enzymes topoisomerase I and II leading to disruption of DNA coiling and prevention of DNA repair after double-strand breakages. In addition, it produces free radicals which cause lipid damage, which is detrimental to the cancer cells.

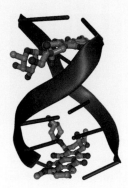

Although it has been successful in tumour growth suppression, doxorubicin is not selective and causes serious damage to healthy cells. Due to the colour and side effects, doxorubicin is also known as the 'red devil'.

Structurally, doxorubicin belongs to the family of anthracyclines, isolated from *Streptomyces* bacteria (Actinomycetes family). These bacteria are known as an excellent source of antibacterial agents. Researchers working within the antitumour screening programme initiated in the 1950s at Instituto Ricerche Farmitalia (FI) and Instituto Nazionale dei Tumori (INT) in Milan, Italy, were the first to show that these bacteria produce potent antitumour drugs such as daunomycin (discovered in 1962). The daunomycin derivative, adriamycin, known today as doxorubicin was obtained in early 1968, and was so promising that the clinical trials started the same year (Cassinelli, 2016), which is unimaginable today.

As can be seen in Figure 6.19, origami-mediated delivery of doxorubicin enhanced its toxicity independent of the shape (Jiang et al., 2012). DNA tubes were equally as toxic as triangles, and much more toxic than doxorubicin itself or doxorubicin combined with scaffold viral DNA (M13).

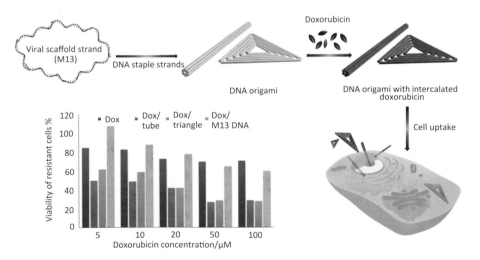

Figure 6.19

DNA origami can be used as a drug carrier. Chemotherapeutic drug doxorubicin incorporated within DNA origami rods and triangles is more efficient for removal of cancer cells than doxorubicin alone. The measure of cell survival is the percentage of cell viability. The higher the viability, the more cells survive and the drug is less efficient.

Adapted with permission from Jiang et al. (2012). © 2012 American Chemical Society.

DNA nanocarrier systems were particularly successful for delivery of chemotherapeutic drugs and therapeutic nucleic acids to multi-resistant cancer cells, cells that develop resistance to many common organic drugs. It seems that the combination of a large biomolecular carrier and a small organic drug evades cell garbage removal mechanisms and minimises evolution of protein pumps that can remove toxic drugs. Use of DNA origami for drug delivery is still in its infancy, but with the application of rational drug design strategies established for other nanocarriers, its potential will increase. Rational design is focused on the development of carriers that have the right combination of surface charge, mechanical properties and drug storing capacity to overcome biological barriers, deliver drug cargo to diseased cells (or pathogens) and undergo controlled release.

Unique mechanical flexibility as well as structural and chemical diversity (in terms of possible applications) of origami nanocarriers might be exactly what the nanocarrier design community is looking for. However, one of the concerns with DNA origami-based drug nanocarriers is their in vivo stability. Premature degradation will minimise the circulation time and the probability of a substantial amount of drug reaching the target. Despite nanocarrier design using origami still being in its infancy, tightly packed DNA structures, as well as the lipid-like origami coatings, have already been shown to increase the stability in blood and other complex biological solutions.

Interesting developments have also been made in the design of **DNA origami nanopores**, which could ease drug trafficking into the cells. Namely, various tube-like nanostructures can be easily prepared using the origami strategy. When modified with lipids or membrane-binding moieties, they can embed within the cell membrane and create artificial channels or pores such as shown in Figure 6.20 (Göpfrich et al., 2016).

Figure 6.20

Origami-based artificial membrane channels. Courtesy of Professor Ulrich Keyser and Dr Kerstin Göpfrich, University of Cambridge.

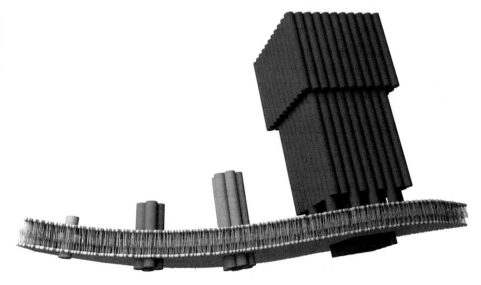

Such systems have already been tested on model membranes and simple cells, but the next step would be making them specific to a particular cell type and enabling selective transport of molecular species tailored to a particular disease.

6.7.3   Biosensors and Movable Devices

Another area in which origami structures have made a significant impact is the design of self-assembled systems that can undergo changes and even make mechanical, robot-like, motion patterns in the presence of external actuators. Initially, such devices had purely theoretical/design value, but they are increasingly interesting for cargo delivery into dynamic cell systems, or in vivo biosensing. One of the first movable origami structures made (featured in Figure 6.16) was one in which the lid of a box can be closed and opened using DNA 'keys' that can be hybridised to carefully positioned protruding arms. In fact, most dynamic origami structures rely on the reversible conformational change introduced by DNA hybridisation. Another way to introduce detectable mechanical change is to employ small molecules (Kuzyk et al., 2016) or plasmonic nanomaterials that can be excited by external stimuli such as light (Figure 6.21a), temperature, magnetic field or by variation in salt concentration (Gerling et al., 2015; Figure 6.21b).

More complex and controllable mechanical devices capable of precise motion over 10–100 nm can also be designed with the help of DNA structuring. To achieve continuous and reversible mechanical movement, each piece of a movable DNA structure needs to be carefully designed to mimic macroscopic machines and motors. These contain joints that enable angular and linear motion and can undergo complex movements with the help of a crank-slider mechanism, all of which were introduced to origami machines (Marras et al., 2015). The latest mechanical devices not only demonstrate the richness of DNA assembly and origami design and push the boundaries of molecular engineering, but can have viable practical applications, in particular as intelligent drug delivery systems or powerful theranostic devices (those that can act both as a diagnostic tool and a therapeutic agent, more on that in Chapter 9). Simple diagnostic sensors that mechanically respond to the presence of a particular DNA or RNA sequence in the cell have successfully been made. It is to be expected that many others will follow.

Science will meet science fiction soon. It is difficult to imagine any other molecule that could be more suitable to be at the intersection than the molecule of life.

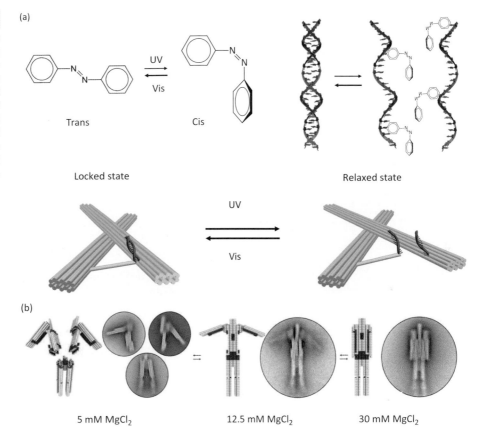

Figure 6.21

Movable origami devices that use a light-induced change of the azobenzene conformation (a), and MgCl$_2$ salt concentration (b) as actuators. (a) From Kuzyk (2016), and (b) Gerling et al. (2015). Reprinted with permission from AAAS.

(a)

Trans   Cis

Locked state   Relaxed state

UV / Vis

(b)

5 mM MgCl$_2$ 12.5 mM MgCl$_2$ 30 mM MgCl$_2$

Key Concepts

DNA barcodes: use of unique DNA sequences to label proteins or antibodies and enable identification of unknown species (also genes) present in low concentrations.

DNA hydrogels: 3D polymeric networks with high water content made entirely of DNA strands.

DNA origami: programmed folding of long DNA strand into desirable shapes with the help of a number of small strands known as **staple strands**.

Phosphoramidite coupling: the most commonly used method for synthesis of short, single stranded DNA known as oligonucleotides.

Protruding arm: single-stranded DNA positioned within 2D nanostructure that can serve as anchor for further immoblisation or assembly.

Sticky ends: short single-stranded sequences added to the ends of DNA structures, complementary to each and used as DNA glue.

Problems

7.1   Taking the volume of each base pair in DNA to be a disc of 2 nm diameter and 0.34 nm in height, how many bases could fit into a nucleus of 3 μm?

7.2   What are the forces that govern the self-assembly of a double helix?

7.4   How many biotinylated DNA strands are needed to bind all available sites in 50 molecules of streptavidin?

7.5   There are around 3.5 billion base pairs within human DNA. Each pair measures approximately 350 pm in length.

   (a) Calculate the length of a stretched DNA from a single human cell.

   (b) The human body contains approximately 50 trillion cells. If the DNA of all of these cells were stretched in one continuous strand, which planet in our Solar System would the strand reach, starting from the Sun?

7.6   Describe three methods that can be used to prepare an antibody–DNA conjugate.

7.7   Cystic fibrosis is a genetic disease caused by a specific gene mutation. The most common mutation is a deletion of three nucleotides as shown below:

   Gene of a healthy patient:
   5′-AAA TAT CAT CTT TCG T
   Gene of the CF-affected patient:
   5′-A AAT ATC ATC CTG

   (a) What is the sequence of the complementary strand that can be employed to design the sensor for cystic fibrosis?

   (b) Design a simple gold nanoparticle colorimetric assay for cystic fibrosis.

7.8   DNA strands were immobilised onto 15 nm gold nanoparticles (Au NPs) in an attempt to design a simple colorimetric assay. UV–Vis spectrometry was employed to determine the number of strands per nanoparticle and the following values were obtained:

   Absorbance (A) at 260 nm = 0.1
   Absorbance (A) at 520 nm = 0.3

   Taking into account that extinction coefficient ε for Au NPs is 4.2×10^8 M^{-1} cm^{-1} and for DNA 126 000 M^{-1} cm^{-1}, calculate the number of DNA strands attached to the nanoparticle.

7.9 Proteases are important classes of enzymes involved in the degradation of proteins. Protease dysfunction is related to various diseases and they are also very important targets for drug testing. Rectangular DNA origami can be used to position different proteases onto a single platform. Describe different steps needed for successful immobilisation onto the origami platform.

Further Reading

Seeman, N. C. (2016). *Structural DNA Nanotechnology*, Cambridge University Press.

Seeman, N. C. and Sleiman, H. F. (2017). DNA nanotechnology. *Nature Reviews*, **3**, 1–23.

Yang, D., Hartman, M. R., Derrien, T. L., et al. (2014). DNA materials: bridging nanotechnology and biotechnology. *Accounts of Chemical Research*, **47**, 1902–1911.

References

Agarwal, K. L., Buchi, H., Caruthers, M. H., et al. (1970). Total synthesis of the gene for an alanine transfer ribonucleic acid from yeast. *Nature*, **227**, 27–34.

Andersen, E. S., Dong, M., Nielsen, M. M., et al. (2009). Self-assembly of a nanoscale DNA box with a controllable lid. *Nature*, **459**, 73–76.

Beaucage, S. L. and Caruthers, M. H. (1981). Deoxynucleoside phosphoramidites: a new class of key intermediates for deoxypolynucleotide synthesis. *Tetrahedron Letters*, **22**, 1859–1862.

Cassinelli, G. (2016). The roots of modern oncology: from discovery of new antitumor anthracyclines to their clinical use. *Tumori*, **102**(3), 226–235.

Chen, C. and Fruk, L. (2013). Functionalisation of maleimide-coated silver nanoparticles through Diels–Alder cycloaddition. *Royal Society of Chemistry Advances*, **3**, 1709–1713.

Douglas, S. M., Marblestone, A. H., Teerapittayanon, S., et al. (2009). Rapid prototyping of 3D DNA-origami shapes with caDNAno. *Nucleic Acids Research*, **37**(15), 5001–5006.

Fruk, Lj., Kuo, C. H., Torres, E. and Niemeyer, C. M. (2009). Apoenzyme reconstitution as a chemical tool for structural enzymology and biotechnology. *Angewandte Chemie International Edition*, **48**, 1550–1574.

Gandor, S., Reisewitz, S., Venkatachalapathy, M., et al. (2013). A protein-interaction array inside a living cell. *Angewandte Chemie International Edition*, **52**, 4790–4794.

Gerling, T., Wagenbauer, K. F., Neuner, A. M. and Dietz, H. (2015). Dynamic DNA devices and assemblies formed by shape-complementary, non-base pairing 3D components. *Science*, **347**, 1446–1452.

Gilham, P. T. and Khorana, H. G. (1958). Studies on polynucleotides: a new and general method for the chemical synthesis of the C5′-C3′ internucleotidic linkage syntheses of deoxyribo-dinucleotides. *Journal of the American Chemical Society*, **80**, 6212–6222.

Göpfrich, K., Li, C-Y., Ricci, M., et al. (2016). Large-conductance transmembrane porin made from DNA origami. *American Chemical Society (ACS) Nano*, **10**, 8207–8214.

Jiang, Q., Song, C., Nangreave, J., et al. (2012). DNA origami as a carrier for circumvention of drug resistance. *Journal of the American Chemical Society*, **134**, 13396–13403.

Katzhendler, J., Cohen, S., Rahamim, E. et al. (1989). The effect of spacer, linkage and solid support on the synthesis of oligonucleotides. *Tetrahedron*, **45**, 2777–2792.

Kuzuya, A., Kimura, M., Numajiri, K., et al. (2009). Precisely programmed and robust 2D streptavidin nanoarrays by using periodical nanometer-scale wells embedded in DNA origami assembly. *ChemBioChem*, **10**(11), 1811–1815.

Kuzyk, A., Yang, Y., Duan, X., et al. (2016). A light-driven three-dimensional plasmonic nanosystem that translates molecular motion into a reversible chiroptical function. *Nature Communications*, **7**, 10591.

Lee, H. S., Dimla. R. D. and Schultz, P. G. (2009). Protein-DNA photocross-linking with a genetically encoded benzophenone-containing amino acid. *Bioorganic and Medicinal Chemistry Letters*, **19**, 5222–5224.

Lee, J. B., Peng, S., Yang, D., et al. (2012). A mechanical metamaterial made from a DNA hydrogel. *Nature Nanotechnology*, **7**, 816–820.

Letsinger, R. L. and Finnan, J. L. (1975). Selective deprotection by reductive cleavage with radical anions. *Journal of the American Chemical Society*, **97**, 7197–7198.

Letsinger, R. L. and Kornet, M. J. (1963). Popcorn polymer as support in multistep syntheses. *Journal of the American Chemical Society*, **85**, 3045–3046.

Letsinger, R. L. and Lunsford W. B. (1976). Synthesis of thymidine oligonucleotides by phosphite triester intermediates. *Journal of the American Chemical Society*, **98**, 3655–3661.

Linuma, R., Ke, Y., Jungmann, R., et al. (2014). Polyhedra self-assembled from DNA tripods and characterised with 3D DNA-PAINT. *Science*, **344**, 65–69.

Marchi, A. N., Saaem, I., Vogen, B. N., Brown, S. and Le Bean, T. H. (2014). Toward larger DNA origami. *Nano Letters*, **14**(10), 5740–5747.

Marras, A. E., Zhou, L., Su, H-J. and Castro, C. E. (2015). A programmable motion of DNA origami mechanisms. *Proceedings of the National Academy of Sciences of the USA*, **112**, 713–718.

Merrifield, R. B. (1963). Solid phase peptide synthesis. I. The synthesis of a tetrapeptide. *Journal of the American Chemical Society*, **85**, 2149–2154.

Michelson, A. M. and Todd, S. R. (1955). Nucleotides part XXXII. Synthesis of a dithymidine dinucleotide containing a 3':5'-internucleotidic linkage. *Journal of the Chemical Society*, **1955**, 2632–2638.

Mirkin, C. A., Letsinger, R. L., Mucic, R. C., and Storhoff, J. J. (1996). A DNA-based method for rationally assembling nanoparticles into macroscopic materials. *Nature*, **382**, 607–609.

Mohsen, M. G. and Kool, E. T. (2016). The discovery of rolling circle amplification and rolling circle transcription. *Accounts of Chemical Research*, **49**(11), 2540–2550.

Park, N., Um, S. H., Funabashi, H., Xu, J. and Luo, D. (2009). A cell-free protein producing gel. *Nature Materials*, **8**, 432–437.

Paunovska, K., Sago, C. D., Monaco, C. M., et al. (2018). A direct comparison of in vitro and in vivo nucleic acid delivery mediated by hundreds of nanoparticles reveals a weak correlation. *Nano Letters*, **18**, 2148–2157.

Peng, H. I. and Miller, B. L. (2011). Recent advancements in optical DNA biosensor: exploiting the plasmonic effects of metal nanoparticles. *Analysts*, **136**, 436–447.

Rothemund, P. W. K. (2006). Folding DNA to create nanoscale shapes and patterns. *Nature*, **440**, 297–302.

Sacca, B. and Niemeyer, C. M. (2012). DNA origami: the art of folding DNA. *Angewandte Chemie International Editon*, **51**, 58–66.

Schaller, H., Weimann, G., Khorana, H. G. and Lerch, B. (1963). The stepwise synthesis of specific deoxyribopolynucleotides (4). Protected derivatives of deoxyribonucleosides and new syntheses of deoxyribonucleotides-3 phosphates. *Journal of the American Chemical Society*, **85**, 3821–3838.

Schreiber, R. (2013). Circular plasmonic DNA nanostructures with switchable circular dichroism. *Nature Communications*, **4**, 2948.

Seeman, N. C. (1982). Nucleic acid junctions and lattices. *Journal of Theoretical Biology*, **99**, 237–247.

Shahbazi, M-A., Bauleth-Ramos, T. and Santos, H. A. (2018). DNA hydrogel assemblies: bridging synthesis principles to biomedical applications. *Advanced Therapeutics*, **1**(4), 1800042.

Shih, W. M., Quispe, J. D. and Joyce, G. F. (2004). A 1.7-kilobase single-stranded DNA that folds into a nanoscale octahedron. *Nature*, **427**, 618–621.

Sinha, N. D., Grossbruchhaus, V. and Koster, H. (1983). A new synthesis of oligodeoxynucleotides methyl phosphonates on control pore glass polymer support using phosphite approach. *Tetrahedron Letters*, **24**, 877–880.

Smith, M., Moffatt, J. G. and Khorana, H. G. (1958). Carbodiimides. VIII. Observations on the reactions of carbodiimides with acids and some new applications in the synthesis of phosphoric acid esters. *Journal of the American Chemical Society*, **80**(23), 6204–6212.

Sprengel, A., Lill, P., Stegemann, P., et al. (2017). Tailored protein encapsulation into a DNA host using geometrically organised supramolecular interactions. *Nature Communications*, **8**, 14472.

Voigt, N. V., Tørring, T., Rotaru, A., et al. (2010). Single-molecule chemical reactions on DNA origami. *Nature Nanotechnology*, **5**, 200–203.

Williams S., Lund, K., Lin C., et al. (2009) Tiamat: a three-dimensional editing tool for complex DNA structures. In A. Goel, F. C. Simmel and P. Sosík (eds.), *DNA Computing. DNA 2008. Lecture Notes in Computer Science*, vol. 5347, Springer.

Zhang, J., Liu, Y., Ke, Y. and Yan, H. (2006). Periodic square-like gold nanoparticle arrays templated by self-assembled 2D DNA nanogrids on a surface. *Nano Letters*, **6**, 248–251.

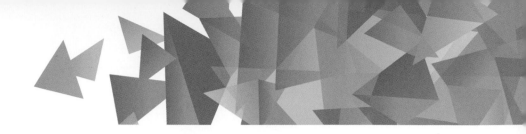

7 Bioinspired Nanotechnology

In Chapter 6 we explored the field of DNA nanotechnology, and the use of nucleic acids to create programmable architectures on a nanoscale. In this chapter, we will look at other biomolecules and biological structures, which inspired the design of novel materials and devices. Although they can operate on a wide range of scales, going from nano to macro, all biosystems have one thing in common: they are the product of millions of years of evolution. They have been adapted to address a particular environmental challenge, such as the emergence of a new predator or the abundance of a particular nutrient or building block. For example, without an increase in the concentration of silicate and carbonate ions in water during the Cambrian period some 500 million years ago, there would have not been a dramatic increase in the number of marine creatures with silica and carbonate hard shells (Peters, 2012).

With the developments of high-resolution microscopy, molecular biology and nanotechnology, we started to understand the diverse roles nanoscale elements play both in determining the structural stability and the functional efficiency of a particular system. With this understanding came the ability to employ biological nanofeatures for the design of new responsive materials and medical tools. Although the field of bioinspired nanotechnology has resulted in innovative approaches to nanodesign, we have just begun to scratch the surface (quite literally).

Hand in hand with our exploration of biological nanoscale features goes the preservation of biological diversity, which is challenged by modern lifestyle. Bioinspired nanotechnology emerged from studies of a limited number of organisms and there is much more we can learn as the number of our study subjects increases. There are still many organisms out there that have not yet been discovered and might have a particular adaptation exceptionally suited for the design of the next generation of light-harvesting devices or wound-healing materials. Our role needs to be not only to study those species we know but also to fight for biodiversity so that we do not lose a chance to learn from those we do not know yet.

In this chapter, we will focus on the main principles of bioinspired nanotechnology. We will start with peptides, continue with proteins and conclude with organelles and whole organisms, all of which were employed either as templates or mimics in design of nanomaterials and nano-based devices (Figure 7.1).

Figure 7.1

Bioinspired nanotechnology. From biomolecules and larger structures to nanoparticles and nanostructured surfaces, images on the right from Li et al. (2007) and Xue et al. (2017).

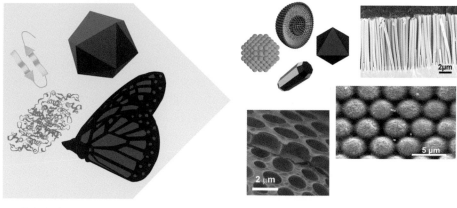

Biological structures   ⟶   Nanomaterials and nanopatterned surfaces

7.1 Self-Assembled Peptide Nanostructures

In Chapter 4 we explored the principles of self-assembly and molecular interactions that lead to the formation of larger and more complex structures. All of the biomolecules engage in some form of self-assembly; lipids assemble into cell membranes, single DNA strands into a double helix, protein units into dimers and larger fibril structures, and carbohydrates, often with the help of proteins, into intricate macroscopic 3D structures such as butterfly wings. One of the most adaptable and versatile building blocks, in terms of new materials engineering, is **self-assembling peptides**.

Although DNA has extensively been used in nanotechnology (see Chapter 6 for more), the major challenge of DNA nanotechnology remains the design of micro- and macro-scale materials, mainly due to the limited availability and cost of the larger amount of DNA building blocks. Peptides, on the other hand, have the advantage that they can be obtained on a larger scale through solid phase synthesis or recombinantly from cells or cell-free systems. For example, Fuzeon, a 36-amino acid peptide used as an HIV inhibitor, is made in near tonne annual quantities using solid phase synthesis (Thayer, 2011). Like oligonucleotides, peptides can also be modified with a range of functional groups and conjugated to larger biomolecules and nanomaterials. In addition, supramolecular structures can be assembled using interactions between distinct structural motifs such as α-helices and β-sheets (Back to Basics 3.7, Chapter 3).

Peptides play a key role in many biological events, particularly those involving signalling and cell–cell communication. They often act as hormones, molecules responsible for the transfer of biochemical information throughout the organism, and can either bind to particular receptors on a cell membrane or penetrate the cell to deliver various molecular effectors. Taking their important role in signalling and communication, it is not surprising that the changes in their structure or concentration have been identified in various diseases. Some of these diseases, such as Alzheimer's disease, are caused by structural changes affecting the self-assembling properties of peptides and the formation of large aggregates. One of the first peptide structures to be correlated to the dangerous aggregate formation was an aromatic dipeptide structure composed of two **phenylalanine units (FF)**. The aggregation of the amyloid fibres involved in Alzheimer's disease seem to be directly linked to phenylalanine dipeptide motif within the protein building block.

Isolated FF dipeptide and its derivatives can self-assemble into a variety of nanoshapes (Figure 7.2) ranging from spherical vesicles and hollow nanotubes to nanofibrils and large nanotubes (Adler-Abramovich and Gazit, 2014). The reason for this lies in the structure of phenylalanine. Besides hydrogen bonding between the backbone amine and carboxylic groups, phenylalanine units also engage in π–π interaction through the aromatic residue. Assembly of nanostructures usually proceeds in several stages. For example, FF-nanotubes originate from cyclic hexamer seeds, which stack into narrow channels that form large sheets, which ultimately coil into tubes with outward-facing hydrophobic residues with length that can reach up to 100 µm

Figure 7.2

Phenylalanine dipeptide readily assembles into various nanosized shapes. (a) Vesicles. Reprinted with permission from Reches and Gazit (2004). © 2004 American Chemical Society. (b) Nanotubes. Reprinted by permission of Springer Nature: Reches and Gazit (2006). (c) Nanowires. Ryu and Park (2009), by permission of John Wiley and Sons. (d) Nanofibres. Huang et al. (2014). https://doi.org/10.1186/1556-276X-9-653. This work is licensed under the Creative Commons Attribution 4.0 International License.

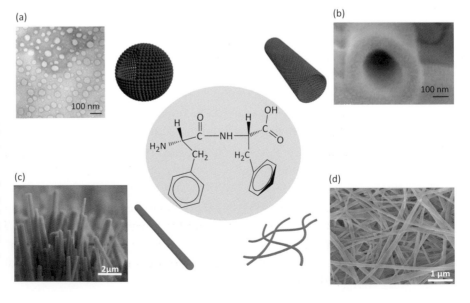

(Silva et al., 2013). Interestingly, the final shape can be controlled by the initial concentration of FF dipeptide. A high concentration of dipeptide ($100\,mg\,ml^{-1}$) leads to the formation of nanotubes, whereas the dilution results in vesicles. The reason for this is a change in the free energy of the system, which makes nanotubes more stable at higher concentration.

Phenylalanine dipeptide contains a single amino acid, and yet it can be used to make a variety of shapes, which can be transformed from one to another by dilution. Other amino acids that contain aromatic residues such as tyrosine and tryptophan have been shown to form nanostructures, as well as a large number of more complex peptides and peptide hybrids. Particularly exciting are **peptide amphiphiles (PA)**, which are usually composed of a few distinct regions; hydrophobic alkyl chain (Figure 7.3, I) linked to amino acids (Figure 7.3, II), β-sheets (Figure 7.3, III) and additional functional group (Figure 7.3, IV).

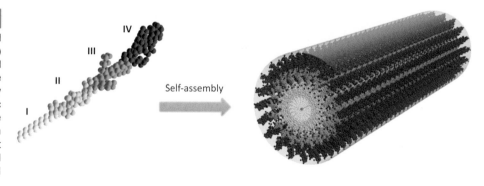

Figure 7.3

Structure of a typical peptide amphiphile (PA) and the assembled nanowire shape. Single PA molecule usually contains a hydrophobic carbon chain (I), peptide chain (II), a peptide chain capable of β-sheet formation (III), and hydrophilic functional group (IV).

The first amphiphilic peptides were described by Matthew Tirrell's group in 1995 (Berndt et al., 1995), and since then structures such as nanofibres, micelles, nanotubes and ribbons were successfully made using PA building blocks. Combination of hydrophobic and hydrophilic structural elements within PA leads to the formation of structures in which the hydrophobic regions are shielded by outward-facing hydrophilic functional groups. The morphology, structure and size of PA shapes can be controlled by varying structural elements such as the β-sheets (III) or the end-functional groups (IV). The versatility of shapes and ease of assembly make amphiphilic peptides particularly interesting for biomedical applications. They have already been successfully used to design materials for drug delivery (Research Report 7.1), bone regeneration, encapsulation of cells and preparation of artificial blood vessels.

Research Report 7.1   Peptides for Drug Delivery

One of the biggest challenges in nanomedicine is the design of **nano-vehicles** that can deliver drugs to specific cells, release them on demand and, depending on the type of disease, allow either a burst or continuous release over time. Peptides are desirable candidates for drug delivery; they are biomolecules, are easily synthesised to contain various functional groups, and can assemble into various shapes. Besides, some peptide sequences are known for their cell-penetrating properties, and others play an important role in cell–cell communication and can be used for targeted delivery.

Effective chemotherapeutic drugs used for cancer treatment are often hydrophobic molecules such as doxorubicin (Back to Basics 6.4). Being hydrophobic they are difficult to deliver within a highly hydrophilic biological environment. To aid the delivery of hydrophobic drugs, vehicles have been used such as micelles or liposomes that have a hydrophobic core to embed the drug, and a hydrophilic shell stable in aqueous environments. Using this principle, Li and coworkers (2014) designed a similar system employing **amphiphilic peptide–doxorubicin conjugate**, which was assembled into a stable nanoparticle (100 nm) with a doxorubicin core and negatively charged surface.

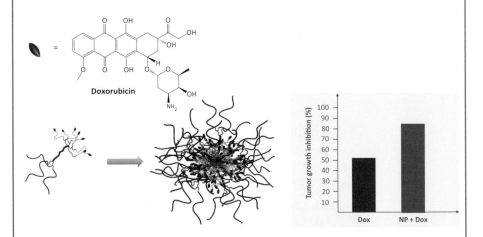

Doxorubicin

The sequence of the amphiphilic peptide was cleverly designed to contain a tetra-peptide sequence (Gly-Phe-Leu-Gly or GFLG), which is a substrate for the enzyme cathepsin. When peptide nanoparticles carrying the drug enter the cancer cell, cathepsin degrades the nanoparticle shell releasing the drug, which then inhibits the tumour growth (Li, 2014).

7.2 Biomineralisation Peptides and Proteins in Nanodesign

7.2.1 Nanostructures in Biomineralisation

Biomineralisation refers to the process by which living organisms produce hierarchically structured organic–inorganic hybrids, often to harden soft organic tissues and in such a way, provide mechanical stability and protection from predators. It is believed that the ability of organisms to utilise their organic molecules to grow hard shells of minerals evolved during the Cambrian period some 500 million years ago. Such an ability resulted in a diversity of biominerals that vary in morphology, composition and function. We know today that there are around 60 different minerals made and used by living organisms adapted to a particular habitat and needs (some biominerals are shown in Back to Basics 7.1). Successful biomineralisation is a result of the

Back to Basics 7.1	Common Biominerals

Most biominerals usually contain elements commonly present in the Earth's crust such as silicon (27.7%), calcium (3.6%) and iron (5%), indicating that organisms have developed strategies to exploit what was abundant in their environment. They usually have elaborate hierarchical structures leading to remarkable hardness and flexibility not found in synthetic materials, and more importantly, they are made under mild conditions such as near-neutral pH and low temperatures. Shown here are some examples of where the common biominerals are found as well as their basic crystal structure.

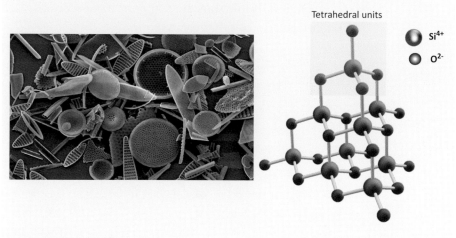

Source: Crespin et al. (2014).

Silica (SiO$_2$) is found in diatoms and marine sponges. All of the silica within sand comes from shells of these organisms discarded after their death. Silica is made of tetrahedral units composed of tetra-coordinated silicon cation.

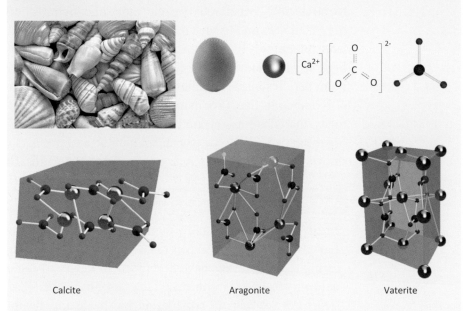

| Calcite | Aragonite | Vaterite |

Source: Mandy Disher Photography/Getty Images.

Calcium carbonate (CaCO$_3$) comes in three polymorphs – calcite, aragonite and vaterite – all characterised by a unique crystal structure. It is found in eggs, mollusc shells, exoskeletons of crustaceans. Calcite crystals found in skeletons of brittle stars are components of specialised photosensory organs considered to be primitive eyes.

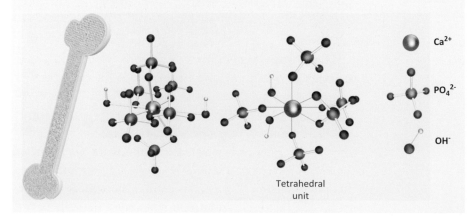

Tetrahedral
unit

Hydroxyapatite ($Ca_{10}(PO_4)_6(OH)_2$) is found in bones and teeth of mammals. Studies have shown that it has piezoelectric properties with a weak electric signal being produced when there is mechanical pressure on the material. It is composed of two types of calcium ions (Ca^{2+}) which differ in number and type of coordination ligands (phosphate PO_4^{2-} and hydroxyl OH^- groups).

Magnetite (Fe_3O_4) has been found in magnetotactic bacteria (left in the figure), in chiton teeth and honey bees and some birds. It is believed that its primary role is to ease the orientation in Earth's geomagnetic field, but there might be other, still unknown, functions. Magnetite is composed of two iron ions (Fe^{3+} and Fe^{2+}) coordinated by oxygen in an octahedral and tetrahedral arrangement.

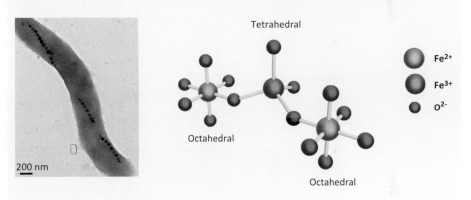

Source: Alphandéry (2014). Creative Commons Attribution Licence CC BY.

synergistic action of different peptides and proteins capable of converting salts into hard mineral structures with ordered micro- and nanopatterns. Such structures are particularly prominent within protecting shells of various sea creatures such as diatoms (Back to Basics 7.1).

The process that utilised ions from water and cascades of biomolecule-driven reactions to precisely grow beautiful shells has fascinated scientists for centuries. In the nineteenth century, Pieter Harting (1812–1885) published essays describing different mineral morphologies which can be formed by mixing organic molecules with calcium, phosphate and carbonate ions (Harting, 1872). However, it was a seminal work *On Growth and Form* (1917) by D'Arcy Thompson (1860–1948) that led to a more scientific understanding of the physiochemical principles behind the variety of biomineral structures. By exploring diatoms, Thompson concluded that the assembly of cells, vesicles and bubbles within the diatom structure act as templates that guide the deposition and further growth of silica structures. The field of biomineralisation went through a renaissance in the second half of the twentieth century thanks to the commercial availability of advanced microscopes. The foundation of the modern biomineralisation theories was laid by Robert J. P. Williams (1893–1988) who studied the exploitation of inorganic elements in biological systems (Williams, 1953). Studies that followed resulted in the understanding of the process in terms of the movement, precipitation and crystal growth of inorganic architectures in an environment composed of various ion-binding proteins and peptides. These early studies inspired Heinz A. Lowenstam (1912–1993), who is considered to be the father of biomineralisation, to propose the theory of **organic matrix-mediated mineralisation** in the 1970s, and prompted the scientific community to look for the proteins and peptides involved in the process.

The mechanism by which biomolecules guide the growth of crystals with remarkable precision and reproducibility is still not fully understood. The studies of biominerals such as calcite (calcium carbonate ($CaCO_3$) polymorph) spikes found in sea urchins have revealed the presence of distinct nanocrystals (Figure 7.4) within the larger structures (Seto et al., 2012).

Figure 7.4

Structure of the sea urchin spike. The spike is composed of calcium carbonate (calcite) and detailed analysis shows it is made by the assembly of nanosized spheric crystals (in (d)). Source: Jong Seto et al. (2012).

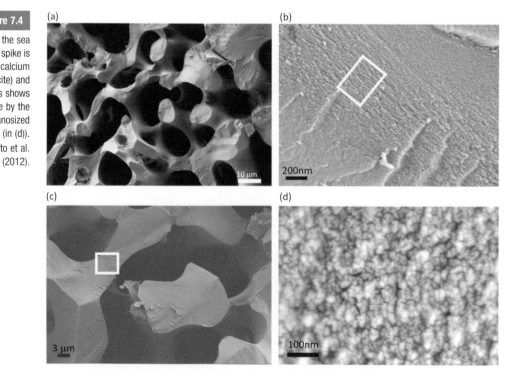

To explain the presence of such nanostructures as well as to understand the calcite biomineralisation, we need to draw on the mechanism of nanocrystal formation and growth we explored in Chapter 1. Two growth phases are particularly important for (nano)crystal formation: the nucleation and the growth through Ostwald ripening. To form highly ordered structures found in a sea urchin, these two processes must occur under the mild conditions and low temperatures tolerated by a living organism. To achieve that, the crystal formation and growth are facilitated by biomolecules, mainly peptides, proteins and polysaccharides. These biomolecules can act as the metal or metal precursor binders, the reducing agents and templates to guide the further growth of bound nuclei. They usually take on all of these roles and act in synergy to create highly hierarchical, macroscopic 3D structures with nano-sized features.

Another clue to how the actual interplay of inorganic and organic elements works in nature came from the studies of nacre, or mother of pearl, found in molluscs (Figure 7.5). Nacre is largely made of $CaCO_3$ mineral **aragonite**. In nature, aragonite is a brittle form of the carbonate, but nacre is around 3000 times tougher than pure aragonite. The reason for that lies in the orientation of the tablet-like units of the aragonite within nacre (Figure 7.5), and different types of self-ordering due to the variations in the growth rates. Studies have shown that the self-ordering in nacre proceeds independently of

Figure 7.5

Structure of nacre from abalone shells: (a) abalone shell. Jure Gasparic/EyeEm/Getty Images; (b) structure of aragonite tablets. Adapted from Barthelat et al. (2007), with permission from Elsevier; (c) scanning electron micrograph of the fractured surface; and (d) the top view of the tablet pattern. (c) and (d) Mao et al. (2017). Reprinted with permission of AAAS.

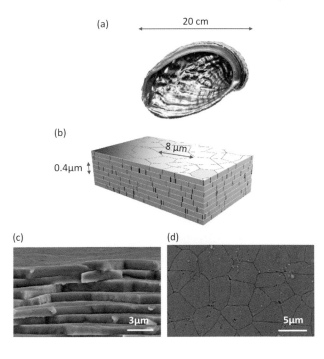

biomolecules and depends solely on the kinetic and thermodynamic parameters. However, it seems that the initial formation of the aragonite tablets is largely influenced by the presence of proteins and other biomolecules in the organic layers. In addition to the hard carbonate phase, a softer, hydrogel-like layer has been identified, which contains a large percentage of polysaccharides and proteins similar to silk fibroin. This hydrogel interacts with other proteins in its immediate surrounding creating a suitable interface for nucleation of $CaCO_3$ nanocrystals. A protein layer formed around the nuclei can be cleaved with the help of protease enzymes exposing the naked crystal core. Once destabilised by removal of the proteins, nuclei can undergo Ostwald ripening that results in the larger aragonite crystals (Evans, 2019).

Studies of the sea urchin spike and mollusc nacre formation have highlighted the importance of nucleation and growth, but also revealed the complexity of the biomineralisation process. Not only does this process involve the formation of inorganic–organic interfaces, which are thermodynamic and kinetic control points, but it also requires a finely tuned interplay of various biomolecular elements.

Despite more than a century of exploration, our understanding of biomineralisation is far from complete, particularly concerning the role of the genetic control and environmental conditions on a final biomineral structure. Two things are clear though: proteins and peptides involved in the initial growth of nanocrystals facilitate the process by taking part in binding and reduction of precursor ions, and by templating the growth of nano- to macroscale with an exquisite precision. It is therefore not surprising that the availability of various molecular tools prompted the use of natural and modified proteins and peptides in the design of novel nanomaterials.

7.2.2   Designer Peptides for Growth of Nanostructures

One of the most successful peptide-based strategies for the controlled growth of nanomaterials is the use of metal ion-binding peptides identified and selected through the **phage-display** libraries (Figure 7.6). At the heart (or better-said the nucleus) of the phage-display selection is the principle of **directed evolution**. In directed evolution, random DNA sequences are generated and inserted into a genome of fast-growing microorganisms or viruses such as **bacteriophages**, which infect bacteria. In bacteria, this altered genetic material can lead to production of mutated proteins. In bacteriophages, the random sequences result in the expression of genetically altered peptides within the viral coat proteins. In short, the small changes in the DNA sequence are directly translated into the structure of the coat peptides and proteins. Once the library of such modified bacteriophages is designed, they are screened for a particular trait. This might be a particular enzymatic activity or the binding to a particular material such as silica. The candidate bacteriophages that stay attached to silica after washing steps are first isolated, then grown into a larger colony and used for identification of the peptide responsible for binding.

Figure 7.6

The phage display process. Library of phage viruses containing different coat proteins/ peptides is created by insertion of random DNA sequences. The phages are then screened for a desired trait by **binding** to a particular surface or an immobilised molecule. Non-binding phages are removed by **washing**, the bound phage(s) **eluted**, and further **amplified** by growth of the colony. Binding phage is usually identified by genome sequencing.

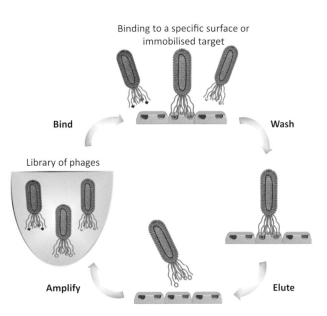

Phage display libraries, first described by George P. Smith in 1985, have resulted in the production of many useful biomolecules such as a whole new class of enzymes previously not found in nature (Arnold, 2018), and an entirely new way to make antibodies (Winter et al., 1994).

Using phage display libraries, peptide sequences were identified that can not only catalyse the reduction of the metal ions but also direct the growth of inorganic crystals (Yu et al., 2003) and aid the preparation of nanomaterials such as noble metal or metal oxide nanoparticles. For example, CCY peptide that contains two cysteines (C) and tyrosine (Y) was identified and successfully employed to make gold, silver and copper nanoparticles. Cysteines act as a metal ion binder, while tyrosine enables mild reduction resulting in small nanoparticles stabilised by a peptide coat. Tripeptide CCY can easily be fused to other peptide sequences, such as those that can bind to a particular cell compartment or a specific protein, resulting in CCY-hybrids being extensively used for biomedical applications. For example, CCY fused to a peptide that targets the nucleus (RGRKKRRQRRR known as the TAT peptide) can be used to prepare small fluorescent silver clusters and study the nucleus binding in different cell lines (Cui, 2011). Other metal-binding/ion-reducing peptides have also been used to generate and deliver a nanoparticle cargo to specific cells (Yang, 2017), and even employed in the design of a new generation of Li-based batteries (Research Report 7.2). Peptide-directed nanomaterial synthesis is considered a 'green strategy' as it involves biodegradable reagents and mild conditions particularly suitable for more sustainable preparation of useful nanoelements.

Research Report 7.2   Virus-Templated Lithium–Oxygen Battery

Li-based batteries, used in laptops, mobile phones and other electronic devices, store and release electrical energy through a reaction that takes place on the electrode materials. For example, rechargeable LiO_2 batteries operate through a reversible reaction between lithium (Li) and oxygen molecules. When Li batteries discharge, Li^+ reacts with reduced oxygen yielding mainly Li_2O_2. On charging, the electrical energy is stored by decomposing Li_2O_2 back into Li^+ and O_2. The anode within a LiO_2 battery is usually composed of materials such as Li-doped graphite, but the design of the cathode is more critical due to a large number of not well-defined processes that take place. Angela Belcher's group from MIT designed a cathode made of nanomaterial-coated viruses using phage display technology (Oh et al., 2013). They used M13 bacteriophage viruses as templates for growth of the catalytic materials that can enable efficient O_2 binding and reduction on a cathode.

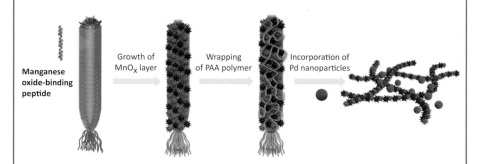

Manganese oxide-binding peptide → Growth of MnO_X layer → Wrapping of PAA polymer → Incorporation of Pd nanoparticles

M13 phages were designed to contain a short peptide sequence using phage display library (Figure 7.6) that can be used as a biotemplate for the production of manganese oxide nanowires. Such wires can be additionally coated with a polyacrylic acid (PAA) polymer that enables binding of the catalytic palladium nanoparticles (Pd NPs). Cathodes made of such phage-

MnO$_x$-Pd NP hybrid showed 45% improvement of the specific capacity in comparison to the bare nanowires, and a life cycle of LiO$_2$ batteries was significantly improved in terms of reversibility of charge–discharge processes and the stability of the whole system. Use of bacteriophages for an electrode design is an excellent example of bionanotechnology, the field that can connect the seemingly impossible to produce a technologically important product.

7.2.3   Nanostructuring Using Biomineralisation Proteins

A significant advance in peptide- and protein-directed material synthesis has been made by the exploration of **silicates**, proteins that build filaments and guide the formation of **silica spicules** in sponges. Spicules are structural elements which can have a range of intricate morphologies, shapes and sizes, such as in the case of one of the most beautiful deep-sea sponges appropriately named the Venus flower basket (Figure 7.7). We know today that these silica structures not only provide mechanical support and protection against predators but also act as light-harvesting lenses and light guides similar to modern optical fibreglass (Aizenberg et al., 2005). Looking deeper into the structure unveils ceramic fibrils (Figure 7.7c) made of interchanging layers of biosilica and organic material (Figure 7.7d and e). Ultimately, silica nanoparticles are revealed when the surface of the spicules is bleached to remove other layers (Aizenberg et al., 2005).

Figure 7.7

Venus basket sponge (a) and its biosilica spicule structure. Science Photo Library/Getty Images. (b) Fragment of the cage structure. (c) Scanning electron micrograph (SEM) fractured and partially etched (with help of hydrofluoric acid) single beam revealing its ceramic fibre-composite structure. (d) SEM of a cross-section through typical spicule. (e) SEM of a fractured spicule revealing an organic interlayer in the middle. (f) Nanoparticulate structures are revealed after the bleaching of biosilica surface. (b–d) Aizenberg et al. (2005). Reprinted with permission from AAAS.

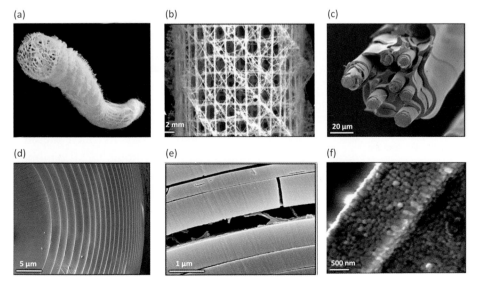

The family of **silicatein proteins** that is involved in the formation of intricate sponge skeletons has three protein members, α-, β- and γ-silicatein with a molecular weight ranging from 27 to 29 kDa (Figure 7.8). Although the repertoire of silicatein roles has still not been fully revealed, they most probably play a dual role in the spicule formation. On the one hand, they are **structure-directing proteins** responsible for the growth of silica nanoparticles into ceramic fibres, and on the other, they act as enzymes which catalyse the formation of silica nuclei. The silicatein structure is similar to the structure of protease enzymes involved in hydrolysis of the peptide bond, and as a result isolated silicateins can aid the **hydrolysis** and **condensation** of tetraethylorthosilicate. Unlike the sol–gel strategy explored in Chapter 2, which requires alkaline conditions and high temperatures, silicateins enable the production of silica nanostructures under significantly milder conditions, physiological temperature and pH, with the help of histidine and serine amino acids present in their catalytic centre (Figure 7.8). It is therefore not surprising that these proteins have been exploited for the preparation of useful structures not found in nature such as gallium oxide semiconducting surfaces, and nanocrystalline $BaTiOF_4$ perovskite minerals employed in the design of the new generation of solar cells.

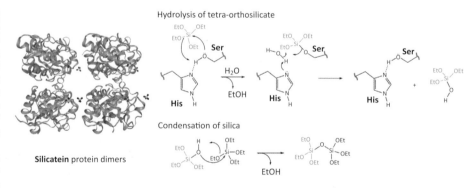

Figure 7.8

Silicatein mediated mechanism of biosilica formation. Proposed mechanism of hydrolysis of tetraethyl-orthosilicate in presence of silicatein protein with the help of histidine–serine catalytic site (Cha et al.,1999). Hydrolysis of silicate reagent is followed by condensation. Structure of silicatein dimers is shown with orange tetraethyl-orthosilicate molecules near the catalytic centres of individual proteins.

The range of silicatein applications can be extended by the preparation of recombinant, genetically altered silicateins. Such altered silicateins have been employed in preparation of spheric noble metal nanoparticles (Figure 7.9a), hybrid nanomaterials such as titanium oxide-coated nanotubes (Figure 7.9b), and line patterns of homogeneous semiconducting gallium oxide (Ga_2O_3) nanoparticles on the glass surface (Figure 7.9d). Equally exciting are applications in tissue engineering (more on tissue engineering in Chapter 9). For example, it has been shown that the activity of the bone mineralising cells is enhanced in the presence of silicatein-coated surfaces and that biosilica can be grown on dental minerals coated with recombinant silicatein, improving the quality of dental implants (Natalio et al., 2010).

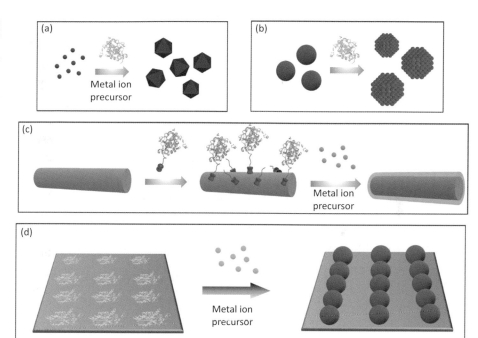

Figure 7.9

Biomineralisation proteins in preparation of nanostructures. Proteins can be used to (a) guide the formation of nanocrystals and (b) change the morphology of the surface. (c) They can also be used to make hybrid nanostructures by guiding the surface layer formation. (d) Some biomineralisation proteins can be patterned onto various surfaces and guide the growth of regular nanocrystal patterns.

In the meantime, many proteins have been isolated and their amino acid sequences identified which are involved in various biomineralisation processes and some are shown in Table 7.1. They are not only employed to prepare nanoparticles from ionic precursors (Figure 7.9a), but they can also be used to change the morphology of the nanoparticle surfaces (Figure 7.9b). For example, **aragonite-associated protein (AP7)** can make the smooth calcium carbonate crystal surfaces rough by directing agglomeration of nanosized particles (Amos and Evans, 2009). Other biomineralisation proteins such as **Mms6 protein** identified in magnetotactic bacteria (Chapter 2) can be used to prepare line patterns of nanoparticles on planar surfaces, which are useful for construction of high-density data storage devices in the electronics industry. Since their discovery in the teeth of chitons, marine invertebrates in the 1960s (Lowenstam, 1962), magnetic iron oxide nanoparticles have been identified in a wider range of organisms including honey bees, fish and birds. As the interest in the role of these bionano particles increases, it will be exciting to see the similarities and differences between the proteins involved in their production across species.

Table 7.1 Some biomineralisation proteins found in nature and their role

Protein	Where is it found?	Function
Calcium carbonate (CaCO$_3$)		
Perlucin	Nacre in shell	Calcite precipitation
MS131, MS60	Nacre in shells	Framework stabilisation
PIF protein family	Nacre in shells, named after *P. fucata* shells	Aragonite crystal formation
Ansocalcin	Eggshell matrix	Template for calcite nucleation
CAP-1	The exoskeleton of crayfish	Crystal growth regulation
N25	Akoya pearl oyster	Modification of the calcium carbonate morphology
Silica (SiO$_2$)		
Silicatein	Sponge spicules	Silica polymerisation
Silaffin	Diatom shells	Silica precipitation
Iron oxide (Fe$_3$O$_4$)		
Mms6	Bacterial magnetite	Control of the crystal size and shape

The most extensively explored biomineralisation proteins are those involved in the construction of various calcium carbonate architectures. Mollusc shells, exoskeletons of crustaceans and eggshells all contain CaCO$_3$, either in one of three crystalline forms (Back to Basics 7.1) or as an amorphous structure. A range of proteins (Table 7.1 lists some of them), peptides and polysaccharides act jointly to provide distinct structures unique to a particular species. In biological systems, carbonate structures have been identified that are several thousand times tougher than their purely inorganic equivalents. As we have seen in the case of nacre, this is often achieved by careful stacking of the nanometre-sized elements.

A slightly different orientation of the small proteins and protein fibre templates can result in structures that differ both in the elasticity and the resilience to mechanical stress. We know today that many of these structures do not only provide mechanical stability and protection from predators but act as the gravity sensors and photosensory organs, which makes them particularly interesting for applications in nanotechnology. It is therefore not surprising that scientists have been trying to employ the principles for biomineralisation in the design of novel materials for application in medicine and manufacturing. However, deciphering the role and structure of biomineralisation proteins is a complex process that involves several steps to isolate and purify the proteins. In biological systems, these proteins are closely bound to inorganic minerals, and to isolate them, the minerals need to be removed. This is often achieved by use of harsh acids, which can damage the proteins and limit the amounts available for further characterisation. It is expected that there are plenty more proteins out there than currently known, many of them having functions that would make them useful for nanostructure design.

Despite tremendous advances in the past decades, translation of the biomineralisation principles to novel material design has not been easy. Besides difficulties in identification of biomolecules involved in the process, there are significant gaps in the fundamental understanding of the underlying principles of biotemplate-guided growth of hierarchical 3D structures. Biominerals are products of cascade reactions controlled both on a biological and physiochemical level. Biology determines the structure of the biomolecule and their catalytic activity, whereas the environmental factors such as ionic strength, pH, temperature and combination of solvents guide the nucleation and growth of the nano- and macro-crystals. The results are remarkable 3D hierarchical structures, the nanotechnological potential of which we have only started to unravel.

7.3   Biotemplate-Assisted Nanodesign

Bottom-up preparation of nanomaterials with controlled and defined geometries on a larger scale is considered as one of the most challenging aspects of nanotechnology (see Chapters 1 and 2). This is particularly true for micro- and macroscopic surfaces with precise nanopatterns, which are often found in nature but very difficult to realise using chemical synthesis and rules of self-assembly. Employing natural templates to guide the preparation of nanomaterials and nanopatterned surfaces might be the answer to that challenge.

Biotemplate-assisted synthesis of nanomaterials makes use of natural self-assembled structures as templates, it is bio-friendly, usually easy to

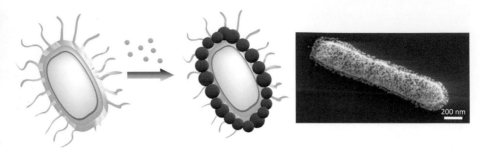

Figure 7.10

Principle of biotemplate-assisted nanomaterial design. Bacteria can be employed to grow and position nanoparticles on their surface. Image shows scanning electron micrograph of Au NPs grown on the surface of live *Bacillus cereus* bacterium.

Berry and Saraf (2005), by permission of John Wiley and Sons.

perform, often cheap, and works under mild conditions (Figure 7.10). Biological templates have an additional advantage over other strategies, and this is their genetic tunability. Proteins, viruses, and microorganisms such as bacteria and yeasts, can all be genetically modified to change their structure, morphology, and functional groups (see phage display technology in Section 7.2.2), which then impacts the properties of the templated nanostructures.

7.3.1   Protein Templates for Nanostructuring

In the previous section, we explored biomineralisation proteins as reducing agents and templates for nanostructure design, but there are other classes of proteins that have been successfully used for the synthesis of nanomaterials. Particularly useful are various enzymes. The inherent catalytic activity of enzymes can be utilised for direct reduction of the metal precursors at the enzyme–solvent interface, and different stages of the nanocrystal growth can be controlled by use of a single **enzyme template**. Nucleation can be achieved near the catalytic centre or on the surface of an enzyme, and the local concentration gradient of nuclei favours the kinetic control of the nanocrystal growth.

Enzyme-driven synthesis has enabled preparation of plasmonic or fluorescent nanoparticles with a protein core (Figure 7.11a) suitable for sensing, porous structures useful for drug delivery and a range of magnetic nanoparticles and hybrid composites. Enzymatic reactions themselves can often be used to tune the conditions, such as pH, and enable precise control of the nanoparticle growth.

For example, urease enzymes can tune the local pH around the enzymes by hydrolysis of urea substrate, which results in the production of ammonia and alkaline environment similar to that required for the condensation step of the sol–gel synthesis (Chapter 2). Such alkaline environment promotes the growth

Figure 7.11

Protein biotemplates for nanomaterial design. (a) Enzymes such as glucose oxidase can control the reduction and growth of spheric nanoparticles. (b) Ring and cage-forming proteins such as ferritin can be employed for the preparation of nanoparticles of controlled size. (c) S-layer proteins form two-dimensional layers that can be used for directed growth of nanoparticle patterns.

(a)

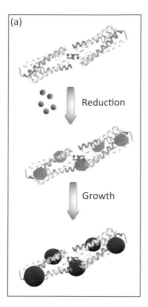

Reduction

Growth

(b)

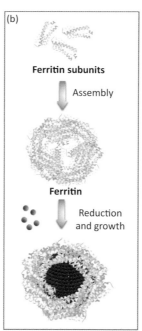

Ferritin subunits

Assembly

Ferritin

Reduction and growth

(c)

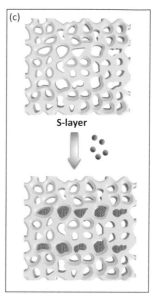

S-layer

of metal oxides such as zinc-oxide semiconducting nanoparticles (de la Rica and Matsui, 2008). Various enzymes such as peroxidases or oxidoreductases have been employed to prepare defect-free nanocrystals at low temperature, minimising the irregularities in the structure caused by thermal stress and aggregation that can often be observed at high temperatures.

Besides enzymes, various **structural proteins**, such as silk fibroin (Research Report 7.3), collagen or flagellin present in bacterial flagella, can be used as nanomaterial templates. Due to their structure, they are particularly suited for the preparation of nanotubes and nanofibres.

Research Report 7.3   Silk Fibroin for Preparation of Nanoparticles

One of the most explored structural proteins in nanotechnology is silk fibroin, the main structural element of the silkworm thread produced by *Bombyx mori* (*B. mori*) silkworm. Silk fibres have a core–shell type structure, with the inner core of fibroin covered by a sericin coating. More detailed analysis of the fibril shows that a mixture of α-helices and β-sheets are interlaced by amorphous regions and held together by hydrogen bonds (Qi et al., 2017).

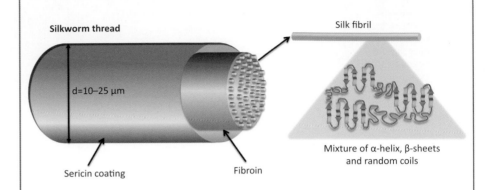

With its unique sequence-specific self-assembly and substrate recognition properties, silk fibroin is one of the most explored structural proteins in nanotechnology. Among other applications, it has been successfully used for the production of nanoparticles. Namely, it has been shown that fibroin can effectively reduce metal precursors through tyrosine residues (Fei et al., 2013). The simple protocol did not involve any harsh solvents or high temperature but relied solely on the strong electron-donating properties of fibroin's tyrosine. Silk fibroin took on the roles of both the metal salt-reducing and nanoparticle-stabilising agent and obtained nano-biocomposite was demonstrated to be useful in the elimination of antibiotic-resistant bacterial strain MRSA.

Source: Reprinted with permission from Fei et al. (2013). © 2013 American Chemical Society.

The reducing potential of silk fibroin was increased significantly by genetic engineering and insertion of amino acids such as cysteine, which are not present in the native protein. Such non-native fibroins were employed to prepare a range of biocompatible gold, silver, palladium and platinum nanoparticles (Das and Dhar, 2014).

The size and shape of the nanocrystals can often be precisely controlled by the use of protein templates which form cage or ring structures (Figure 7.11b). The most prominent example of such a template is the iron storage protein **ferritin**. Ferritin forms a hollow structure with a 7 nm cavity by a controlled assembly of 24 protein units. Such a structure is particularly suited for the preparation of small nanocrystals and has been successfully employed for the synthesis of iron and cobalt oxide nanocrystals. Ferritin is particularly interesting as each protein unit can be genetically modified to contain peptide structures useful to guide and control the metal ion binding and nanocrystal growth. For example, insertion of a cysteine-rich peptide can direct the growth of small plasmonic nanocrystals that have an affinity to thiols. Double-ring structures with an interior cavity formed by the heat shock chaperonin proteins, as well as other supramolecular protein structures can be used to make bimetallic nanocrystals or metal oxide rods. Often these ring or cage structures can further assemble into two-dimensional arrays resulting in patterns that guide assembly of metallic or magnetic nanoparticles. Two-dimensional crystal arrangements of proteins and glycoproteins also occur naturally and have been found on the surface of many bacteria. So-called **S-layers** (for the surface layer, Sleytr et al., 1999) are composed of identical protein subunits ranging from 40 to 200 kDA assembled into highly repetitive nanosized surface structures (Figure 7.11c). Depending on the type of bacteria, they often display different lattice symmetries with nanosized pores usually in the range of 2 to 8 nm in diameter. S-layers can be employed as templates to prepare arrays of various nanoparticles using physical deposition or chemical reduction methods. Both native and genetically modified S-layers can be obtained to act as anchoring surfaces for various types of nanostructures. For example, they can be coated onto silicon chips or gold electrodes and used for the preparation of conductive nanoarrays (Freeman, 2017).

7.3.2 Nanostructure Design Using Microbial and Viral Templates

Microorganisms and viruses are usually fast-growing organisms, easily obtained in larger amounts, well-studied and simple enough to be genetically altered in a predictable way. The cell wall of microorganisms such as bacteria contains functional groups such as amines, phosphates and carboxylic groups, all of which are suitable for metal binding and nanocrystal nucleation. Besides often having intricate nanoscale patterns spread over the microscale surface area, microorganisms also possess detox machinery composed of intracellular oxidoreductases and various surface-bound proteins, many of which have metal-reducing or metal-binding ability. Many microorganisms, particularly bacteria, are known to harvest toxic heavy metals and make them less harmful by converting them into stable complexes or nanocrystals and have been explored for use in environmental remediation (Ayangbenro and Babalola, 2017), but also as a mild strategy for nanoparticle preparation (Chapter 2). As biotemplates, microorganisms can be used whole or in part; their larger structural elements can be isolated and used individually (Figure 7.12). For example, bacterial flagella used for movement and communications between bacteria can serve as templates to guide the growth of the metallic nanofibres.

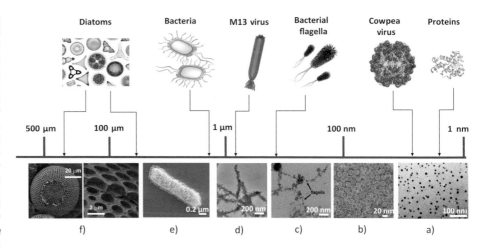

Figure 7.12

Scales of microbial and viral templates and nano designs obtained using biotemplate-assisted synthesis. (a) Avidin templated silver nanoparticles (Mor et al., 2011). (b) Cowpea mosaic virus (CPMV) as a template for iron–platinum nanoparticles (Shah et al., 2009). (c) Magnetite wires prepared using engineered flagellar filaments of *Salmonella* bacteria (Bereczek-Tompa et al., 2017, published by The Royal Society of Chemistry). (d) M13 virus as a template for perovskite nanomaterial synthesis (Nuraje et al., 2012, by permission of John Wiley and Sons). (e) Gold nanoparticle assembly on *Bacillus cereus* bacterium (Berry and Saraf, 2005). (f) Diatom structure (reprinted by permission from Springer Nature: Brunner et al., 2009).

While bacteria are usually spherically or cylindrically shaped organisms, **viruses** have much more diverse structures both in terms of the size and shape, including intricate structural protrusions (Back to Basics 7.2). Some of them are also not dangerous for humans and animals, can be easily genetically manipulated and, together with their unique structural features, are excellent templates for the design of nanostructured hybrids, nanoparticles and nanowires, and hollow structures suitable for drug delivery. Most commonly used viral templates are bacterial viruses such as bacteriophages and plant viruses such as rod-shaped tobacco mosaic virus (TMB, Back to Basics 7.2) and spherical cowpea viruses (cowpea mosaic virus, CPMV; see Research Report 7.4). Besides the ease of modification, the advantage of viruses is that they can be prepared on a larger scale (several grams and more) easing the manufacture of homogeneous nanocrystals or nanostructured surfaces.

Back to Basics 7.2   Structural Diversity of Viruses

Viruses are infectious agents that reproduce only in living cells and are made of a nucleic acid core (either DNA or RNA) protected by a protein shell often referred to as capsids.

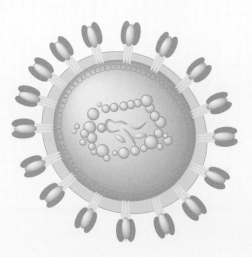

They come in a variety of shapes and sizes. The largest virus to date, *Pithovirus sibericum* identified in Siberian permafrost in 2014, is 1.5 μm long, between 10 and 100 times larger than an average virus.

Viruses can be divided into four distinct shape-based classes. **Spheric** or **icosahedral** viruses of different sizes are usually made of an icosahedral arrangement of proteins within the capsid which protects the core nucleic acid. **Rod-shaped** or **helical** viruses which have a helical arrangement of capsid proteins are often found in plant viruses such as tobacco mosaic virus. **Enveloped** viruses are characterised by an intricate coat around the helical or icosahedral core. Such structure is found in many viruses pathogenic for humans such as HIV, human influenza virus or rabies. Finally, there is a class of **complex** viruses, which do not have a single defined structure. They are either composed of multiple structural elements or have irregular shapes. Such as bacteriophages made of the icosahedral capsid and helically shaped body with attached leg-like protrusions, or worm-shaped ebola or amphora-shaped mega viruses.

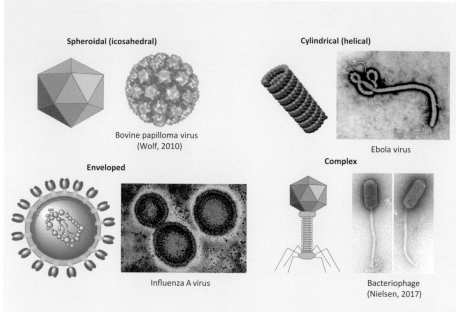

Spheroidal (icosahedral)

Bovine papilloma virus
(Wolf, 2010)

Cylindrical (helical)

Ebola virus

Enveloped

Influenza A virus

Complex

Bacteriophage
(Nielsen, 2017)

Source: (Influenza A virus) BSIP/Contributor/Universal Images Group Editorial/Getty Images; (Ebola virus) Callista Images/Getty Images.

Two routes are usually taken to obtain nanostructures; viruses can either be used as nano-confined reactors enabling the growth of nanocrystals within their capsid or nanostructures can be growth on the surface (Figure 7.13).

Figure 7.13

Different routes for the preparation of metal nanomaterials using viral templates. (a) An inner cavity can be used as a confined nanoreactor to control the size of nanocrystals. Viral capsid can be modified to enable either (b) binding and reduction of precursors or (c) further self-assembly into, for example, nanowires, or both assembling properties.

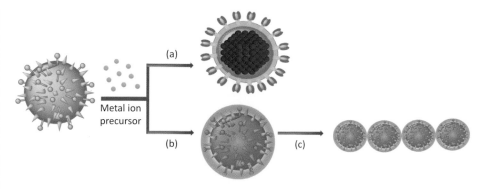

Metal ion precursor

(a)

(b)

(c)

Surface-coated viral templates can often be further assembled into larger structures affording precise surface patterning. For example, CPMV virus can be engineered to contain a large number of cysteine groups in capsid proteins, which can act for the precise positioning of gold nanoparticles on the surface of the virus (Fontana et al., 2014). Such assemblies are particularly well-suited for the preparation of strongly plasmonic systems (Research Report 7.4) and application in biosensor design and surface-enhanced Raman (Chapter 5).

Research Report 7.4	Plasmonic Metamaterials from Cowpea Mosaic Virus

Precisely controlled three-dimensional assemblies of plasmonic nanoparticles often lead to materials with electromagnetic and optical properties not found in nature. Materials with unusual properties derived from their structural features rather then chemical compositions are known as metamaterials (the prefix meta indicates something beyond what is found in nature).

By engineering the arrangement of nanoelements, architectures can be achieved that have a negative refractive index and unnaturally bend light, that reflect light resulting in invisibility cloaks or trap acoustic waves. Despite the huge potential and exciting properties, the main challenge with metamaterials is their manufacture. Traditionally, top-down lithographic methods are employed, but bottom-up assembly is simpler and cheaper.

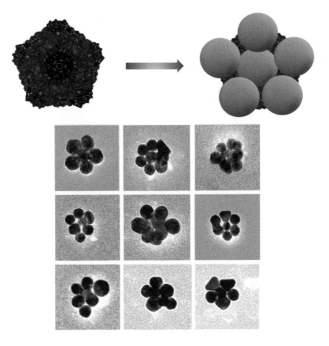

Source: Fontana et al. (2014), by permission of John Wiley and Sons.

Introducing: **cowpea mosaic virus (CPMV)**. It has an icosahedral capsid 30 nm in diameter (Lin et al., 1999), which is stable over a broad range of temperatures, pH and organic solvents, and is easily engineered to afford various surface groups. It is an excellent biotemplate for otherwise very difficult polyhedric assembly of nanoparticles. In their paper, Fontana et al. (2014) engineered the CPMV capsid proteins to contain cysteine groups, which can strongly bind gold nanoparticles. Using CPMV as a template, they could achieve the assembly of gold nanoparticles (either 18 or 30 nm) in five-fold symmetry guided by the morphology of the viral template (Fontana et al., 2014). Not only did such a strategy lead to precisely assembled structures, but they have also shown 10-fold enhancement of the local electromagnetic field, opening a new route to the design of templated plasmonic metamaterials.

Although there are some giant viruses and large bacteria, the largest microorganisms are diatoms and they range from 2 μm to 0.5 mm in diameter. Their intricate nanopatterned silica shells have been used as templates to create various nanopatterned surfaces, ranging from plasmonic metals to magnetic oxide and titanium dioxide layers. However, rather than as direct templates, diatoms and larger biological structures such as insect wings are more often used as a design inspiration and used within the field of **biomimetic nanodesign**.

7.4   Biomimetic Nanodesign

Nature is excellent in designing highly adaptable structures. In a desert, insects are found that have shells made of hydrophilic materials that can harvest even the tiniest amounts of water vapour to prevent dehydration, while in water-rich environments, plants have evolved highly hydrophobic leaves to prevent water accumulation. Skin and insect wings might possess precisely patterned structure to prevent the growth of pathogenic microorganisms or to ease sunlight harvesting, and vibrant colours are often a product of the nanopatterned arrangement of polysaccharides and proteins.

Nanotechnology has looked into a small number of these architectures for inspiration, but a few have already made it into commercial products. By mimicking lotus leaf structures, hydrophobic self-cleaning paints were developed, while powerful self-adhesive materials were designed based on the surface pattern of gecko lizard feet (see Section 7.4.2 and Figure 7.15).

The advancement of **biomimetic nanodesign** was made possible by the development of advanced electron microscopy and its applications to study natural structures. However, biomimicking is not a new concept; in the fifteenth century, Leonardo da Vinci (1452–1519) studied bird flight in an attempt to design a flying machine. However, although being around for centuries, the field of biomimicry was given its official name and definition by Jack Steele (1924–2009) in the 1960s. The words *bio* from the Greek root meaning life, and *'mimicry'* or *'to mimic'* to copy, perfectly describe the field in which biological structures are used as an inspiration to prepare functional materials and devices.

Earlier, while exploring biomineralisation, we have seen that structures in nature are assembled hierarchically; nanosized elements are produced, guided by the genetic information and then assembled into larger structures that can perform functions necessary for survival and reproduction. Although our knowledge of the underlying molecular biology and chemistry of life has increased tremendously in the past hundred years, our understanding of the assembly of biological elements into functional units is still limited. Therefore, instead of thinking about the design of nanostructures from scratch, often it is worth looking into nature and what kind of solutions it has developed to tackle challenges ranging from energy and nutrients supply to protection from predators and pathogens.

In the next sections, we will cover the main routes to mimicked nanodesign and look at some successfully mimicked biostructures and their applications. This field is truly in its infancy, but the diversity and functional beauty of biostructures as well as the need for sustainable manufacturing of useful materials, are attracting an increasing number of researchers, engineers and investors.

7.4.1 Biomimetic Catalysts: Enzyme-Like Nanostructures

In 1970 Ronald Breslow (1931–2017) coined the term **artificial enzymes** to describe the design of new catalysts which could mimic the principles of natural enzymes using alternative materials. But, if the enzymes are so diverse and specialised and effective as we mentioned in Chapter 3, why not simply use them instead of designing a whole new class of enzyme-like materials? The reason for the development of artificial enzymes lies in the practical challenges of the use of natural enzymes, which are active within a very narrow temperature, pH and solvent range, and are often not suitable for applications outside biological systems. To apply them to industrial-scale reactions one needs to extract them and purify them in large amounts, which is not only time-consuming and expensive, but often simply not possible. And finally, recycling them out of solution and preserving them for continuous use is a technical challenge. This is not to say that enzymes have not been used by the chemical and pharmaceutical industry. Indeed, we can even buy them in a supermarket as they are components of products such as washing powders. However, out of a large family of enzymes, there are only a few families that are extensively used, most notably lipases, proteases, amylases and a few peroxidases.

Biomimetic catalytic systems based on polymers, carbohydrates, metal complexes, antibodies (catalytic antibodies) and nucleic acids (RNA- and DNAzymes) have been prepared and used to catalyse some of the reactions previously driven only by enzymes. With the development of nanomaterials, a new class of artificial enzymes has emerged, referred to as **nanozymes**.

Nanozymes use nanomaterials either as catalytic centres or as carriers of catalytic centres. The term was first used to describe the RNase activity (RNA cleavage) of a thiol protected gold cluster and Zn(II) complex in 2004 (Manea, 2004). In the meanwhile, the field has expanded and several nanomaterials and bionano hybrids have been developed that mimic the activity of natural enzymes, mainly oxidoreductases and some hydrolases involved in ester cleavage.

The most explored enzymes are metal oxide nanoparticles such as a magnetic iron oxide or ceria (CeO_2) nanoparticles. These nanoparticles are often characterised by the presence of the mixed-valence ions (Ce^{3+} and Ce^{4+} in CeO_2 nanomaterials) and oxygen vacancies, which enable switching between the oxidation states, leading to an inherent redox activity. Metal oxide nanomaterials have been shown to have catalase, superoxide dismutase, oxidase and peroxidase activity (Figure 7.14), all of which involve radical species intermediates. It should be noted at this stage that the molecular mechanism of the catalytic activity of many nanozymes, apart from the widely explored nanoceria, is not clear.

Figure 7.14

Range of enzyme-like activities shown by nanoparticle-based enzymes. Superoxide dismutase turns superoxide radical into peroxide and oxygen, catalase degrades hydrogen peroxide into water and oxygen. Oxidases convert a range of substrates into products in the presence of oxygen, while peroxidases employ peroxide.

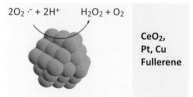
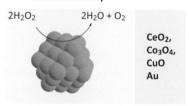
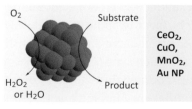
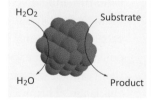

One of the most interesting discoveries in the field of nanozymes was the intrinsic **peroxidase activity of magnetic iron oxide nanoparticles** (Gao et al., 2007). Peroxidases catalyse the oxidation of substrates in the presence of hydrogen peroxide (H_2O_2, Figure 7.14), and play a number of important biological roles such as acting as detox enzymes (glutathione peroxidase) and being the first line of defence against pathogens (myeloperoxidase). In addition, peroxidases such as horseradish peroxidase or HRP are a valuable bioanalytical tool used in various bioassays. Iron oxide nanoparticles have been shown to have activity comparable to that of HRP, which is considered one of the strongest peroxidases. It is believed that such activity comes from the ability to coordinate a large number of substrates to the large nanoparticle surface. Initially, there were concerns that the high catalytic activity was not due to the structure and size of the nanocrystals, but that it rather stems from various iron ions leached into the solution. This was shown not to be the case, as the concentration of leached ions was found to be much too low to account for high activity.

In the meantime, other nanoparticles such as Au, CuO and Pt NPs, as well as carbon nanotubes, have all been shown to have peroxidase activity, although not as high as iron oxide, and have been used in the design of various bioassays. A decade after the discovery of peroxidase activity of iron oxide nanoparticles, not only has the field of nanozymes expanded to include a wider class of materials, but different strategies are continuously introduced to tune and improve their catalytic activity (Wei and Wang, 2013).

Catalytic properties are size-dependent. In most cases, smaller NPs have higher activity than larger ones mainly due to a higher surface-to-volume ratio. Shape and morphology such as the presence of a particular crystal plane play an important role as well, as does the surface coating. Introduction of various functional groups such as enzyme cofactors or charged groups to the surface of a nanocore can significantly improve the catalytic properties of a nanozyme. Although the catalytic activity of nanozymes is often still much lower than that of their natural counterparts, nanomaterials have their own set of advantages. Besides tunable size and easily tailored surfaces, they are characterised by high stability and tolerance of harsh environments, making them suitable for applications in industrial reactors. Nanomaterials also have intrinsic properties, which can be employed to introduce properties not found in natural enzymes. For example, iron oxide nanoparticles cannot only be used to perform enzyme-like reactions but can be easily removed from the solution using magnets and in such a way improve the recycling and reuse of the catalyst. Other materials such as quantum dots (Research Report 7.5) or semiconducting metal oxides, like titanium oxide, produce reactive oxygen species in aqueous solution upon irradiation. These reactive species engage in a catalytic cascade meaning that such semiconducting enzymes can be activated on demand by irradiation. The number of nanoparticle-based enzymes is continuously increasing and the current challenge is to design artificial enzymes that can catalyse stereoselective reactions important for the synthesis of various pharmaceutically relevant chiral drug molecules.

Nanomaterials make nanozymes more robust than native enzymes by extending the storage time, by increasing the tolerance to high temperatures and organic solvents often needed to improve the reaction yields. They also introduce new properties such as on-demand activation and extraction, improving the reuse of the catalysts, and in such a way reducing the cost of the catalytic process. Despite these advantages there are issues still to be resolved such as their large-scale production and relatively low specificity and selectivity in comparison to the native enzymes. Development of new surface modification strategies and hybrid materials will likely resolve these issues in the years to come.

Research Report 7.5   Peptide–Quantum Dot Hybrid As a Powerful Nanozyme

Nitrate reductase is an important enzyme found in plants, algae and fungi that catalyses the first step of nitrate assimilation, a reduction of the nitrate into nitrite using nicotinamide adenine dinucleotide (NADH) as a sacrificial electron donor:

$$NO_3^- + NADH \rightarrow NO_2^- + NAD^+ + OH^-$$

Nitrates are the most significant source of nitrogen in crop plants and nitrate reductase activity is an important control point in carbon and nitrogen metabolism and protein production. However, nitrates can have a pretty damaging effect if overused, and their presence in water can cause rapid and uncontrollable growth of algae and fungi (some of which are toxic). Therefore, the control of the nitrate amount by its reduction into other species is an important process in water remediation.

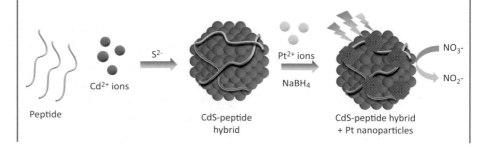

Using peptide-driven synthesis by employing cysteine-modified short peptide (22 amino acids) and cadmium (Cd^{2+}) and sulphide (S^{2-}) ions, CdS–peptide nano hybrid was prepared onto which Pt NPs were grown using the $NaBH_4$ aided reduction of Pt^{2+} salts (see Chapter 3). Ultimately, bionano hybrids 13 nm in diameter were obtained, which had remarkable on-demand nanozyme activity. Cadmium sulphide is a semiconductor with a bandgap which can be overcome by irradiation with UV light (250 nm). Upon radiation, photoexcited electrons are produced which can aid the reduction of nitrate in the solution. Not only could the nanozyme be activated by light, but the activity was 23-fold higher than that of the enzyme under the same conditions. (Slocik et al., 2008).

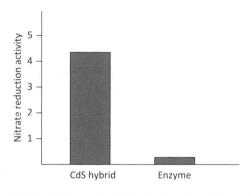

Source: Reprinted by permission of Slocik et al. (2008), by permission of John Wiley and Sons.

7.4.2 Nanostructured Superhydrophobic Materials and Adhesive Surfaces

Superhydrophobic materials are defined by the way water interacts with the surface and the type of wetting (Back to Basics 7.3).

Back to Basics 7.3   Superhydrophobicity and Surface Wetting

Interaction of the water droplet with the surface is usually explained in terms of the contact angle (θ). For a surface to be superhydrophobic the contact angle needs to be as high as possible, usually higher than 150°:

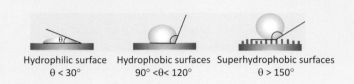

Hydrophilic surface   Hydrophobic surfaces   Superhydrophobic surfaces
$\theta < 30°$ $90° < \theta < 120°$ $\theta > 150°$

Any rough surface can interact with water in two ways; a water droplet can either penetrate completely into the rough surface (homogeneous wetting or Wenzel state) or there is another liquid layer or air trapped within the protrusions resulting in heterogeneous wetting (Cassie–Baxter state).

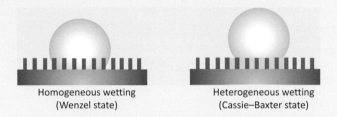

Homogeneous wetting   Heterogeneous wetting
(Wenzel state)   (Cassie–Baxter state)

In nature, heterogeneous wetting is preferred due to the wetted area being smaller than for homogeneous wetting, ensuring that the contact angle is higher. This ultimately means that the water will slide off the surface easier and hydrophobicity is increased.

Leaves of lotus plants, which grow on freshwater surfaces, were long known for their self-cleaning properties. However, the origin of this property was fully understood in the 1990s after extensive characterisation with the help of scanning electron microscopy (Barthlott, 1990). The self-cleaning ability of lotus leaves was shown to be a result of their **super-hydrophobicity**, stemming from a rough surface produced by an array of protrusions made of chitin core coated with wax crystals and sizes ranging from 200 nm to 1 μm (Figure 7.15a). Such a double-pillar structure composed of two distinct nanosized elements (chitin and wax), described in the 1990s, has been mimicked numerous times in order to achieve superhydrophobic surfaces. Traditionally, the most commonly employed technique to prepare such surfaces was soft lithography (Chapter 2, Back to Basics 2.1), which employs the leaf to cast a negative template out of polymer. Such a template can then be used to transfer the nanostructured pattern onto various materials. The simpler approach developed recently involves the bottom-up assembly of microspheres, which are then coated with polymer nanofibres or carbon nanotubes to create nanosized features (Figure 7.16a). Lotus leaf-inspired materials are used in various commercial products, most notably self-cleaning paints for car manufacturing and architecture.

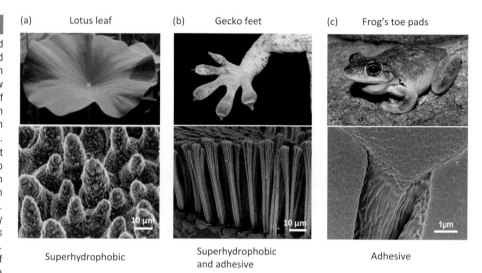

Figure 7.15

Micro- and nanostructured biosurfaces as an inspiration for new materials. (a) Lotus leaf is made of chitin protrusions coated in wax nanocrystals. Adapted from Ensikat et al. (2011). (b) Gecko lizard feet contain keratin hair-like structures with nanostructured endings. ePhotocorp/iStock/Getty Images and Dr. Travis Hagey (bottom image). (c) Hexagonal arrays of epithelial cells are separated by narrow channels crossed by densely packed keratin nanofibres. Xue et al. (2017).

Another widely explored example of the superhydrophobic surface is based on the structure of **gecko lizard feet** (Figure 7.15b). Gecko lizards are found throughout the world in warm climates. They are known as exceptional climbers, which we now know is due to the presence of hair-like microstructures called **setae** on the surface of their feet. Setae are made of keratin and each is composed of hundreds of nanostructured spatula 100 to 200 nm in diameter (Figure 7.16b). Due to their structures, setae are not only superhydrophobic but also adhesive towards the water, which might seem as counterintuitive at first. However, the adhesion is a consequence of the change in the setae orientation, the tilting of their protruding ends. Such a change in the orientation impacts the van der Waals interactions between the water droplet and the nanopillar-filled edges, causing them to adhere.

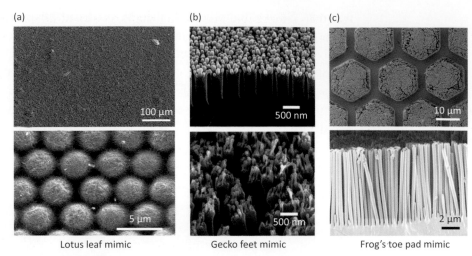

Figure 7.16

Examples of biomimicked superhydrophobic and adhesive nanosurfaces. (a) Polystyrene beads coated with carbon nanotubes mimic the rough surfacc of the lotus leaf. Reprinted with permission from Li et al. (2007). © 2007 American Chemical Society. (b) Polystyrene nanohairs with rough endings mimic the gecko feet (Lee et al., 2012). (c) Polydimethylsiloxane hexagonal micropillars with embedded polystyrene nanohairs mimic the frog toe pad (Xue et al., 2017).

Lotus leaf mimic   Gecko feet mimic   Frog's toe pad mimic

The structure of Gecko feet was successfully mimicked using various polymer materials such as polystyrene (Lee et al., 2012) or polyimide, and by introducing flexible endings such as shown in Figure 7.16b. Gecko feet-like materials are used in applications that require strong adhesion with minimal destructive force, such as robotic fingers for picking up and moving of fragile manufactured goods, and in the design of materials that remain adhesive and dry under water.

Adhesive surfaces were also found in **amphibians' toe pads** (Figure 7.15c). It was long believed that the strong adhesive action of toe pads in frogs is a consequence of the mucous secretion from the glands on the bottom of the pads. However, electron microscopy and AFM studies have shown that this is not the case. Rather than being smooth, the epithelial surface of the toe pad is made of hexagonal arrays of soft epithelial cells separated by narrow channels, which are crossed with hard keratin nanofibres ranging from 300 to 400 nm in height and diameter (Figure 7.15c). Although the interplay of the composition and morphology of these epithelial structures is still to be fully explained, similar artificial structures were recently designed in the lab. For example, a combination of poly(dimethylsiloxane) (PDMS) micropillars with interior structure made of polystyrene nanopillars (Figure 7.15c) resulted in increased friction and adhesion due to the toe pad-like hierarchical assembly (Xue et al., 2017). A similar principle has been used to design devices in which strong but non-destructive adhesion is required such as in safety razors or surgical graspers (Research Report 7.6).

Superhydrophobic and adhesive surfaces that stem from protruding and pillar-like nanostructures are not the only clever designs found in nature.

Another remarkable adaptation employs structural patterns that can trap water, and in such a way, repel other liquids and surfaces. Such a design can be found in the walls of some insect-eating plants, which are completely wettable due to micropatterns that trap water. Trapped water forms a continuous surface film on the plant, which prevents insects from making contact with the surface and causing them to slip down into the plant where they are digested. Using this principle, surfaces were prepared containing the pattern of nanopores filled with a lubricant, resulting in a super-slippery surface that can minimise the anti-fouling and, in particular, the formation of dangerous bacterial biofilms (Wong et al., 2011).

| **Research Report 7.6** | Frog's Toe Pad Structure As Inspiration for Surgical Graspers |

A surgical grasper is one of the most popular surgical instruments, but often responsible for tissue trauma and damage, particularly in soft tissue such as bladder and bowels. This is due to a strong holding force needed to prevent slipping of the soft tissue and mediocre friction properties at the interface of the grasper and the soft tissue in wet conditions.

The mature spotted-leg tree frog (*Polypedates megacephalus*) was used as an inspiration for a new design of the grasper's surface to minimise tissue damage. The surgical environment is filled with fluids and the conditions similar to those found in the tree frog's habitat. Despite wet conditions, frogs exert exceptional adhesive force onto the soft surfaces without slipping or tearing either their toe pads or the surface they attach to. The reason for this lies in the intricate hexagonal pillar structure of their surface epithelial layer:

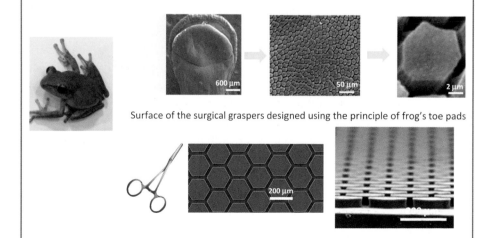

Surface of the surgical graspers designed using the principle of frog's toe pads

These hexagonal pillars were mimicked using poly(dimethylsiloxane) (PDMS) polymer. Exploration of sizes and heights of the pillars showed that slimmer pillars exhibit more friction and stronger direction-dependent properties as well as low tissue deformation and damage (Chen et al., 2015).

Although the grasper surface was coated in micrometre pillars, further improvement in properties could be achieved by introducing nanosized structures. This would require overcoming some manufacturing obstacles such as finding the right type of starting materials and the most afford-able technique to achieve hierarchical macrosized materials with nanopatterns.

7.4.3 Nanostructured Colour

Across the natural world colour has evolved to be a means of communication, serve as camouflage and be involved in sensing. When somebody mentions colours, we immediately think of molecular structures such as various organic and inorganic dyes, which contain chromophores that can absorb light of particular wavelengths. However, in Chapters 1 and 2 we also learned that some nanoparticles appear coloured either due to the interaction of light with their surface electrons (plasmonic nanoparticles) or based on the quantum confinement that impacts the band energy and transfer of electrons from ground to the excited state (quantum dots). In nature, there are many examples where the colour is not a result of either of these phenomena but entirely based on the intricate structuring of biomolecules, which guides their interaction with light. Such structure-guided colours are called **structural colours**. They are the consequence of the interaction of light with the periodic arrangements of hierarchical biostructures which are composed of nanoscale elements. Structural colours do not fade, usually have a shiny, metallic hue and are often **iridescent**. Iridescence refers to an ability of certain surfaces to change the colour with the angle at which the surface is viewed or illuminated. The most common example of iridescence is a soap bubble, which has an intricate interplay of colours which change depending on which side you are viewing it. The phenomenon of iridescence is the result of different optical effects such as interference, diffraction or scattering as light interacts with the periodically repeating features within the structure known as **photonic crystals** (Back to Basics 7.4).

Back to Basics 7.4   Photonic Crystals

Photonic crystals are characterised by periodically ordered dielectric structures. The periodic variation of the dielectric constant strongly affects the propagation of light. This is particularly prominent at wavelengths that are comparable to those corresponding to the size of the periodic features, which can range from several nanometres to a few micrometres.

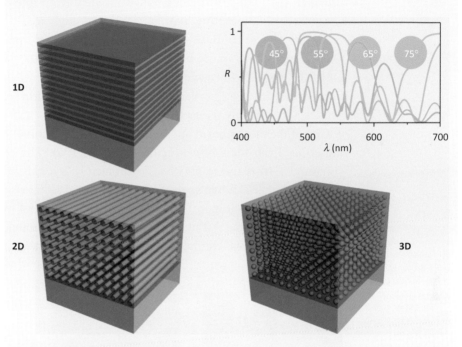

Source: adapted from Dumanli and Savin (2016).

Periodicity of photonic crystals can be in one dimension (1D), in which case the crystals can be considered as a periodic multi-layer. Such photonic crystals were already explored by Lord Rayleigh (1842–1919) in 1887. Resulting reflectance spectrum for 1D photonic crystals will exhibit a set of peaks (shown in the figure). However, in most cases, photonic crystals are more complex two- (2D) or three- (3D) dimensional structures. As a consequence, there is no simple model to predict the reflectance peak wavelengths, and extensive computational modelling is needed to predict their spectra. These complex photonic crystals are widespread. For example, 2D-photonic crystals are responsible for the colour of bird feathers, whereas 3D-photonic crystals are common in insects.

Natural photonic crystals are composed mainly of proteins such as keratin and polysaccharides such as cellulose and chitin. Besides being responsible for the appearance of colour, the photonic crystals also evolved to respond to different levels of irradiation enabling the organism to make the most of the ambient light. Some organisms thrive under bright sunlight, while others, particularly those living in dim environments found on a rainforest floor, needed to adapt to the low intensity of incoming light. Photonic crystals found in the animal and plant kingdom vary from one-dimensional crystals composed of alternating parallel layers of high and low refractive index materials (Back to Basics 7.4) to two- and three-dimensional structures. One- dimensional photonic crystals are found in the skin of cephalopods and fish as well as in jewel beetles, 2D photonic crystals provide colour to bird feathers, while 3D photonic crystals are common in the scales of many beetles and butterfly wings (Figure 7.17).

One of the most studied and mimicked structural colours is the blue colour of butterflies from the *Morpho* genus (Figure 7.17a). The colour of their wings (Figure 7.17b) is the result of a hierarchically layered structure composed of microsized scales known as the cover and ground scales (Figure 7.17c) and their nanosized features (Figure 7.17d). The wings are made of long chitin fibrils with a diameter of 3 nm. Within the fibrils, chitin units are held together by strong hydrogen bonds, which makes wings and insect shells exceptionally tough.

Figure 7.17

Blue structural colour of *Morpho* genus butterflies. (a) *Morpho peledies* butterfly found in Mexico. (b) Close-up of the *Morpho* butterfly wings. (c) The microscopic structure of the wing composed of layers of ground and cover scales. (d) Scanning electron micrograph of ground scales shows periodically repeating nanoscale structures composed of ridges. Brown layers in (a) are composed of melanin, which absorbs the light, resulting in dark brown colour (also found in the underside of the wings). NISE Network. Content licenced under Creative Commons Attribution Non-Commercial Share Alike 3.0 United States (CC BY-NC-SA 3.0 US).

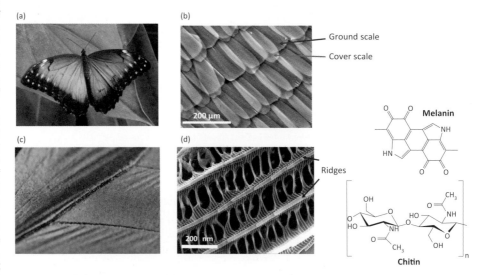

If we looked at the wings, we would notice that they shift through different hues of blue depending on the angle of the viewing, showing a copper colour when viewed side-on and brown when viewed from underneath. Such iridescence is the result of the structure of the ground scales, which are composed of ridges, each containing six to eight layered lamellae 200 nm apart (Figure 7.18a and b). The cross-section of these ridges shows that the lamellae are irregular and shaped like a Christmas tree (Kinoshita et al., 2002). The branches of the tree structures have exactly the right spacing between them to strongly reflect blue light. Ultimately, the colour of the wings and the changes of colours from blue to copper as the angle of viewing is changed are the consequence of several optical phenomena. The blue colour is the result of constructive **interference** and **diffraction** from the irregularly shaped, but regularly spaced, lamellar structures. Irregular heights cause **accidental interference** of the **scattered light**, which manifests as glittering speckles, whereas the brown underside of the wing stems from **absorption of light** by the pigment melanin.

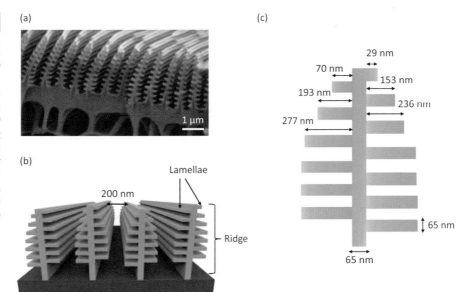

Figure 7.18

Nanostructures are responsible for the structural colour of *Morpho* butterfly wings. The Christmas tree-like ridges (a) are composed of 6 to 8 layers of lamellae 200 nm apart (b). Different sizes of the ridges are responsible for various optical phenomena such as reflection, diffraction and constructive interference (c). Zhang (2015).

The structure of butterfly wings has been mimicked extensively to design photonic crystals from various (bio)polymers and to prepare structural colours (Figure 7.19), antibacterial surfaces and sensing devices. Structural colours not only have significantly decreased environmental impact (dye-making and dying are among the most polluting processes) but also do not fade and photobleach with time or under increased pH or temperature.

Structural arrangements similar to butterfly wings are found also in other insects. In coloured bird feathers, the 2D photonic crystals are made of sponge-like structures composed of protein keratin and air bubbles (Parnell

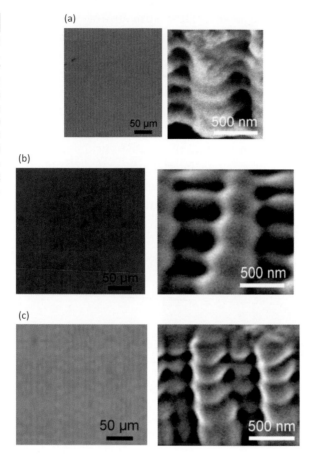

et al., 2015). In plants, on the other hand, brilliant colours are the result of structuring within cells. The most brilliant blue structural colour known is found in the marble berries of *Pollia condensata* (Figure 7.20a) and stems from the reflection of helically stacked cellulose fibrils, which form multi-layers in the cell walls of the outmost layer of the fruit (Vignolini et al., 2012).

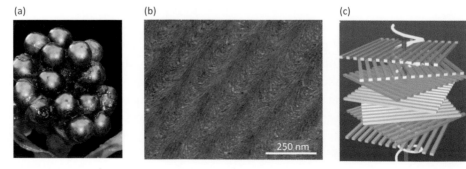

Multi-scale hierarchical architectures that result in photonic crystals have many potential applications, in particular for the design of sensors that can change colour as a consequence of nanoscale interactions or changes. Such sensors have been designed to monitor food and water quality by notifying the presence of pathogens, detecting heavy metals and changes to pH or humidity. Particularly exciting are developments in the design of actuators for applications in robotics (Research Report 7.7). With the advancements in artificial intelligence and robot design, it can be expected that soft, responsive nanostructured materials that can be achieved by mimicking living systems will be a desirable alternative to the non-responsive polymers and metals in use at the moment.

Research Report 7.7 | Bioinspired Structural Colours As Actuators

Structural colour materials can modulate electromagnetic waves and control the propagation of photons due to the energy of their photonic bandgap (PBG). Swelling or shrinking of a structural colour material can lead to a change in PBG, resulting in the change of colour. Such behaviour can be utilised in the design of hydrogel materials, which can change the PBG by swelling in water and in such a way, act as humidity sensors. However, the disadvantage of current bioinspired, responsive structural colour materials is that they require an external stimulus (temperature, addition of water, application of pressure) to introduce the colour change.

Fu and colleagues recently took another approach and developed structural colour hydrogel with an autonomic regulation capability inspired by the colour shift mechanism of chamelcons (Fu et al., 2018).

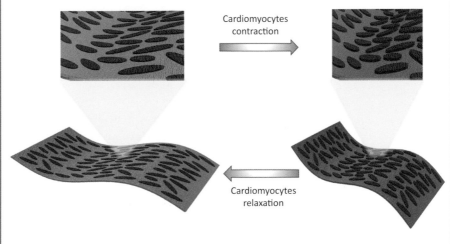

Source: Fu et al. (2018). Reprinted with permission from AAAS.

They assembled heart muscle cells on the synthetic inverse opal hydrogel films, which changes the colour as the cells beat. These hydrogel films were fabricated by replicating silica colloidal crystal templates obtained either by self-assembly of silica nanoparticles on the glass slides or by micropatterning the silicon wafers to form ordered colloidal crystal arrays. Either way, patterns were obtained which were filled with liquid methacrylate gelatine and polymerised by UV light to form hybrid hydrogels. The free-standing inverse opal-structured hydrogel films (150 µm thick) were then obtained by etching the silica nanoparticles out of the hybrid hydrogel with 2 wt% hydrofluoric acid. The high biocompatibility and plasticity of the hydrogels allowed a facile attachment and growth of cardiomyocytes and their stable autonomic beating. Volume and morphology changes of both cardiomyocytes and hydrogel during the beating process led to the change in the photonic bandgap and, as a consequence, continuous change of colour.

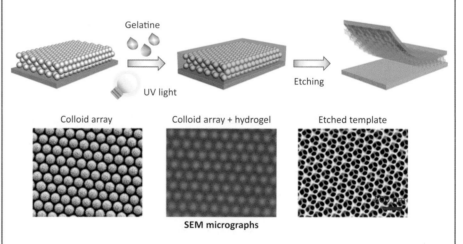

Source: Fu et al. (2018). Reprinted with permission from AAAS.

Such an autonomus change was utilised to design a soft robotic device that mimicked the shape of *Morpho* butterflies. Due to the anisotropic laminar organisation of cardiomyocytes, the hydrogel film in the shape of a butterfly appears to swing its wings in the cell medium resembling the flying butterfly.

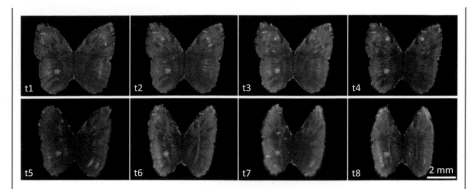

Finally, to demonstrate the potential of such hybrid photonic crystals, a heart-on-chip device was designed by combining the biohybrid materials with microfluidics. A colour change was observed at the different sites of the microfluidic chip, as the beating of cardiomyocytes changed under stress or a change of the liquid flow. In the future, such a device could be used to study the impact of environmental changes or drugs on cardiac tissue.

Key Concepts

Biomimetic nanodesign: use of biomolecules and structures as an inspiration or a blueprint for design of nanomaterials and nanopatterned surfaces with unique mechanical and physiochemical properties.

Biomineralisation: a process by which living organisms make hierarchical structures composed of organic and inorganic elements. Biomineralisation results in hybrid materials that span different scales; they contain nanosized elements assembled and structured over micro- and macroscale.

Biotemplate-assisted synthesis: use of whole organisms, usually microorganisms, or their components (organelles or biomolecules) to guide or facilitate the synthesis of nanomaterials.

Nanozyme: nanoparticle-based catalyst that can mimic the activity of natural enzymes. Such are for example iron oxide nanoparticles that can mimic peroxidase activity or ceria nanoparticles that can act as superoxide dismutase.

Peptide amphiphiles: peptides composed of two or more distinct regions with affinity towards either polar (such as water) or non-polar solvents.

Amphiphiles are particulary well-suited for design of nanomaterials such as nanofibres, nanotubes and nanovesicles.

Phage display: a method by which peptides are selected from a library prepared by directed evolution that have a desired trait such as binding to a particular surface or molecular species. In bionanotechnology, phage display libraries are useful for finding peptide structures that have high affinity for a particular nanomaterial.

Structural colour: colour that is a result of the structural motifs, rather than presence of organic pigments. It stems from the interaction of light with the periodic arrangements of (nano)structured elements. Natural structural colours can be found across the animal and plant world, and have been used as an inspiration for design of colours resistant to photobleaching and biosensors that use colour change as a reporting method.

Superhydrophobicity: property of some surfaces, which makes them highly hydrophobic (water-repelling). It stems from hydrophobicity combined with surface roughness. Superhybrophobic materials are self-cleaning and the commercial design was inspired by lotus leaf structure.

Problems

7.1   What is the difference between α-helix and β-sheets peptide motifs?

7.2   Which of the following peptides are amphiphilic and why? Which motif is contained within amphiphilic peptide?
(a) Gly-Ala-Ala-Val-Val-Gly-Lys-Lys-Arg
(b) CH_3-$(CH_2)_6$–His-His-Lys-Arg-Arg-Val
(c) CH_3-$(CH_2)_6$–Val-Val-Iso-Thr-Iso-Iso-Arg-Arg-Lys

7.3   What are the forces that guide assembly of amphiphilic peptides into nanovesicles?

7.4   Peptide amphiphile was prepared in order to afford the assembly of peptide nanotubes. Cysteine residues were built into the structure to enhance the stability of the resulting structure. How do cysteines improve the overall stability?

7.5   Peptide nanotubes are used for delivery of a chemotherapeutic drug to the cancer cells. They will be administered intravenously and need to be protected from white blood cells, which will be done by PEGylation. Which amino acids do you need to introduce to the peptide to enable attachment of carboxy and amino PEG groups?

7.6   Why are phosphorylated amino acids such as phosphoserine often added to the surface of protein fibres used to make artificial bones?

7.7   Why is nacre almost 3000 times stronger than the mineral aragonite from which it is made?

7.8   What is the biggest obstacle to translating the principles of biomineralisation to large-scale production of nanomaterials?

7.9   Which bioinspired strategy(ies) could you employ to design antibacterial surfaces to make surgery tables for use in hospitals?

7.10   A phage display is performed to find a peptide sequence that binds to silica nanoparticles. To achieve that, silica nanoparticles were added to the library of peptides in a plastic vial. After several rounds in the presence of silica nanoparticle a peptide was isolated and its sequence determined. A control was run without the added silica nanoparticles. When the peptide sequence of the control was compared to that with added silica nanoparticles they were identical. What is the peptide likely binding to? How could you improve the design of your experiment?

7.11   The coat of a 50 nm virus was genetically modified to contain cysteine-rich peptides in order to enable binding of small gold nanoparticles (10 nm) and create regular assemblies of gold patterned viral nanoparticles. However, only large and irregular assemblies were formed. What is the reason for this and what needs to be done to avoid formation of large assemblies?

7.12   Propose the design of non-fading, biodegradable food packaging that can sense the presence of bacterial pathogens.

7.13   Name some examples of photonic crystals found in nature.

Further Reading

Freeman, A. (2017). Protein-mediated templating on the nanoscale. *Biomimetics*, **2**, 14–29.

Garg, P., Ghatmale, P., Tarward, K. and Chavan, S. (2017). Influence of nanotechnology and the role of nanostructures in biomimetic studies and their potential applications. *Biomimetics*, **2**, 1–25.

Guyon, L., Lepeltier, E. and Passirani, C. (2018). Self-assembly of peptide-based nanostructures: synthesis and biological activity. *Nano Research*, **11**(5), 2315–2335.

Hendricks, M. P., Sato, K., Palmer, L. C. and Stupp, S. I. (2017). Supramolecular assembly of peptide amphiphiles. *Account of Chemical Research*, **50** (10), 2440–2448.

Mendes, A. C., Baran, E. T., Reis, R. L. and Azevedo, H. S. (2013). Self-assembly in nature; using the principles of nature to create complex nanomaterials. *WIRE's Nanomedicine and Nanotechnology*, **5**(6), 582–612.

Reches, M. and Gazit, E. (2006). Designed aromatic homo-dipeptides: formation of ordered nanostructures and potential nanotechnological applications. *Physical Biology*, **3**(1), 10–19.

Rica, R. D. L. and Matsui, H. (2010). Applications of peptide and protein-based materials in bionanotechnology. *Chemical Society Reviews*, **39**, 3499–3509.

Sotiropoulou, S., Sierra-Sastre, Y., Mark, S. S. and Batt, C. A. (2008). Biotemplated nanostructured materials. *Chemistry of Materials*, **20**, 821–834.

Wu, J., Wang, X., Wang, Q., et al. (2019). Nanomaterials with enzyme-like characteristics (nanozymes): next-generation artificial enzymes (II). *Chemical Society Reviews*, **48**, 1004–1076.

References

Adler-Abramovich, L. and Gazit, E. (2014). The physical properties of supramolecular peptide assemblies: from building block association to technological applications. *Chemical Society Reviews*, **43**, 6881–6893.

Aizenberg, J., Weaver, J. C., Thanawala, M. S., et al. (2005). Skeleton of *Euplectella* sp: structural hierarchy from the nanoscale to the macroscale. *Science*, **309**, 275–278.

Alphandéry, E. (2014). Applications of magnetosomes synthesized by magnetotactic bacteria in medicine. *Frontiers in Bioengineering and Biotechnology*, **2**(5).

Amos, F. F. and Evans, J. S. (2009). AP7, a partially disordered pseudo C-RING protein, is capable of forming stabilised aragonite in vitro. *Biochemistry*, **48**, 1332–1339.

Arnold, F. H. (2018). Directed evolution: brining new chemistry to life. *Angewandte Chemie International Edition*, **57**(16), 4143–4148.

Ayangbenro, A. S. and Babalola, O. O. (2017). A new strategy for heavy metal polluted environments: a review of microbial biosorbents. *International Journal of Environmental Research and Public Health*, **14**(1), 94–97.

Barthelat, F., Tang, H., Zavattieri, P. D., Li, C.-M. and Espinosa, H. D. (2007). On the mechanics of mother-of-pearl: a key feature in the material hierarchical structure. *Journal of the Mechanics and Physics of Solids*, **55**, 306–337.

Barthlott, W. (1990). Scanning electron microscopy of the epidermal surface in plants. In D. Claugher (ed.), *Scanning Electron Microscopy in Taxonomy and Functional Morphology*, vol. 41, Clarendon Press, pp. 69–94.

Bereczk-Tompa, E., Vonderviszt, F., Horvath, B., Szalai, I. and Posfai, M. (2017). Biotemplated synthesis of magnetic filaments. *Nanoscale*, **9**, 15062–15069.

Berndt, P., Fields, G. B. and Tirrell, M. (1995). Synthethic lipidation of peptides and amino acids: monolayer structure and properties. *Journal of the American Chemical Society*, **117**, 9515–9522.

Berry, V. and Saraf, R. F. (2005). Self-assembly of nanoparticles on live bacterium: an avenue to fabricate electronic devices. *Angewandte Chemie International Edition*, **117**, 6826–6831.

Brunner, E., Gröger, C., Lutz, K., et al. (2009). Analytical studies of silica biomineralisation: towards an understanding of silica processing by diatoms. *Applied Microbiology and Biotechnology*, **84**, 607–616.

Cha, J. N., Shimizu, K., Zhou, Y., et al. (1999). Silicatein filaments and subunits from a marine sponge direct the polymerisation of silica and silicones in vitro. *Proceedings of the National Academy of Sciences of the USA*, **96**, 361–365.

Chen, H., Zhang, L., Zhang, D., Zhang, P. and Han, Z. (2015). Bioinspired surface for surgical graspers based on the strong wet friction of tree frog toe pads. *American Chemical Society Applied Materials and Interfaces*, **7**, 13987–13995.

Crespin, J., Yam, R., Crosta, X., et al. (2014). Holocene glacial discharge fluctuation and recent instability in East Antarctica. *Earth and Planetary Science Letters*, **394**, 38–47.

Cui, Y., Wang, Y., Liu, R., et al. (2011). Serial silver clusters biomineralised by one peptide. *ACS Nano*, **5**(11), 8684–8689.

Das, S. and Dhar, B. B. (2014). Green synthesis of noble metal nanoparticles using cysteine-modified silk fibroin: catalysis and antibacterial activity. *RSC Advances*, **4**, 46285–46292.

De la Rica, R. and Matsui, H. (2008). Urease as a nanoreactor for growing crystalline ZnO nanoshells at room temperature. *Angewandte Chemie*, **47**, 5415–5417.

Dumanli, A. G. and Savin, T. (2016). Recent advances in the biomimicry of structural colours. *Chemical Society Reviews*, **45**, 6698–6724.

Ensikat, H. J., Ditsche-Kuru, P., Neinhuis, C. and Barthlott, W. (2011). Superhydrophobicity in perfection: the outstanding properties of the lotus leaf. *Beilstein Journal of Nanotechnology*, **2**, 152–161.

Evans, J. S. (2019). Composite materials design: biomineralisation proteins and the guided assembly and organisation of biomineral nanoparticles. *MDPI Materials*, **12**, 581–591.

Fei, X., Jia, M., Du, X., et al. (2013). Green synthesis of silk fibroin-silver nanoparticle composites with effective antibacterial and biofilm-disrupting properties. *Biomacromolecules*, **14**, 4483–4488.

Fontana, J., Dressick, W. J., Phelps, J., et al. (2014). Virus-templated plasmonic nanoclusters with icosahedral symmetry via directed self-assembly. *Small*, **10**(15), 3058–3063.

Freeman, A. (2017). Protein-mediated templating on the nanoscale. *Biomimetics*, **2**, 14–29.

Fu, F., Shang, L., Chen, Z., Yu, Y. and Zhao, Y. (2018). Bioinspired living structural colour hydrogels. *Science Robotics*, **3**, 8580–8587.

Gao, L., Zhuang, J., Nie, L., et al. (2007). Intrinsic peroxidase-like activity of ferromagnetic nanoparticles. *Nature Nanotechnology*, **2**, 577–583.

Harting, P. (1872). *Recherches de morphologie synthetique sur la production artificielle de quelques formations calcaire organiques*, van der Post.

Huang, R., Wang, Y., Qi, W., Su, R. and He, Z. (2014). Temperature-induced reversible self-assembly of diphenylalanine peptide and the structural transition from organogel to crystalline nanowires. *Nanoscale Research Letters*, **9**, 653–666.

Kinoshita, S., Yoshioka, S. and Kawagoe, K. (2002). Mechanism of structural colour in the Morpho butterfly: cooperation of regularity and irregularity in an iridescent scale. *Proceedings: Biological Sciences*, **269**, 1417–1421.

Lee, D. Y., Lee, D. H., Lee, S. G. and Cho, K. (2012). Hierarchical gecko-inspired nanohairs with a high aspect ratio induced by nanoyielding. *Soft Matter*, **8**, 4905–4910.

Li, N., Li, N., Yi, Q., et al. (2014). Amphiphilic peptide dendritic copolymer doxorubicin nanoscale conjugate self-assembled to an enzyme-responsive anti-cancer agent. *Biomaterials*, **35**(35), 9529–9545.

Li, Y., Huang, X. J., Heo, S. H., et al. (2007). Superhydrophobic bionic surfaces with hierarchical microsphere/SWCNT composite arrays. *Langmuir*, **23**, 2169–2174.

Lin, T., Chen, Z., Usha, R., et al. (1999). The refined crystal structure of cowpea mosaic virus at 2.8Å resolution. *Virology*, **265**, 20–34.

Lowenstam, H. A. (1962). Magnetite in denticle capping in recent chitons. *Geo Science Association Bulletin*, **73**, 435–438.

Manea, F., Houillon, F. B., Pasquato, L. and Scrimin, P. (2004). Nanozymes: gold-nanoparticle-based transphosphorylation catalyst. *Angewandte Chemie International Edition*, **43**, 6165–6169.

Mao, L.-B., Gao, H.-L., Yao, H.-B., et al. (2017). Synthetic nacre by predesigned matrix-directed mineralisation. *Science*, **345**, 107–110.

Mor, G., Vernick, S., Moscovich-Dragan, H., Dror, Y. and Freeman, A. (2011). Novel biologically active silver-avidin hybrids. *Journal of Physical Chemistry C*, **115**(46), 22695–22700.

Natalio, F., Link, T., Müller, W. E. G., et al. (2010). Bioengineering of the silica-polymerizing enzyme silicatein-alpha for a targeted application to hydroxyapatite. *Acta Biomaterialia*, **6**, 3720–3728.

Nielsen, T. K., Carstens, A. B., Browne, P., et al. (2017). The first characterised phage against a member of the ecologically important sphingomonads reveals high dissimilarity. *Scientific Reports*, **7**, 13566.

Nuraje, N., Dang, X., Qi, J., et al. (2012). Biotemplated synthesis of perovskite nanomaterials for solar energy conversion. *Advanced Materials*, **24**, 2885–2890.

Oh, D., Qi, J., Lu, Y-C., et al. (2013). Biologically enhanced cathode design for improved capacity and cycle life for lithum-oxygen batteries. *Nature*, **4**, 2756–2764.

Parnell, A., Washington, A. L., Mykhaylyk, O. O., et al. (2015). Spatially modulated structural colour in bird feathers. *Scientific Reports*, **5**, 18317.

Peters, S. E. and Gaines, R. R. (2012). Formation of the 'Great Unconformity' as a trigger for the Cambrian explosion. *Nature*, **484**, 363–366.

Qi, Y., Wang, H., Wei, K., et al. (2017). A review of structure construction of silk fibroin biomaterials from single structures to multi-level structures. *International Journal of Molecular Sciences*, **18**, 237–258.

Reches, M. and Gazit, E. (2004). Formation of closed-cage nanostructures by self-assembly of aromatic dipeptides. *Nano Letters*, **4**, 581–585.

Reches, M. and Gazit, E. (2006). Controlled patterning of aligned self-assembled peptide nanotubes. *Nature Nanotechnology*, **1**, 195–200.

Ryu, J. and Park, C. B. (2009). Synthesis of diphenylalanine/polyalanine core/shell conducting nanowires by peptide self-assembly. *Angewandte Chemie International Edition*, **48**(26), 4820–4823.

Seto, J., Ma, Y., Davis, S. A., et al. (2012). Structure-property relationship of a biological monocrystal in the adult sea urchin spine. *Proceedings of the National Academy of Sciences of the USA*, **109**(10), 3699–3704.

Shah, S. N., Steinmetz, N. F., Aljabali, A. A., Lomonossoff, G. P. and Evans, D. J. (2009). Environmentally benign synthesis of virus-templated, monodisperse iron-platinum nanoparticles. *Dalton Transactions*, **40**, 8479–8480.

Silva, R. F., Araujo, D. R., Silva, E. R., Ando, R. A., and Alves, W. A. (2013). L-Diphenylalanine microtubes as a potential drug-delivery system: characterisation, release kinetics and cytotoxicity. *Langmuir*, **29**(32), 10205–10212.

Sleytr, U. B., Messner, P., Pum, D. and Sara, M. (1999). Crystalline bacterial cell surface layers (S layers): from supramolecular cell structure to biomimetics and nanotechnology. *Angewandte Chemie International Edition*, **38**(8), 1034–1054.

Slocik, J. M., Govorov, A. O. and Naik, R. R. (2008). Photoactivated bio template nanoparticles as an enzyme mimic. *Angewandte Chemie International Edition*, **47**, 5335–5339.

Thayer, A. M. (2011). Making peptides at large scale. *Chemistry and Engineering*, **89**(22), 21–25.

Thompson, D. A. W. (1917). *On Growth and Form*, 1st edn, Cambridge University Press.

Vignolini, S., Rudall, P. J., Rowland, A. V., et al. (2012). Pointillist structural color in Pollia fruit. *Proceedings of the National Academy of Sciences of the USA*, **109**(39), 15712–15715.

Wei, H. and Wang, E. (2013). Nanomaterials with enzyme-like characteristics (nanozymes): next-generation artificial enzymes. *Chemical Society Reviews*, **42**, 6060–6093.

Williams, R. J. P. (1953). Metal ions in biological systems. *Biological Reviews of the Cambridge Philosophical Society*, **28**, 381–415.

Winter, G., Griffiths, A. D., Hawkins, R. E. and Hoogenboom, H. R. (1994). Making antibodies by phage display technology. *Annual Review of Immunology*, **12**, 433–455.

Wolf, M., Garcea, R. L., Grigorieff, N. and Harrison, S. C. (2010). Subunit interactions in bovine papillomavirus. *Proceedings of the National Academy of Sciences of the USA*, **107**(14), 6298–6303.

Wong, T.-S., Kang, S. H., Tang, S. K. Y., et al. (2011). Bioinspired self-repairing slippery surfaces with pressure-stable omniphobicity. *Nature*, **477**, 443–447.

Xue, L., Sanz, B., Luo, A., et al. (2017). Hybrid surface patterns mimicking the design of the adhesive toe pad of tree frog. *American Chemical Society Nano*, **11**, 9711–9719.

Yang, W., Guo, W., Chang, J. and Zhang, B. (2017). Protein/peptide-templated biomimetic synthesis of inorganic nanoparticles for biomedical applications. *Journal of Materials Chemistry B*, **5**, 401–417.

Yu, L. T., Banerjee, I. A. and Matsui, H. (2003). Direct growth of shape-controlled nanocrystals on nanotubes via biological recognition. *Journal of the American Chemical Society*, **125**, 14837–14840.

Zyla, G., Kovalev, A., Grafen, M., et al. (2017). Generation of bioinspired structural colours via two-photon polymerisation. *Scientific Reports*, **7**, 17622.

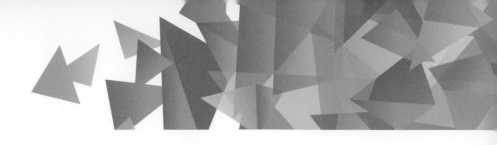

8 Bionanotechnology in Biosensor Design

Bionanotechnology has the potential not only to improve existing medical processes but also to introduce entirely new tools and materials. Advances have already been made, in particular, in design of probes and biosensors for advanced diagnostics, targeted drug nanocarriers and environment-responsive materials for tissue engineering. We need to keep in mind that at the core of all of these applications is the fundamental question of the nature of the interaction of nanomaterials and nanostructured surfaces with biological systems. The exploration of these interactions is strongly embedded within the field of nanomedicine, but it is also a part of nanotoxicology, a field that studies the environmental impact of new materials. Some strategies, findings and policy actions concerning the regulation of use of nanomaterials will be covered in the last chapter.

In this chapter we will have a look at the principles of biosensors and the ways bionano strategies have impacted the field.

8.1   Biosensors and Nanosensors

Biosensors are integrated devices which can convert a molecular recognition event into a detectible physiochemical signal. Generally, a **biosensor** contains a **biological recognition element** that interacts with a target bio(molecular) species, and a **transducing element** for signal detection (Figure 8.1).

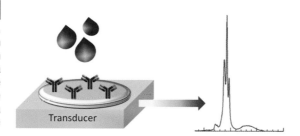

Figure 8.1

Biosensor design. Biological recognition elements interact with the target resulting in a physiochemical change which can be transformed into a readable signal with the help of a transducer.

Biological recognition elements
Antibodies
Enzymes
Nucleic acids
Membrane proteins

Transducer
Electrical/electrochemical
Optical
Gravimetric
Magnetic

Most biosensors use biomolecules such as nucleic acids (DNA or, less often, RNA) and proteins (enzymes, antibodies, protein receptors) as recognition elements, and a range of detection strategies (optical, electrochemical, gravimetric or a combination of these). Biosensors are commonly grouped into different types based on the method of detection, but at the most basic level they can be considered as **label based** and **label free**. For example, the FRET strategy we discussed in Chapter 5 is often used for design of sensing devices but requires the addition of a fluorescent label and is considered a label-based strategy. Surface plasmon resonance (SPR), on the other hand, based on measuring the changes in plasmon resonance of a thin gold film, usually does not require any labels and it is known as label-free strategy.

The first biosensor was developed in 1962 by Leland C. Clark (1918–2005), the inventor of the oxygen electrode, and his coworkers (Clark and Lyons, 1962). Clark's biosensor employed the enzyme glucose oxidase as a biological recognition element, and measured the depletion of oxygen in the presence of glucose with the help of the oxygen electrode. The biosensor field advanced significantly after the commercial success of this biosensor, which was put on the market by Yellow Spring Instruments in 1975. New read-out strategies and various recognition elements were developed, and at the end of the 1990s a new era of biosensors began with the introduction of nanomaterials.

A good biosensor is efficient, specific, portable and easy-to-use at the point of care, usually in hospitals or directly by patients. Biosensors which either require large and expensive read-out instruments and special storage facilities or have a short shelf life will be limited in both accessibility and commercial success.

One of the many challenges in biosensor development is finding ways to efficiently capture the signal that reports on particular biological events or interaction with the **analyte** component in an unknown mix. These events can be anything from a particular gene mutation, changes in enzymatic activity, presence of specific pathogens or disease biomarkers. As you can guess from the diversity of these events, they also involve very different interacting species, and transducers need to be designed that can convert the interactions into a detectable signal. Traditionally, electrochemical transducers have been most widely used, although the introduction of nanomaterials into sensor design resulted in sensitive transducers that can detect minute optical, magnetic or mechanical changes.

The earliest examples of **nanosensors** were colorimetric sensors based on plasmonic nanoparticles such as gold, which were developed in the 1990s and used for detection of particular DNA sequences or the presence of heavy metals. Plasmonic nanomaterials were soon followed by carbon nanotubes and graphene and a range of fluorescent nanomaterials such as quantum dots. The use of nanomaterials has enabled a significant reduction of the biosensor size, resulting in the use of smaller sample volumes, improved sensitivity and faster measurements. For example, the characteristic property of double layer capacitance at the interface of electrode and surrounding electrolyte, decreases with the size of electrodes. The introduction of nanosized electrodes into electrochemical biosensors significantly improved the speed of measurements, going down to nanosecond range.

To illustrate different types of nano-based biosensors, we have classified them according to the type of the read-out – **optical** (fluorescence, FRET, SERS, SPR), **electrochemical** (impedance, field effect transistors, amperometric) and **mechanical** (cantilever-based, QCM).

8.2   Nano-Enhanced Electrochemical Biosensors

Electrochemical biosensors are based either on the detection of electron exchange between molecules involved in a biological event or the detection of the local changes in electronic properties caused by binding/interaction of particular species with the transducer. Change of voltage, current or conductance/resistivity proportional to the amount of the analyte is monitored, using techniques such as amperometry, voltammetry, potentiometry or impedance (Figure 8.2). **Amperometry** monitors current over time while the potential is kept constant. The current is a result of an electrochemical reduction or oxidation and it is directly proportional to the concentration of the electrochemical species in the solution. In **voltammetry**, on the other hand, potential is not kept constant, which results in varying current. Both amperometry and voltammetry have been extensively used in the design of biosensors either to monitor enzymatic activity, determine the concentrations of protein markers or study interactions with small analytes. Potentiometric biosensors, particularly those based on nanoparticle labels, have not only been extensively used to explore enzymes, but also to detect DNA, small molecules such as ATP (see Back to Basics 3.3) and various pathogens (Ding and Qin, 2020). **Potentimetry** measures the potential across an interface, often a polymeric membrane, and uses a stable and well-defined electrode as a reference (Bratov et al., 2010). One of the most prominent types of potentiometric sensors are ion-selective electrodes such as a well-known pH-electrode, which can be found in almost every (bio) chemistry lab.

Figure 8.2

Electrochemical biosensors. Analyte interacts specifically with the recognition element immobilised onto a working electrode, and the interaction results in electron transfer. The main strategies to measure the electron transfer processes are amperometry, voltammetry, impedance and potentiometry, such as the use of field effect transistors.

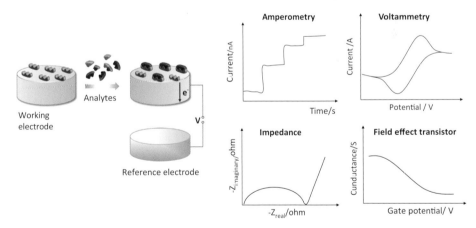

In 1975, Lorenz and Schulze introduced **impedance** or **electrochemical impedance spectroscopy (EIS)**. It measures the current response after the application of a small sinusoidal varying potential to an electrochemical cell (Lorenz and Schulze, 1975). By measuring the current over the range of frequencies of the applied potential (typically 100 kHz to 1 mHz), impedance can be obtained, which contains the information on resistivity and conductivity of the materials. Impedance spectroscopy has been particularly useful to study electrochemical changes stemming from biorecognition events at the surfaces of modified electrodes.

The simplest electrochemical biosensors consist of a working and reference electrode (Figure 8.2), although more widely used are the three electrode systems with an additional counter or auxiliary electrode. In an ideal scenario, the electron exchange during a monitored bioprocess can be directly transduced into current. This is the case with many enzymatic reactions, although design of such **enzyme-based biosensors** usually requires the immobilisation of enzymes in the close proximity of the electrode surface so that the electron transfer can occur (Figure 8.3a). However, the direct electron transfer to the electrode in enzyme-based sensors is often not possible if the enzyme's catalytic centre is shielded by a thick non-conductive protein shell. This can be overcome by use of **mediators**, small organic compounds which are oxidised at the electrode and often reduced at the enzyme site and act as efficient electron shuttles (Figure 8.3b). Commonly used mediators include quinones, organic conducting salts, dyes, ruthenium complexes and iron complexes such as ferrocene and ferricyanide derivatives.

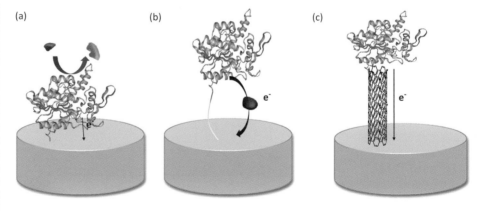

Figure 8.3

Enzyme-based biosensors. (a) Immobilisation of enzymes onto electrodes can result in direct transfer of electrons. (b) Often direct transfer is not possible and mediators are required for electron shuttling. (c) Conductive nanomaterials can be used to design effective electron transfer interface between enzymes and electrodes.

(a)   (b)   (c)

The use of mediators can be avoided by the design of effective electron transfer interfaces made of conductive nanomaterials (Figure 8.3c; Patolsky et al., 2004). Nanostructures such as carbon nanotubes can enable electron transport but also provide enough surface area for immobilisation of a large number of enzymes, thus significantly increasing the sensitivity of the biosensor (Research Report 8.1).

Research Report 8.1 | Carbon Nanotube-Based Electrochemical Glucose Biosensor

One of the most interesting and relevant biosensors is the one capable of the fast, reliable and cheap detection of glucose levels in blood. It is, therefore, not surprising that this sensor is often used as a proof-of-concept to test either novel materials or read-out strategies. At the heart of the glucose biosensing is the oxidation of glucose into D-glucono-1,5-lactone and H_2O_2 in the presence of glucose oxidase (GOx):

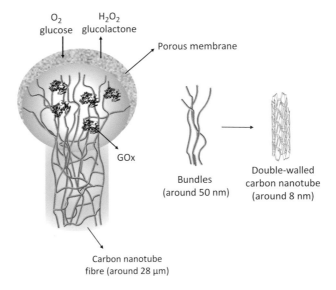

To design a new generation of the electrochemical glucose biosensor, carbon nanotubes can be employed to provide direct communication between the GOx enzyme with the electrode, and produced H_2O_2 monitored.

As the amount of H_2O_2 produced is proportional to the amount of oxidised glucose, the obtained signal can directly be used to assess the glucose levels in the reaction mix or blood. Glucose oxidase can be attached to the carbon nanotube mediator either covalently or by adsorption.

Zhu and colleagues designed a sensitive biosensor using adsorption of GOx onto carbon nanotube brushes composed of carbon nanotubes with loose ends. Porous polymer membrane deposited around the nanotube brush prevents the leakage of the enzyme, but allows for transport of glucose and H_2O_2 (Zhu et al., 2010). Such a design takes advantage of carbon nanotube conductivity and the large surface area of brush structures that enables adsorption of a large number of enzymes.

Many biological interactions such as DNA hybridisation or antibody–antigen binding are based on the affinity of the probe towards the analyte and referred to as **affinity biosensors** (Figure 8.4).

(a)

(b)

(c)

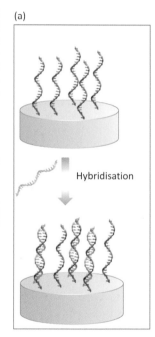

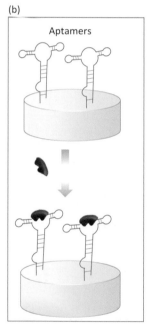

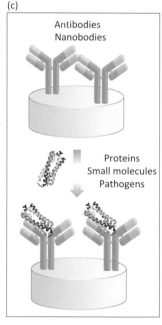

Affinity biosensors. This family of biosensors is based on a specific and usually reversible binding event between the analyte and the biological recognition element. Biological recognition elements can be: (a) nucleic acids that undergo hybridization; (b) aptamers; and (c) antibodies/nanobodies that specifically interact with a wide range of molecules species and whole cells.

Such affinity interactions are not accompanied by a detectable electron exchange. However, most of the biomolecules carry electrostatic charges and their interaction involves a change in electric potential. Such a change is exploited for the design of **field effect transistor (FET) biosensors**. In a broader sense, FET can be considered as an impedance technique. A FET device is composed of two electrodes (**source and drain**) positioned onto semiconducting material and separated by a gap (Figure 8.5a). Electrical field potential is varied at the third electrode known as the **gate** and used to control the conductivity of this gap. In a biosensor, the gate electrode is replaced by biochemically sensitive surface which is in contact with the solution of analyte (Figure 8.5b). Any bio-interaction between the analyte and a probe results in a change of electric potential, which can be directly linked to the concentration of the analyte.

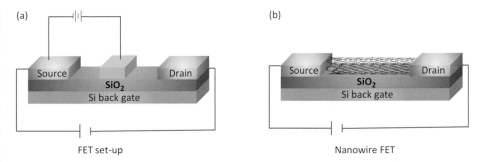

Figure 8.5

FET biosensors. (a) A typical design consists of source and drain electrode separated by a gap and a third electrode known as the gate. (b) Sensitive nano-FET devices employ nanomaterials such as carbon nanotubes to bridge the gap.

The first FET sensors were developed in the 1970s to measure the concentration of ions (Bergveld, 1970), followed by sensors for antigen–antibody interactions (Souteyrand et al., 1994) and DNA hybridisation (Souteyrand et al.,1997). A significant advance in FET technology was made by the introduction of nanoelements such as nanowires to bridge the source and the drain of the planar FET (Figure 8.5b). When a probe, for example an antibody, is immobilised onto the surface of nanowires, minute changes in conductance upon an antigen binding can be detected with high sensitivity and reproducibility (Research Report 4.7 in Chapter 4). Carbon nanotubes have been often used as a FET element, although the main challenge with their use is the lack of purity as they often come as a mixture of semiconducting and metallic nanotubes, which leads to decreased sensitivity of the sensor. Successful alternatives to carbon nanotubes have been silicon nanowires, which can be grown chemically in high purity and easily modified (Research Report 8.2). In the meanwhile FET have been used for design of label-free, sensitive and selective sensors for detection of nucleic acids, biomarkers and pathogens, and silicon nanowires have also been adapted for in vivo sensing, in particular, detection of neuronal activity.

Research Report 8.2	Silicon Nanowire FET Biosensors

Silicon nanowire (SiNW) FET biosensors were pioneered by Charles M. Lieber and his group in the early 2000s (Patolsky et al., 2006). The first silicon nanowire biosensor was a solid state FET device that used boron doped silicon nanowires modified with 3-aminopropyltriethoxysilane

(APTES). Due to surface modification with APTES, NWs can be protonated and deprotonated with the increase of pH resulting in a linear increase of conductance.

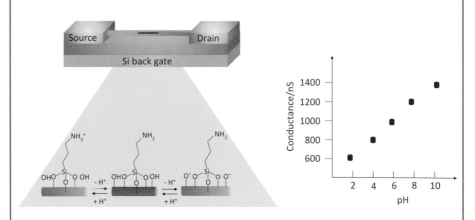

After this initial proof of concept, SiNWs were functionalised with biotin to provide a biotin–streptavidin (STV) sensor (more on streptavidin in Chapters 3 and 4).

The conductance increased upon the streptavidin addition as a consequence of binding of negatively charged protein to the SiNW surface, and streptavidin was detected in concentration down to 10 pM. Other protein biosensors followed resulting in precise time- and concentration-dependent detection (Patolsky, 2006).

8.3   Optical Bionanosensors

Optical biosensors use optical transducer elements such as a spectrometer to convert the biological interaction into a signal. The most interesting developments in optical bionanosensors have been inspired by the introduction of fluorescent nano-labels and plasmonic nanoparticles to monitor the changes in localised surface plasmon resonance (LSPR).

8.3.1   Plasmonic Nanosensors

Plasmonic nanoparticles are characterised by the ability to convert a photon into collective plasmon oscillations (Back to Basics 1.2 in Chapter 1). The theory behind such behaviour was postulated in 1908 by Gustav Mie

(1868–1957) to explain the interaction of an incoming wave with a spherical colloidal particle (Mie, 1908). Depending on the type and shape of the metallic nanoparticle, a photon of a specific wavelength can be absorbed resulting in a specific colour. The changes in plasmon can often be detected by inspecting the colour of plasmonic nanoparticles, which is the principle of **plasmonic nanosensors** or **LSPR biosensors** (Research Report 8.3).

Research Report 8.3	Colorimetric Detection of Influenza A Virus

Influenza viral infection caused by influenza virus A has been responsible for influenza pandemics across the globe, affecting not only humans but also a range of animal species. In order to deal with the annual epidemics and prevent the virus spread, it is necessary to detect the disease in the early stage when it is still asymptomatic. Type A viruses are classified based on the type of haemagglutinin (HA) and neuraminidase (NA) proteins within their coat. For example, avian flu virus H7N9, which killed 40% of infected patients in China in 2013, is composed of HA type 7 and NA type 9. Haemagglutinin protein is a major component of influenza viruses and has a key role in initiating viral infection by binding to sialic acid present on the surface of the cells (Gallagher et al., 2018). Detection of HA protein can be used to design sensitive virus biosensors. One such design combined Au nanoparticles and the interaction between anti-HA antibody and 500 HA proteins on the surface of a virus, affording cheap and fast detection of small amounts of H3N2 virus.

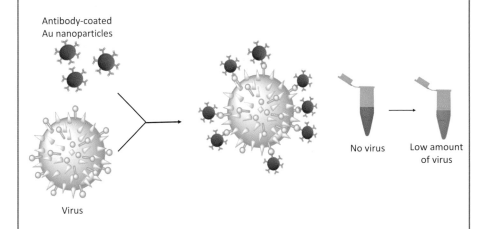

Gold nanoparticles of 13 nm were coated with anti-HA antibody and allowed to incubate with the virus, which resulted in Au NPs binding onto the viral coat. The assembly of Au NPs on a viral coat resulted in a shift of the surface plasmon resonance peak at 520 nm, and noticeable colour change. Detection was done in one step and resulted in the specific detection of as few as 8 HA proteins, which is much less than a single virus contains in a 250 µl sample (Liu, 2015).

A number of colorimetric sensors based on gold nanoparticles have already been commercialised and used in home pregnancy tests and commercial kits for detection of various enzymes and proteins (Aldewachi, 2018).

Localised surface plasmon resonance biosensors are in many ways similar to SPR biosensors (see Chapter 5), although they do not employ complex optical designs and use nanoparticles instead of planar gold surfaces. Generally, when an analyte binds to a surface of a plasmonic nanoparticle, this induces a change of the refractive index, which in turn shifts the LSPR peak frequency ($\Delta\lambda$) described as:

$$\Delta\lambda = m(\Delta n)\left[1 - \exp\left(\frac{-2d}{l_d}\right)\right],\qquad(8.1)$$

where m is a refractive index sensitivity, Δn is a change in refractive index induced by the analyte binding, d is the adsorbate layer thickness and l_d is the electromagnetic field decay length.

As can be seen from Equation 8.1, the difference in wavelength can be directly correlated to the change of refractive index and the size of the analyte determined by d. Electromagnetic field decay length l_d depends on the nanoparticle size, and is determined by the distance from the surface within which the analyte binding can induce the change in plasmon. For 50–100 nm nanoparticles, l_d will be 5–10 nm. Conveniently that corresponds to the of many proteins including antibodies, making these plasmonic nanoparticles suitable for affinity sensor design (Figure 8.6).

Sensitivity of LSPR biosensors has been improved by use of single nanoparticles of a particular geometry such as gold nanorods, or by employing a combination of nanomaterials such as graphene oxide and gold nanoparticles for enhanced biosensing with multiple read-outs (Chiu, 2018). Despite a number of commercial LSPR biosensors being available, they are not suitable for cell and in vivo sensing due to their low stability in complex biological fluids.

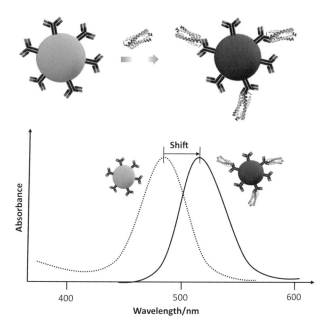

8.3.2   FRET Biosensors

Optical biosensors that have been crucial for studies of bio-interactions within cells are FRET biosensors. In Chapter 5 we discussed the principles of FRET and how it can be used as a tool for detection of nanoscale interactions. The performance of FRET biosensors depends on the choice of the donor and acceptor dyes as well as the type of the attachment to the molecules of interest. It is important to remember that FRET can only occur when the intermolecular distance between donors and acceptors is smaller than 10 nm, which makes it very sensitive for the detection of binding between molecules, cleavage events and conformational changes within a single molecule (Figure 8.7a–c).

Fluorescence resonance energy transfer biosensors based on organic dyes have the advantages of simple preparation and low cost, but they are limited by weak signals, poor resistance to photobleaching, short fluorescence lifetime and, often, low chemical stability. Some of them can also be toxic to the cell, making them unsuitable for intracellular applications. On the other hand, fluorescence protein-based FRET biosensors permit experiments in living cells, can be fused to a range of proteins, but are large in size and often plagued by a spectral cross-talk due to broad excitation/emission spectra. These drawbacks of organic fluorescent species prompted the use of nano-particles, which often have strong and stable fluorescence and high quantum

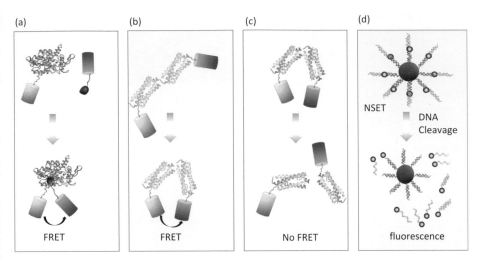

Figure 8.7

FRET based biosensors. Different biological events can be explored using the change in fluorescence of fluorophore donors and acceptors in close proximity such as (a) binding of a ligand to a protein, (b) conformational change within a single protein or (c) enzyme cleavage. Nanomaterial surface energy transfer (NSET) can lead to fluorescence quenching when flurophore is in the close proximity of the nanomaterial surface. The fluorescence can be restored when the fluorophore is cleaved from the surface.

yields. A number of nanoparticle classes, most prominently semiconductor quantum dots (QDs), graphene quantum dots (GQDs), upconversion nanoparticles (UCNPs), gold nanoparticles (AuNPs) and graphene oxide (GO), have been used in the design of FRET biosensors either by replacing conventional fluorescent dyes and proteins, or acting as quenchers.

The use of gold nanoparticles is not based on their fluorescence, but rather the ability to quench the fluorescently labelled probe. Spherical Au NPs, unlike fluorescent dyes, have no defined dipole moment. As a result, the energy transfer to Au NPs is independent of the donor orientation which leads to the **fluorescence quenching**. The distance between donors and Au NPs for quenching to occur was shown to be in the range of 70–100 nm, which is almost 10 times longer than distances that can be monitored by conventional FRET. Another frequently used nano-quencher is graphene oxide (GO), a derivative of graphene, which contains carboxylic, hydroxyl and epoxy groups. Such heterogeneous structure makes GO a universal quencher for almost all fluorophores used in FRET within the distance of 30 nm. Biosensors based on the use of nanomaterials as fluorescence quenchers rather than conventional acceptors are sometimes referred to as **nanomaterial surface electron transfer** (NSET) biosensors (Figure 8.7d).

In addition to their multiple roles as fluorophores and quenchers, nanomaterials have large surface areas, which enable immobilisation of large numbers of molecules, thus facilitating the 'single-to-multiple' FRET. As a consequence, the replacement of organic fluorescent dyes by nanoparticles can result in high-energy transfer efficiency, a long-range working distance, longer fluorescence lifetime, stronger signal and tunable spectra, which can minimise the cross-talk between donors and acceptors.

8.3.3 Surface-Enhanced Raman Scattering Biosensors

Another type of optical biosensor, which benefitted from developments in nanomaterial design are **surface-enhanced Raman scattering (SERS) biosensors**. In SERS, plasmonic nanomaterials, such as silver or gold nanoparticles, are used as Raman signal enhancers of molecular species attached or adsorbed to their surface (Chapter 5). One of the first demonstrations of SERS biosensing potential was the detection of a target DNA strand with the help of gold nanoparticles immobilised with complementary DNA (Cao, 2002). In recent years, SERS has been particularly successful for the design of very sensitive biosensors for detection of low amounts of cancer biomarkers or pathogen microorganisms or viruses (Research Report 8.4).

Research Report 8.4	SERS Nanosensor for Detection of Multiple Antibiotic-Resistant Pathogens

Because of the overuse of antibiotics, bacterial pathogens such as MRSA, *Pseudomonas, E. coli* and *Mycobacterium tuberculosis* develop drug resistance which results in the rise of untreatable bacterial infections. To avoid public health issues arising from antibiotic-resistant bacteria, efficient methods for isolation and detection of pathogens are crucial. Conventional methods employ growing bacterial cell cultures and colony counting, and DNA and immunology-based assays, which are time-consuming, expensive and require specialist equipment. This can be overcome by development of sensitive biosensors, as demonstrated by researchers from the University of Strathclyde. They designed a nanobiosensor, which enabled both the isolation and detection of pathogenic bacteria with the help of magnetic separation and SERS – a **SERS nanosensor.**

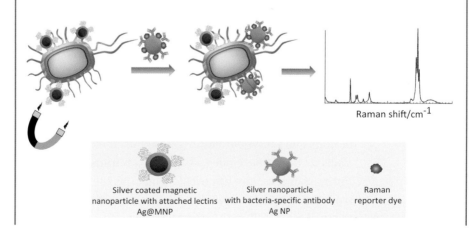

Raman shift/cm^{-1}

Silver coated magnetic nanoparticle with attached lectins Ag@MNP

Silver nanoparticle with bacteria-specific antibody Ag NP

Raman reporter dye

The biosensor employed silver-coated magnetic nanoparticles (Ag@MNPs) functionalised with lectin (Concanvilin A), which binds specifically to sugar groups present on the surface of three different strains of bacteria. By applying the magnetic field, nanoparticle-captured bacteria can be separated from the sample matrix. After separation, SERS active silver nanoparticles (Ag NPs) functionalised with a unique Raman reporter and antibodies specific to each strain are added to concentrated and separated bacteria. Three Raman reporters are used, each functionalised together with a specific antibody, to act as reporters for *E. coli*, *Salmonella typhi* and MRSA strains respectively. Once functionalised, bacteria can be identified using SERS. The assay was successfully applied to detect the bacteria strains individually as well as to distinguished them in the mix of all three. There were 10^4 to 10^1 colony-forming units per ml (CFU/ml) detected, which is below the recommended limits currently required for clinical diagnostics ($\geq 10^3$ CFU/ml). Besides sensitivity and use of a portable Raman instrument for the read-out, the advantage of the SERS biosensor is a very fast analysis time (~1 h). In comparison, the culture-based method can take up to seven days for results to be obtained (Kearns et al., 2017).

Optical biosensors are extensively used and continuously being improved and adapted to various systems. There is a large number of publications and books (see this chapter's Further Reading) dedicated to their design and applications, with only a short overview given here to illustrate the basic principles.

8.4   Mechanical Nanosensors

Mechanical nanosensors employ nanosized materials either as transducers of mechanical force which can be linked to the mass change into a detectable signal, or enhancers of the mechanical response. In Chapter 5 we already talked about quartz crystal microbalance (QCM) principle and use in sensor design. The **QCM biosensor** is based on the use of piezoelectric materials (see Back to Basics 5.9), such as quartz, to translate mechanical stress related to the mass change into electrical signal. QCM biosensors have benefitted largely from use of nanomaterial labels such as gold nanoparticles for signal enhancement (Research Report 5.3 in Chapter 5).

For example, antibody-coated gold nanoparticles have been used as 'heavy' reporter probes to enhance the detection of pathogen bound on the QCM electrode (Figure 8.8a), or as secondary nanoparticle-labelled antibody for detection of cancer biomarkers.

Figure 8.8

Mechanical nanosensors. (a) Quartz microbalance can be used to detect small changes in mass resulting from specific binding of the antibody-labelled gold nanoparticles to the immobilised bacteria. (b) Cantilever biosensor modified with single-stranded DNA, can be used to detect the hybridisation event through mechanical motion. Fritz et al. (2000). Reprinted with permission from AAAS.

(a)

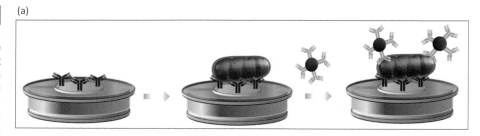

(b)

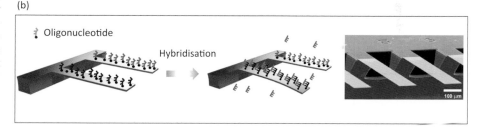

Another class of nanosensors that monitors mechanical changes was developed as early as 2000 to detect the hybridisation of DNA and it is based on use of **cantilever-like nanosensors** (Fritz et al., 2000). Small silicon cantilever of nanometre thickness can be functionalised with single-stranded DNA, and double helix formation in the presence of the complementary strand causes the displacement of the cantilever (Figure 8.8b). Such displacement can be detected as a deflection of the incoming laser beam similar to atomic force microscopy.

Cantilever biosensors can be manufactured in different sizes and from different materials, although gold and silicon/silicon nitrate are the most commonly employed due to the well-explored strategies of surface biofunctionalisation. Displacement caused by the interaction of a probe and an analyte can not only be detected by deflection of the laser beam but also using piezoelectric effect.

If the analyte is uniformly distributed along the resonant cantilever, the change is frequency **Δf** is related to the mass of the attached species (Tamayo, 2013):

$$\frac{\Delta f}{f_0} \cong -\frac{1}{2}\frac{m}{m_c}, \tag{8.2}$$

where f_0 is the resonant frequency of the system, m is the mass of the attached species and m_c is the mass of the cantilever. The ratio of $f_0/\Delta f$ is known as the *quality factor* (Q) which tells us more about the sharpness of the resonance peak of the cantilever and relates the oscillation frequency to energy dissipation of the given system. Nanoscale cantilever beams can have Q to about 100 when they are oscillating in air, and the Q factor is a good value to estimate the quality of the cantilever sensor design, and the expected amplitude of deflection.

Cantilever biosensors have benefitted from the development of new strategies for production of small geometries but also from advances in biofunctionalisation strategies and combination with other detection techniques (Research Report 8.5).

Research Report 8.5 | Hybrid Mechanical and Plasmonic Nanobiosensor

Sensors capable of detecting low concentrations of biomarkers in blood could be used in the early detection of diseases such as cancer. To achieve high sensitivity, often a combination of transducers needs to be employed. Kosaka et al. (2014) combined mechanical and optoplasmonic transduction for detection of cancer biomarkers carcinoembryonic antigen (CEA, ~190 kDa) and prostate specific antigen (PSA, ~32 kDa) in blood. The hybrid biosensor was composed of antigen specific antibody anchored to the surface of the cantilever. Once the biomarker is bound to the surface antibody, a secondary antibody tethered to a 100 nm diameter gold nanoparticle (mass around 10 fg) binds onto the capture biomarker.

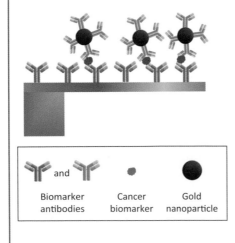

Biomarker antibodies | Cancer biomarker | Gold nanoparticle

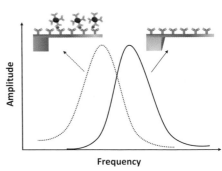

Gold nanoparticles act both as a mass and plasmonic label. To detect the signals (weight and plasmonic shift) a silicon cantilever, 500 μm long, 100 μm wide and 1 μm thick, which exhibits a fundamental resonance frequency of 5.08 ± 0.18 kHz, was used. The mass loading leads to a decrease of the resonance frequency of the silicon cantilever. The opto-plasmonic transduction of the captured biomarker is monitored via the enhanced light scattering of the gold nanoparticles caused by their localised plasmon resonances. For the particles bound to the microcantilever, there is a coupling of the optical cavity modes and the localised surface plasmon modes at the characteristic frequencies, which results in formation of hybrid plasmonic supermodes. Ultimately, these can be used to achieve the detection limit of 1×10^{-16} g ml^{-1} for PSA biomarker, which is at least seven orders of magnitude lower than that routinely used in clinical tests (Kosaka et al., 2014).

The limits of detection of cantilever biosensors are in the range of several attograms ($1\,\text{ag} = 10^{-18}$ g) which is a significant improvement over 1 ng detected by QCM or 1 pg detected by surface plasmon resonance. In addition to mass and surface stress, such nanosensors can also be used to determine the viscoelasticity and Young modulus, which is a measure of elasticity. Due to development in the field of mechanobiology, we know that elasticity and other mechanical properties play an important role in cell development and growth, and that their changes can be directly related to various diseases. Sensors capable of detecting mechanical and other physiochemical changes in biological systems, in particular within the cells and tissues, and reporting in real time will comprise the next generation of nanobiosensors – **in vivo nanosensors**.

8.5   In Vivo Nanosensors

The ultimate biosensor should be able to monitor biochemical changes continuously over a prolonged period of time, in real time and in vivo. These requirements can be met through the design of injectable, implantable or circulating nanosensors. Although the concept of in vivo nanosensors has the potential to change healthcare practices by enabling personalised approaches, there are only few reports to date of successful biosensors. The challenges faced by the field are similar to those encountered in drug delivery systems, which we will discuss in the next chapter, namely, biocompatibility, selectivity, prolonged circulation, immunogenic response and continuous monitoring. In addition, in case of the biosensors, the signal has to be robust, and there should be a minimal need for recalibration, and the removal of it should be possible.

The most clinically relevant biosensor remains an implantable sensor for continuous glucose monitoring. It was approved by the US Food and Drug Administration in 2018 for use by patients with diabetes. In vivo nanosensors are still mostly in a research stage of development. One of the first nanoscale sensors for in vivo use, demonstrated in 2013, used the changes in fluorescence of single-walled carbon nanotubes to monitor the level of nitric oxide in mice (Iverson et al., 2013). Different types of nanosensors based on optical measurements (sometimes referred to as optode nanosensors) were also developed, but they can only be implanted in skin due to the limited penetration depth of the light (several millimetres).

Unlike implantable biosensors, injectable nanosensors could provide continuous monitoring of changes in blood and inform the physicians on the impact of a particular drug or treatment. However, this would require the design of transducers that are not limited by the penetration depth of light, using, for instance, photoacoustic detection (Research Report 8.6), or electrochemical nanosensors made of biocompatible sensing surfaces (Jo et al., 2011).

Research Report 8.6   Photoacoustic Imaging of the Distribution of an Injected Drug

In photoacoustic imaging, ultrasound signals are produced as a consequence of the photoacoustic effect when photons are absorbed by a molecule. Photoacoustics can be used to either monitor natural molecules such as haemoglobin, or dye- and nanoparticle-probes (gold nanorods, IR absorbing carbon nanotubes). Many fluorescent dyes can be used as photoacoustic probes, the advantage of photoacoustics being deeper tissue penetration and 3D imaging. These advantages were employed in designing injectable nanosensors for monitoring drug levels in tissue by Cash et al. (2015). They explored the distribution of lithium, commonly used in the treatment of bipolar disorders. Lithium has a narrow therapeutic window (0.6–1.2 mM) and a low toxic dose (2 mM), requiring continuous monitoring.

The in vivo photoacoustic nanosensor – injected into the skin tissue of mice – was based on the use of lithium selective crown ether ionophore (embedded within a 27 nm nanoparticle composed of a polymer cocktail commonly referred to as **optode**). As lithium ions are bound to the ionophore (IO) within nanoparticles, chromoionophore (CH$^+$) embedded in the nanoparticles is deprotonated, which changed the optical properties and the photoacoustic response of the nanosensor. Additive (R$^-$) balanced the charge inside the sensor. The changes in the photoacoustic response across the mice tissue allowed for precise detection of Li distribution.

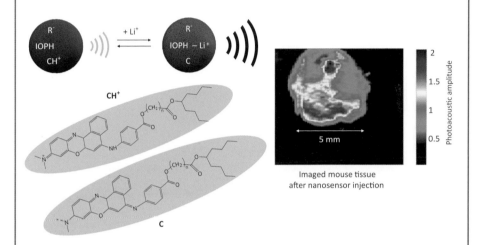

Imaged mouse tissue
after nanosensor injection

Not only 3D distribution was achieved but a fast response was obtained (within 15 s), and the nanosensor was reversible and selective to lithium over other ions such as commonly present sodium (Cash et al., 2015).

Although in vivo nanosensors are still reported rarely, their development will benefit from design of new nanomaterials and nano hybrids. Besides the read-out technology, it will be crucial to develop biocompatible materials such as nanocomposite hydrogels or biopolymer coats. Advances in in vivo nanosensors go hand-in-hand with developments of nanosized drug delivery systems, which we will discuss in the next chapter. Ultimately two concepts – diagnostic and therapeutic actions – can be merged into **theranostic devices**, which could provide diagnostic information and enable tailored delivery of therapeutics (Chapter 9). Such devices are made possible by development of biofunctionalised nanomaterials and have a huge potential to become important tools for personalised medicine.

Key Concepts

Affinity biosensor: an analytical device based on measurements of the changes stemming from biomolecular binding.

Biosensor: an integrated analytical device that uses biological recognition elements to bind to or react with the target (analyte), and convert such an event into a readable signal with the help of a transducer.

Cantilever-like nanosensors: use mechanical movements of silicon cantilever caused by an interaction of immobilised probe molecules with labelled or unlabelled analytes.

Enzyme-based biosensor: a sensor that employs enzymes to produce a readable signal proportional to the concentration of an analyte.

Field effect transistor (FET) biosensor: a device that measures minute changes in conductance induced by the binding of molecules.

Fluorescence quenching: a phenomenon in which some molecules and nanoparticles engage in a distance-dependent energy transfer that results in quenching of fluorescence.

In vivo nanosensors: implantable, injectable or ingestible analytical devices (either nanosized or containing nanosized elements) that can be used for in vivo continuous monitoring of analytes.

Nanosensor: a sensing device that employs nanomaterials to facilitate the detection of an analyte.

Plasmonic nanosensor: a sensor that employs changes in localised plasmonic resonance peak of plasmonic nanoparticles to explore biomolecular interactions.

SERS nanosensor: an analytical device that employs plasmonic nanoparticles to enhance the Raman signal of an intrinsically Raman active or Raman-dye labelled analyte.

Problems

8.1 Name the main components of the biosensor and explain what is the difference between a biosensor and a bionanosensor.

8.2 Group the following sensors into label free or label based:
   (a) quantum dots modified with HIV virus antibody used for HIV detection in blood;
   (b) SPR-based detection of cystic fibrosis gene;

(c) gold nanoparticle-based colorimetric assay for the detection of pathogenic bacteria in water;

(d) QCM-based sensor for antibody–antigen interaction;

(e) carbon-nanotube FET detection of toxic gasses;

(f) FRET biosensor for interaction of a model drug with a ribosome.

8.3 Why is it important to take into account the nature of the chemical bond between the enzyme and electrode when designing enzyme-based electrochemical nanosensors?

8.4 Glucose oxidase is a dimeric globular protein with approximate diameter of 5 nm. How many enzymes could be immobilised onto a single walled carbon nanotube with diameter of 2 nm and length of 500 nm?

8.5 What is the role of mediators in the design of enzyme biosensors and which nanomaterials could be used as a suitable alternative to chemical mediators?

8.6 Describe, with a drawing, the basic surface plasmon resonance (SPR) set-up for detection of breast cancer antigen present in the blood serum of patients (consult Chapter 5 for details on SPR). How could nanoparticles be employed to enhance the signal?

8.7 The specific receptor Rec1 is expressed in lung cancer cells and could be used for specific targeting of these cells. A FRET sensor using a fluorescent protein EYFP (l_{ex} = 520 nm, l_{em} = 540 nm) and CdSe quantum dots (l_{ex} = 380 nm, l_{em} = 510 nm) was designed to screen model nanobodies and find the one that is binding specifically to Rec1.

(a) Describe the principle of such FRET biosensor.

(b) Which strategies can be used to label Rec1 and a nanobody?

(c) Consulting Chapter 5 calculate what is the separation (in nm) between CdSe quantum dot and EYFP if the FRET efficiency (E_{FRET}) is 60% and the Föster distance R_0 for this system is 6 nm.

8.8 Cystic fibrosis (CF) is a genetic disease caused by a specific gene mutation. The most common mutation is a deletion of three DNA nucleotides coding for phenylalanine in the CF gene:

5′-AAA TAT CAT **CTT T**CG T (DNA sequence of the healthy patient)

5′-AAA TAT CAT CCG T (DNA sequence of the CF-affected patient)

(a) Design a biosensor based on gold nanoparticles for detection of the CF mutation, clearly stating which DNA sequences need to be attached to the nanoparticle(s) (remember that convention says you need to write the sequences from 5′ to 3′).

(b) Which read-out method can be used for detection?

(c) Which control measurements do you need to perform to ensure there are no false positive and false negative results?

8.9   Proteases are enzymes responsible for protein degradation. They are also important drug targets, and one such potential drug *LF42* is predicted to bind proteases from breast cancer cells by binding to the catalytic site of the enzyme. Such irreversible binding deactivates proteases in the cancer cells, leading to accumulation of protein garbage and eventual cell death. Design a mechanical nanosensor to test the activity of the drug using one of the strategies mentioned in this chapter. Which controls need to be performed to ensure the results are valid?

8.10 A small protein adsorbs onto the surface of a rectangular silicon beam (length = 100 mm, thickness = 500 nm). The elastic modulus is 100 GPa and Poisson's ratio $v = 0.22$. The binding alters the surface stress by 5×10^{-4} N m^{-1}. Equation 8.3 describes the relationship between a beam's deflection, z, and the differential surface stress ($\Delta\sigma$):

$$\Delta z = \frac{C\, l^2(1-v)\Delta\sigma}{E_{\mathrm{m}} t^3}, \tag{8.3}$$

where C is a geometrical constant and for a rectangular beam $C = 3$, l is the length, v is Poisson's ratio and describes the tendency of the material to get thinner as it elongates, E_{m} is the elastic modulus of the beam material and t is the thickness of the beam. Use Equation 8.3 to calculate by how much the beam deflects upon the adsorption of the protein.

8.11 What are different types of in vivo nanosensors? What are the biggest challenges in the design of in vivo sensors and how could they be overcome?

Further Reading

Doucey, M-A. and Carrara, S. (2019). Nanowire sensors in cancer. *Trends in Biotechnology*, **37**, 86–99.

Duque, J. S., Blandon, J. S. and Riascos, H. (2017). Localised plasmon resonance in metal nanoparticles using Mie theory. *Journal of Physics Conference Series*, **850**, 012017.

Holzberger, M., Goff, A. L. and Cosnier, S. (2014). Nanomaterials for biosensing applications: a review. *Frontiers in Chemistry*, **2**, 63.

Kimmel, D. W., LeBlanc, G., Meschievitz, M. E. and Cliffel, D. E. (2012). Electrochemical sensors and biosensors. *Analytical Chemistry*, **84**(2), 685–707.

Rogers, K. R. (2000). Principles of affinity-based biosensors. *Molecular Biotechnology*, **14**(2), 109–129.

Rong, G., Corrie, S. R. and Clark, H. A. (2017). In vivo biosensing: progress and perspectives. *ACS Sensors*, **2**(3), 327–338.

Ruckh, T. T. and Clark, H. A. (2014). Implantable nanosensors: toward continuous physiologic monitoring. *Analytical Chemistry*, **86**(3), 1314–1323.

Tamayo, J., Kosaka, P. M., Ruz, J. J., Paulo, A. S. and Calleja, M. (2013). Biosensor based on nanomechanical systems. *Chemical Society Reviews*, **42**, 1287–1311.

Toumazou, C. and Georgiou, P. (2011). Piet Bergveld: 40 years of ISFET technology: from neuronal sensing to DNA sequencing. *Electronics Letters*, **47**(26), S7.

Unsser, S., Bruzas, I., He, J. and Sagle, L. (2015). Localised surface plasmon resonance biosening: current challenges and approaches. *Sensors*, **15**, 15684–15716.

FRET

Chen, N-T., Cheng, S-H, Liu, C-P., et al. (2012). Recent advances in nanoparticle-based Forster resonance energy transfer for biosensing, molecular imaging, and drug release profiling. *International Journal of Molecular Science*, **13**(120), 16598–16623.

Gambin, Y. and Deniz, A. A. (2010). Multicolor single-molecule FRET to explore protein folding and binding. *Molecular Biosystems*, **6**, 1540–1547.

Ma, L., Yang, F. and Zheng, J. (2014). Application of fluorescence resonance energy transfer in protein studies. *Journal of Molecular Structure*, **1077**, 87–100.

References

Aldewachi, H., Chalati, T., Woodroofe, M. N., et al. (2018). Gold nanoparticle-based colorimetric biosensors. *Nanoscale*, **10**, 18–33.

Bergveld, P. (1970). Development of an ion-sensitive solid-state device for neurophysiological measurements. *IEEE Transactions on Bio-Medical Engineering*, **1**, 70–71.

Bratov, A., Abramova, N. and Ipatov, A. (2010). Recent trends in potentiometric sensor arrays: a review. *Analytical Chimica Acta*, **678**, 149–159.

Cao, Y. C., Jin, R. and Mirkin, C. A. (2002). Nanoparticles with Raman spectroscopic fingerprints for DNA and RNA detection. *Science*, **297**, 1536–1540.

Cash, K. J., Chiye, L., Xia, J., Wang, L. V. and Clark, H. A. (2015). Optical drug monitoring: photoacoustic imaging of nanosensors to monitor therapeutic lithium in vivo. *ACS Nano*, **9**(2), 1692–1698.

Chiu, N-F., Chen, C-C, Yang, C-D, Kao, Y-S. and Wu, W-R (2018). Nanoparticle-grapene oxide based label free immunoassay. *Nanoscale Research Letters*, **13**, 152.

Clark, L. C. and Lyons, C. (1962). Electrode systems for continuous monitoring in cardiovascular surgery. *Automated and Semiautomated Systems in Clinical Chemistry*, **102**(1), 29–45.

Ding, J. and Qin, W. (2020). Recent advances in potentiometric biosensors. *Trends in Analytical Chemistry*, **124**, 115803.

Fritz, J., Baller, M. K., Lang, H. P., et al. (2000). Translating biomolecular recognition into nanomechanics. *Science*, **288**, 316–318.

Gallagher, J. R., McCraw, D. M., Torian, U., et al. (2018). Characterization of hemagglutinin antigens of influenza virus and within vaccines using electron microscopy. *Vaccines*, **6**(2), 31.

Iverson, N. M., Barone, P. W., Shandell, M., et al. (2013). In vivo biosensing via tissue-localisable near-infrared-fluorescent single-walled carbon nanotubes. *Nature Nanotechnology*, **8**(11),873–880.

Jo, A., Do, H., Jhon, G-J., Suh, M. and Lee, Y. (2011). Electrochemical nanosensor for real-time direct imaging of nitric oxide in living brain. *Analytical Chemistry*, **83**, 8314–8319.

Kearns, H., Goodacre, R., Jamieson, L. E., Graham, D. and Faulds, K. (2017). SERS detection of multiple antimicrobial-resistant pathogens using nanosensors. *Analytical Chemistry*, **89**, 12666–12673.

Kosaka, P. M., Pini, V., Ruz, J. J., et al. (2014). Detection of cancer biomarkers in serum using a hybrid mechanical and optoplasmonic nanosensor. *Nature Nanotechnology*, **9**, 1047–1053.

Liu, Y., Zhang, L., Wei, W., et al. (2015). Colorimetric detection of influenza A virus using antibody-functionalised gold nanoparticles. *Analyst*, **140**, 3989–3995.

Lorenz, W. and Schulze, K. D. (1975). Application of transform-impedance spectrometry. *Journal of Electroanalytical Chemistry*, **65**, 141–153.

Mie, G. (1908). Beiträge zur Optik trüber Medien, speziell kolloidaler Metallösungen. *Annalen der Physik*, **4**(25), 377–445.

Patolsky, F., Weizmann, Y. and Willner, I. (2004). Long-range electrical contacting of redox enzymes by SWCNT connectors. *Angewandte Chemie*, **43**, 16–18.

Patolsky, F., Zheng, G. and Lieber, C. M. (2006). Fabrication of silicon nanowire devices for ultrasensitive, label-free, real-time detection of biological and chemical species. *Nature Protocols*, **1**, 1711–1724.

Souteyrand, E., Martin, J. R. and Martelet, C. (1994). Direct detection of biomolecules by electrochemical impedance measurements. *Sensors and Actuators B: Chemical*, **20**(1), 63–66.

Souteyrand, E., Cloarec, J. P., Martin, J. R., et al. (1997). Direct detection of the hybridisation of synthetic homo-oligomer DNA sequences by field effect. *Journal of Physical Chemistry B*, **101**(15), 2980–2985.

Zhu, Z., Song, W., Burugapalli, K., et al. (2010). Nano-yarn carbon nanotube fiber based enzymatic glucose biosensor. *Nanotechnology*, **21**(16), 165501.

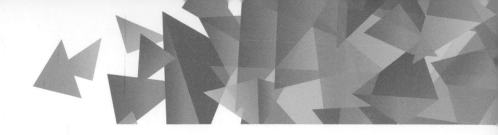

9 Bionanotechnology Meets Medicine

Nanomedicine, like conventional medicine, has two aims: to diagnose the disease, as accurately and as early as possible, and to deliver the most efficient treatment possible. Unlike conventional medicine, it uses nanomaterials and nanotools to achieve this. We saw in Chapter 8 the way in which nanotechnology advanced the field of biosensors, and we now look at some of the concepts behind the design of drug nanocarriers and nanocomposites for tissue engineering, as well as some challenges that still need to be overcome. In the core of bionanotechnology is the exploration of interactions between engineered nanomaterials with biomolecules and cells. Such studies are not only important to help the design of biocompatible materials, but also to assess the environmental impact of man-made nanosized structures. Nanotoxicology has emerged as an independent research discipline that studies the toxicology of nanostructures, which as we have seen in previous chapters have a unique set of properties due to their small size. Some of the protocols to assess the toxicological profile of new nanomaterials, as well as existing regulations and risk assessments, will be briefly covered in the last part of the chapter.

9.1 Nano-Based Therapeutics

A particular advantage of nanotechnology is that it provides tools and materials to ease the engineering of tailored nanodrugs or drug nanocarriers (Figure 9.1). Such nanotherapeutics aim to improve the stability of the active compound in biological fluids, minimise the immune response and prolong the blood retention. As we have seen in Chapter 4, this can often be done by

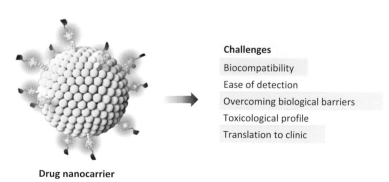

Figure 9.1

Drug nanocarriers represent a new generation of smart drug systems. Bionanotechnology can help to overcome some challenges associated with their design.

Challenges

Biocompatibility

Ease of detection

Overcoming biological barriers

Toxicological profile

Translation to clinic

Drug nanocarrier

the addition of the chemical moieties or proteins to the surface that enhance the stealth of the delivered materials. But there are also additional features that make nanotherapeutics 'smarter', such as targeting of the diseased cells and controlled release of the active cargo by use of internal (enzymes, pH change) or external (acoustic waves, light, magnetic field) stimuli. In short, nanotechnology can help us to achieve novel drug formulations that 'seek, deliver and destroy'; they seek the pathogens or diseased cells and deliver the drug selectively and in such a way aid their death and removal.

Although there is a huge interest in the development of nanotherapeutics, in particular, drug nanocarriers, there are several challenges to overcome before their implementation in a clinical setting (Figure 9.1). Even when suitable nanostructures are designed such that the loading and release of drugs as well as continuous monitoring can be achieved, the limited accumulation of such nanostructures in diseased tissue might hinder their therapeutic applications. Lack of accumulation is directly linked to the limited mass transfer of nanostructures across various **biological barriers** (Blanco et al., 2012). These barriers – such as blood vessels, epithelial barrier in intestines, blood–brain barrier (BBB, Back to Basics 9.1) and cell membranes – effectively sort out circulating molecular species, particles and even whole cells into those to be removed and those to be used in the normal course of biological functioning of the body.

Back to Basics 9.1	The Blood–Brain Barrier

The blood–brain barrier (BBB) was first described by German physician Paul Ehrlich (1854–1915), who injected a dye into rats and noticed that the dye stained all organs except the brain. The barrier is made of tightly packed cells that prevent the entry of many molecular species that occurs regularly through free diffusion in most organs. The only exception is molecules such as nutrients (for example, glucose) and proteins such as insulin, which are used by the brain (Wong et al., 2013).

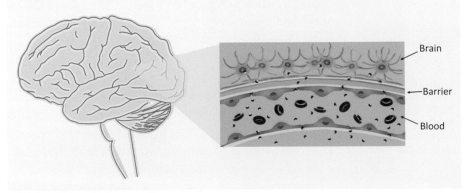

Molecules that enter the brain must have a sufficient lipid solubility, and be a particular size. No matter what the solubility, the larger the molecule, the more difficult it will be for it to cross the BBB. Small molecules vital for the brain usually have specific transporter proteins to carry them across the BBB, through **carrier-mediated transport**. Proteins usually bind to the receptors, which pull them across the barrier in a process known as **receptor-mediated transcytosis**. Some ionic proteins (e.g. cationic albumin) bind to and penetrate the BBB using electrostatic interactions (**absorptive-mediated transcytosis**).

The blood–brain barrier makes the design of efficient drugs to diagnose and treat neurological diseases particularly challenging. Some successes have been achieved using a 'Trojan horse' approach, in which a contrast agent or drug is attached to BBB-penetrating molecules. These can be monoclonal antibodies, which bind to the receptor proteins on the barrier, penetrating peptides or even whole cells.

There are also other ways of reaching the diseased brain parts. Direct injection or the surgical implantation of drug-releasing materials has been used to treat aggressive types of brain cancers, but these are extremely invasive and expensive.

In some cases, non-invasive drug delivery through the nose has been successful. Inhalation mimics the route by which some viruses or highly addictive molecules such as cocaine get into the brain, but the efficiency of the process is strongly dependent on the drug formulation (Gaenger and Schindowski, 2018).

Each of these mechanical barriers works closely together with the dynamic **garbage removal system** of the body, composed of cleaner/scavenger cells such as macrophages or the brain's glial cells, enzymes that degrade toxic species, or ionic and molecular pumps built into a cell membrane that aid removal of the species from the cell's interior. All of these natural barriers need to be taken into account during the design of nanotherapeutics to prevent their deactivation and premature clearance.

Material design and active cargo encapsulation or addition are the first steps in the formulation of novel nanotherapeutics. But before the new formulation can be put into clinical use and applied to patients, its quality, efficacy and toxicity need to be assessed using relevant biological models, and finally clinical studies using a well-defined group of patients and healthy controls. Commonly, the first step in the assessment of the toxicity and efficiency is to use **cell cultures**. A cell culture describes the process by which cells of interest are grown under controlled conditions in an artificial environment. The two-dimensional cell cultures used traditionally are nowadays being replaced with more biologically relevant 3D cultures grown within hydrogel scaffolds (Back to Basics 9.2). Particularly interesting, for studies of drug efficiency and assessment of nanocarriers for chemotherapeutics used in cancer treatment, are cancer organoids, 3D tissue mimics composed of several cancer and healthy cell lines (Drost and Clevers, 2018).

Back to Basics 9.2 Two- and Three-Dimensional Cell Cultures

Cell culture is defined as the process of growing cells in a favourable artificial environment under controlled conditions such as precise pH, osmotic pressure, temperature (usually 37 °C). Two-dimensional cell culture describes adherent cells that grow as a monolayer attached to a flat surface, usually the bottom of a culture flask or a Petri dish. Three-dimensional cell culture refers to a system in which cells grow and interact with the surrounding extracellular framework in three dimensions. A more detailed comparison of 2D and 3D cell cultures is given in the table (adapted from Kapalczynska et al., 2018).

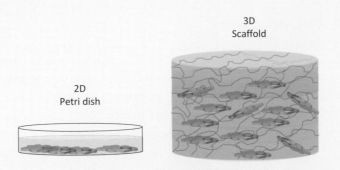

Primary cells or different cell lines can be used in cell cultures. Primary cells are directly isolated from a particular tissue, whereas cell lines are permanently established and can proliferate indefinitely given the right conditions.

	Type of culture	
	2D	3D
Time of culture formation	Minutes to hours	Hours to days
Characteristics	High performance and reproducibility	Worse performance and reproducibility
In vivo imitation	Do not mimic the natural structure of the tissue or tumour mass	In vivo tissues and organs and in 3D form
Cell interactions	Deprived of cell–cell and cell–extracellular environment interactions and no 'niches'	Proper interactions of cell–cell and cell–extracellular environment, 'niches' are created
Characteristics of cells	Changed morphology and way of divisions; loss of diverse phenotype and polarity	Preserved morphology and way of divisions, diverse phenotype and polarity
Access to oxygen, nutrients, metabolites and signalling molecules	Unlimited (in contrast to in vivo)	Variable (as in vivo)
Cost of maintaining	Cheap, commercially available	More expensive and time-consuming
Difficulty	Simplicity of culture	Culture more difficult to carry out

Three-dimensional cell cultures can be further divided into scaffold and scaffold-free cultures, with scaffold referring to natural or synthetic materials to which cells can adhere. Commonly used scaffolds are hydrogels, due to their mechanical properties which can be tuned to resemble the structure of tissues.

Organoids are synthetic organ mimics produced from embryonic stem cells or induced pluripotent stem cells, which are embedded within the 3D hydrogel matrix and stimulated to grow into particular tissue cells. Cancer organoids are particularly useful for studying cancer development and drug efficiency. Organoids are often used interchangeably with spheroids, although today spheroids refer more to 3D systems composed of established cell lines, whereas organoids contain primary cells.

9.2 Drug Nanocarriers and Therapeutic Nanomaterials

The role of drug **nanocarriers** is to protect a drug from premature degradation and removal by biological cleaner systems and thereby enhancing the efficiency of the drugs by prolonging the circulation times, improving the cell penetration if possible and enabling targeted delivery. Some nanocarriers such as liposomes and various polymers have already been approved for clinical use. Figure 9.2 shows Doxil, a liposomal formulation of the chemotherapeutic drug doxorubicin which has been used for the treatment of AIDS and Kaposi's sarcoma since 1995. Doxil is based on the encapsulation of the chemotherapeutic drug within the nanocarrier. However, therapeutic cargo can also be conjugated to the surface of the carrier (Figure 9.3). To be biologically relevant, nanocarriers need to be made of biocompatible material stable in biological fluids in terms of degradation and aggregation and have extended circulation half-time so they reach diseased cells before ending up in cleaner cells and being degraded or excreted. Nanocarriers also need to exhibit high differential uptake efficiency in the target, diseased cells in comparison with healthy cells, and desirably, have a long shelf life (Peer et al., 2007).

Taking all of this into account, it is not surprising that despite the significant advances in nanotechnology in the past 30 years, the number of

Figure 9.2

Doxil structure. The first approved nanocarrier for clinical use is based on the encapsulation of chemotherapeutic drug doxorubicin within a liposomal nanocarrier.

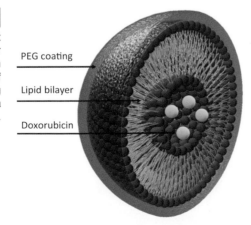

PEG coating

Lipid bilayer

Doxorubicin

Figure 9.3

Two routes to nanocarrier design. Drug cargo can be conjugated to the surface or encapsulated within the nanocarrier. Various functional groups can be added to the surface to ease the detection or attachment of the nanocarrier to the cell.

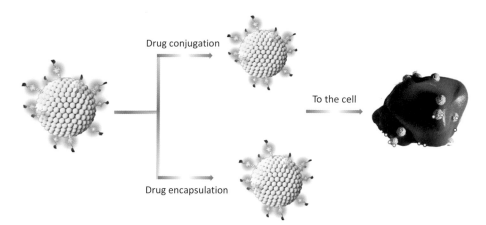

Figure 9.3

Two routes to nanocarrier design. Drug cargo can be conjugated to the surface or encapsulated within the nanocarrier. Various functional groups can be added to the surface to ease the detection or attachment of the nanocarrier to the cell.

nanoformulated drugs approved for clinical use is still limited. Besides liposomes, several nanostructured materials ranging from biocompatible polymers to porous inorganic nanoparticles have been employed for nanoformulation (Back to Basics 9.3), with varying levels of success.

Back to Basics 9.3   Types of Drug Nanocarriers

Lipids are employed to design **liposomal nanocarriers** which generally have long circulation times, can accumulate in tumours and can be designed for controlled release of drugs under increased temperature or under pH changes.

Many liposomal formulations have been approved for clinical use, including Doxil, doxorubicin-loaded liposomes.

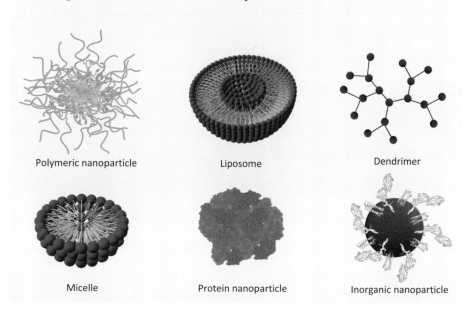

Polymeric nanoparticle   Liposome   Dendrimer

Micelle   Protein nanoparticle   Inorganic nanoparticle

Polymer nanostructures are easily synthesised and widely used in nano-medicine (see Back to Basics 2.4). Polymers can be either conjugated to the drug and used directly as enhancing drugs, or they can be employed to prepare nanoscale aggregates or particles that encapsulate drugs and enhance the accumulation in, and controlled release from, diseased cells. Particularly interesting is the use of biodegradable polymers such as poly-saccharide hyaluron, as there is an enzyme system in place that enables efficient removal of the material, once the drug is delivered. There are many polymer–drug formulations that have been approved for clinical use, including for treatment of haemophilia, rheumatoid arthritis, hepatitis and other conditions.

The subclass of polymer nanodrugs is **dendrimer nanoparticles**. Dendri-mers are polymeric species with iterative monomers arranged concentric-ally around the central core. Drugs can be encapsulated within the dendrimer cavities or attached to the surface, and dendrimers have been extensively explored for the delivery of nucleic acids.

Micelles are assembled from smaller molecular units that possess hydro-phobic and hydrophilic units. They usually have a hydrophobic internal core, which is particularly useful for the encapsulation of drugs that have poor solubility in water. Many micellar antitumour formulations are in the final stages of clinical trials, and the micellar formulation of the hormone oestradiol is approved for the treatment of menopause-associated symptoms.

Nanocrystals are nanosized crystals of drugs. They are composed of 100% drugs and there is no other carrier material. The only modification which is required is the addition of the surface molecules such as PEG that stabilise the drug particles and increase their solubility and circulation time (Junghanns and Müller, 2008).

Inorganic nanoparticles such as iron oxide and mesoporous silica nanoparticles have been approved for medical uses, mainly imaging, although many different compositions are in clinical trials. Noble metals such as gold and silver are also being explored for the delivery of toxic anti-tumour agents or as antimicrobials (Research Report 9.1).

Early **protein nanoparticles** exploited the properties of proteins such as albumin found in abundance in blood serum. Clinically available nano-drug, Abraxane is composed of 130 nm albumin nanoparticles conjugated with a chemotherapeutic drug Paclitaxel. Protein nanoparticles are non-toxic and can be degraded by the action of native enzymes. In addition, the high content of hydroxyl, amino and carboxyl groups makes them suitable for chemical modification. Besides albumin, proteins such as sericin and fibroin from silk, gelatin, collagen and a range of viral proteins are used as building blocks.

To date around 50 nanotherapeutics are used for therapy, or are undergoing clinical trials for various indications. Although nanomaterials have been employed for the removal of various pathogens either alone or in combination with drugs (Research Report 9.1), the majority of nanoformulated drugs have been developed for cancer therapy (Back to Basics 9.4).

An important issue, which still has not been resolved and is plagued by contradicting literature reports, is the understanding of the impact of nanocarriers' size, shape and charge on the efficiency of the drug delivery into solid cancer tissues known as **tumours**. What we know is that 100 to 150 nm nanocarriers enable longer circulation times, but nanocarriers smaller than 100 nm are often needed to penetrate tumour vasculature. The effect of the charges is much more difficult to understand, as the charge acts in synergy with the shape and mechanical properties of the material.

What has been observed up to now is that positively charged nanocarriers are readily taken up by macrophages and as a consequence, might have a shorter circulation time. However, compared to neutral or negatively charged nanocarriers, those that are positively charged transverse the cell membrane easier and can escape from the membrane-bound vesicles involved in the transport across the membrane (see Back to Basics 9.4 for more).

As the number of studies concerning the behaviour of nanomaterials in the biological system grew, it became clearer that it is not easy to rationalise their design. Nevertheless, lots of insight on uptake and transport of nanocarriers, particularly into tumour tissue and cancer cells, have been gained, which is having an impact on their therapeutic applications.

Research Report 9.1	Nanomaterials As Potent Antibacterial Agents

Antimicrobials, derived from Greek words *anti* (against), *micro* (little) and *bios* (life), are agents that act against microorganisms such as bacteria (antibacterial), viruses (antiviral), fungi (antifungal) and protozoa (antiprotozoal). Due to the overuse of some antibiotics, several antibiotic-resistant bacteria such as the methicillin-resistant *Staphylococcus aureus* (MRSA) have emerged, which pose a significant risk to public health (see Research Report 8.4). Centres for Disease Control (CDC), USA, predicted that there will be more deaths from antibiotic-resistant bacteria than from all cancers combined by 2050. Similar to other drugs, ideal antibiotics should have selective toxicity, high solubility and stability in body fluids, non-allergenic properties and should not lead to the development of resistance.

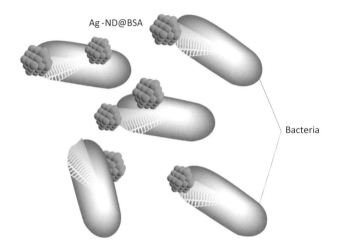

Various types of antimicrobial-active nanoformulations have been developed, based on the inherent or induced toxic activity of nanomaterials. For example, Chang and colleagues (2019) prepared silver–nanodiamond hybrids coated with bovine serum albumin, the most common serum protein. Such nanohybrids (Ag-ND@BSA) were 100–200 nm in size and showed an excellent colloidal stability in bacterial culture. To test their general toxicity, three cell lines were studied: human fibroblasts, lung adenocarcinoma epithelial cells and breast adenocarcinoma cells. These showed that more than 80% of the cells were still viable after treatment with high amount of Ag-ND@BSA (500 μg mL^{-1}) after 24 h cell incubation.

The antibiotic activity was explored using *E. coli* and *S. aureus* bacteria. At a concentration of 250 μg mL^{-1}, nanohybrids showed a long-term bactericidal effect up to 36 days after the treatment most probably due to the action of released silver ions.

Such high antibacterial activity was employed to design antibacterial wound dressings by embedding AgND@BSA within a polysaccharide hydrogel, which can be directly applied to the skin (Chang et al., 2019).

Back to Basics 9.4 | Cancer

Cancer is a term that encompasses a group of diseases characterised by loss of normal cellular function resulting in uncontrolled cell growth. In some cases, these cells grow into tumours, solid structures characterised by high heterogeneity and their blood and lymph system.

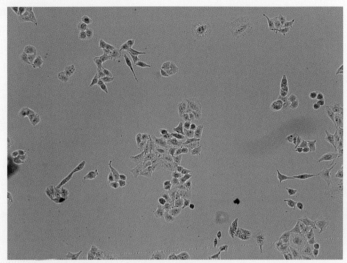

Microscopic image of lung cancer A549 cell line. Courtesy of Andrew Baker, University of Cambridge.

Cancer is considered to be the second leading cause of death worldwide, responsible for 9.6 million deaths per year, and that number could reach more than 13 million per year by 2030 according to the World Health Organization.

Survival rates vary across different cancer types and depend on the stage at diagnosis, available treatments, and a range of patient-specific factors. For many types of cancers, survival rates have significantly improved in the past decades, but some types such as brain, lung (shown in the figure is the lung cancer A549 cell line) and pancreatic cancer continue to respond poorly to available treatments.

Current chemotherapeutic strategies to treat cancer suffer from limited selectivity and do not distinguish between cancerous and healthy cells, leading to severe side effects. The new generation of smart chemo-therapeutics should afford targeted and more efficient delivery, and the use of nanocarriers is being considered as one of the routes to achieve that.

9.2.1   Passive Targeting and EPR Effect for Delivery of Nanotherapeutics

In many cases, drug–nanoparticle conjugates reach their target through passive targeting, which involves a non-specific accumulation of nanosized species due to the increased permeability of the membrane or blood vessels in diseased tissue. Such physiological changes have been observed both during bacterial infections and in cancer tissue. The blood vessel permeability observed in tumours is known as **enhanced permeation and retention (EPR) effect** (Matsumura and Maeda, 1986). The initial discovery of this phenomenon was made during clinical trials involving therapeutic polymer poly (styrene-co-maleic acid)-neocarzinostatin (SMANCS), which can non-covalently bind protein albumin when injected into the blood. Large protein–polymer conjugates formed, accumulated in tumours and remained there over a prolonged period, which was attributed to the fenestration of imperfect tumour blood vessels (Back to Basics 9.5). Nowadays, it is clear that the EPR effect is much more complex than initially thought, and it is a result of many biological processes such as vessel formation (angiogenesis), the heterogeneous nature of the tumour and presence of various enzymes in the tumour tissue (Bertrand et al., 2014).

The EPR effect can not only be used to explain enhanced tumour penetration, but also prolonged retention of species once they are there. Extracellular fluid in normal tissue is continuously drained to the lymphatic vessels, which allows for the renewal of the fluids and recycling of solutes back into the circulation.

Back to Basics 9.5	Fenestration of Tumour Blood Vessels

Tumour tissue is a fast-growing assembly of cancer and tissue cells, with an extracellular matrix that acts as a scaffold. Tumours also have their own blood vessels that supply nutrients and oxygen. When a tumour reaches a certain size, the normal blood vessels in its vicinity cannot provide everything needed to sustain its growth. As cells start to die, they release growth factors that trigger the production of new blood vessels from surrounding capillaries, in a process known as angiogenesis. **Angiogenesis** promotes the rapid development of new, irregular blood vessels that contain fenestrations, pores that allow the passage of long-circulating large molecular species. The pores are usually from 200 to 1200 nm in size depending on the tumour type and its environment.

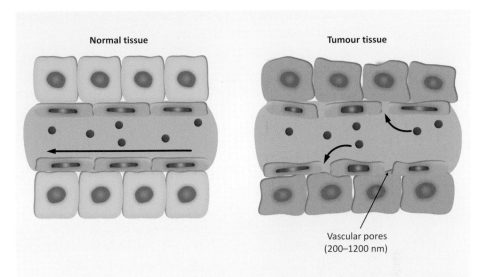

Normal blood vessels typically possess tight junctions that prevent the entry of particles into the tissue. However, some organs that require a fast and frequent exchange of nutrients and other molecules such as kidney, small intestine and endocrine glands are also fenestrated.

The presence and large size of pores in tumour tissue is attributed to several factors such as increased levels of nitric oxide and VEGF (vascular endothelial growth factor).

In tumours, this process is disrupted and there is minimal uptake of interstitial fluid (the thin layer of fluid surrounding the cells) so that larger particles do not readily get back into the circulation. Whereas smaller molecules, those smaller than 4 nm, can diffuse back to the blood, large species such as nanocarriers or macromolecules cannot. As a result, they are retained within the tumour. However, it should be kept in mind that tumours are highly heterogeneous, composed of various cells and intercellular structures and as a result, the EPR effect is not uniform across the tissue. For example, it has been observed that lymphatic activity in the interior of the solid tumours can differ from that on the margins, leading to an uneven distribution of nanocarriers across the tumour.

Two main strategies can be used to modulate the EPR effect and improve the uptake of designed nanostructures. The EPR effect can be increased either by changing the biology of the tumour or by changing the physicochemical properties of the nanomaterials. Besides various growth factors, inhibitors of growth factors or enzymes have been shown to impact the permeability of the blood vessels. However, there is less agreement on the impact of the nanocarrier shape, size and charge, and the recommendation is to test and optimise every new formulation.

9.2.2   Active Targeting of Nanocarriers

Active targeting is often referred to as **ligand-mediated cell targeting**, and it is based on the modification of the nanocarrier's surface so that it contains ligands that can specifically bind to the receptors on the cell surface. Some active targeting strategies, however, do not involve direct binding to the cell receptors but use strategies that ease the cell membrane penetration, or the interaction with specific enzymes within the cell or in the cell's microenvironment. The choice of the targeting ligands depends on the type of targeted cell, carriers' building blocks and possible surface modification strategies. Pathogens such as bacteria and viruses are often characterised by unique cell receptors, which can be used to develop **receptor-specific antibodies** or **aptamers**. As we have seen in Research Report 8.3, the influenza virus can be targeted using the antibody specific to the haemagglutinin receptor on the surface of the virus. Similarly, targeted cells might also possess receptors for peptides or small molecules such as vitamins or carbohydrates, which can then be used as targeting molecules and attached to the surface of the nanocarriers (Figure 9.4).

Figure 9.4

Classes of targeting species used in the design of nanocarriers and nanodrug systems. Antibodies and aptamers can be produced that target particular receptors on the surface of the target cell, peptides can aid active targeting by easing the cell penetration by binding to the surface receptors, whereas small molecules, such as vitamins, interact predominantly with the protein receptors on the cell surface.

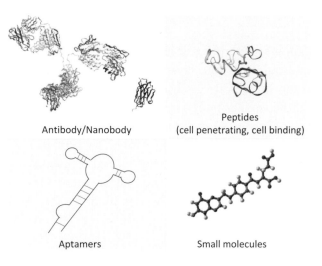

Antibody/Nanobody

Peptides
(cell penetrating, cell binding)

Aptamers

Small molecules

There are two major challenges in achieving active targeting. One is the identification of the target and the suitable ligand, and the other is the identification of the strategy for ligand attachment (for more on that see Chapter 4). It is important to remember that the choice of functionalisation strategy for clinically relevant nanocarriers also depends on the route of drug administration. Ingestion requires a different formulation than an injection of the nanocarrier, as it involves the exposure to very low stomach pH. Inhalation, on the other hand, requires well-dispersed and stable formulations, which are not easily cleared from the lungs, this is often difficult to achieve due to the multiple pulmonary clearance mechanisms.

The identification of specific targets also poses a huge challenge, particularly in the case of cancer. This is a result of similarities between cancer and healthy cells, and a vast number of potential target candidates. Nevertheless, some receptors such as folic acid receptors, surface glycoproteins and epidermal growth factor receptor (EGFR) are overexpressed in specific cancer cells and successfully employed for active targeting.

Regardless of the target cell and the type of nanomaterial, active targeting aims to improve the interaction of nanocarrier or nano-based drugs with that cell, and increase the internalisation of the active compound to achieve efficient therapies with fewer undesirable side effects.

9.2.3   Cell Uptake Mechanisms

Small hydrophobic molecules are often capable of diffusion through the lipid bilayer membrane of cells, but engineered nanocarriers usually require active uptake. Cell uptake of nanoparticles is achieved via the membrane trafficking process known as **endocytosis**. Although universal in eukaryotic cells, endocytosis in prokaryotes such as bacteria was identified only recently (Lonhienne et al., 2010). Endocytosis is a process of macromolecule and nanoparticle uptake through the formation of the membrane buds or vacuoles inside the cells. Depending on the size and the type of the species and the cells, endocytosis can be divided into several distinct processes (Figure 9.5).

Figure 9.5

Endocytosis pathways of cell entry. Phagocytosis is a process of ingestion of large particles and structures, pinocytosis of smaller particles and molecules. Pinocytosis can be divided into clathrin- and caveolin-dependent, and clathrin- and caveolin-independent process. In micropinocytosis, large particles are engulfed together with a significant amount of the extracellular liquid. Some species can enter the cell by diffusion.

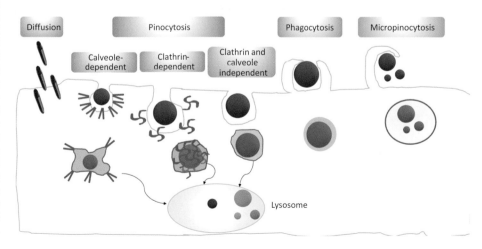

Large particles and structures, as well as whole cells, can be ingested through **phagocytosis** (from Greek for *phagein* 'to eat' and *kytos* 'hollow cell'). In mammals such as humans, phagocytosis is usually performed by specialised cells called phagocytes and initiated by opsonisation, which is the binding of opsonin proteins to the surface of injected nanoparticles (see Chapter 4). In terms of nanoparticle delivery, opsonisation is a process that should be minimised as it results in the fast clearance of nanoparticles and their accumulation in the liver and spleen. Smaller particles and molecules within the extracellular fluid are taken up by **pinocytosis** (from the Greek *pino* 'to drink') during which a cell surrounds the particle and then encloses it within a membrane-built vesicle.

The main process by which cells get nutrients and building blocks such as lipids is **clathrin-dependent endocytosis** during which vesicles with a diameter of 100–150 nm are formed in the membrane areas rich in the protein **clathrin** (usually 0.5–2% of the cell surface). The clathrin unit has a three-legged structure called triskelion which aids membrane folding into an architecture suitable for the transport of species. Once inside the cell, the clathrin coat is shedded and the naked vesicle is first fused with an endosome to be delivered to the enzyme-containing lysosome.

Cell uptake and the fate of the nanoparticle depend on the cell type and the physicochemical properties of the nanomaterials; their composition, size, shape and surface properties. Positively charged and lipid nanoparticles were shown to employ clathrin-dependent endocytosis to get into a cell. Such a pathway is often not suitable for nanoparticles that carry drug cargo susceptible to enzyme degradation such as proteins or nucleic acids, as they usually end up in enzyme-rich lysosomes. To avoid ending up in lysosomes, pathogens such as viruses and bacteria use **caveolae-dependent endocytosis**, to get into the host cells. Caveolae are flask-shaped membrane invaginations lined with the protein caveolin and are usually 50–80 nm in size.

Cells deprived of caveolin and clathrin take up nanoparticles using **clathrin- and caveolae-independent endocytosis**. Folate-modified nanoparticles are known to be internalised using this mechanism, which is initiated by binding of the folate to the folate receptor on the surface of the cell. Nanomaterials that enter the cell through this pathway might escape the internalisation into the lysosome, and be released directly into the cytoplasm. Larger nanoparticles use the process of **micropinocytosis**, characterised by the formation of membrane extensions that create large vesicles (0.2–5 μm), which can trap large particles regardless of the presence of the specific receptors.

Although cell uptake of a large number of nanoparticles has been explored, there is little consensus over general rules that could be applied to the design of materials to ensure efficient delivery into cells. Studies on nanoparticle uptake are most commonly conducted using cell cultures, which often do not translate into in vivo models. For example, the transport of nanoparticles through the body is often accompanied by the formation of the **protein corona**, a layer of proteins such as serum albumin, commonly found in blood. Protein corona has long been considered to be an obstacle to nanoparticle delivery as it impacts their size and surface properties. However, it was shown lately that instead of hindering the delivery, controlled formation of a protein layer on the surface of nanoparticles can have a positive effect on a nanoparticle delivery and lower the uptake by cleaner cells (Research Report 9.2).

Research Report 9.2	Mesoporous Nanoparticles Coated with a Protein Corona Shield

A layer of proteins that rapidly forms upon exposure of nanoparticles to biological fluid is referred to as a protein corona. Such a protein layer has a significant impact on the properties of nanoparticles such as size, charge, specific targeting, circulation time and the level of macrophage uptake. Although PEGylation (Chapter 4) is often used to reduce the macrophage uptake, the targeting agents attached to PEG linkers can often act as hot spots for corona formation.

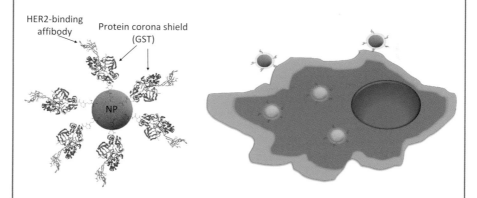

To overcome these issues, Jun Yang Oh and colleagues (2018) used a protein corona as a functional coat which can be added to the nanoparticle before administration. This was achieved by attaching recombinant fusion protein GST-HER2-Affb (GST is glutathione-*S*-transferase and HER2-Affb is HER2 affibody, a small protein specific for HER2 receptor) to glutathione (GSH) functionalised mesoporous silica nanoparticles that act as a drug carrier. Attachment of the fusion proteins through interaction between GSH molecules on the surface of the nanoparticle and GST fraction of the fusion protein resulted in the formation of a protein layer around the nanoparticle core (final size 270 nm).

Such protein–nanoparticle hybrids showed no significant binding of serum proteins, which commonly form undesirable protein coronas around unmodified silica nanoparticles. Besides, studies with macrophages showed significantly reduced uptake in comparison with non-modified controls proving that GST-HER2-Affb can be used as a protein corona shield.

When targeting efficiency was explored using a breast cancer cell line with overexpressed HER2 receptor (SK-BR3), drug-loaded silica nanoparticles with a protein corona shield were uptaken through receptor-mediated endocytosis and showed high antitumour efficiency (Oh et al., 2018).

Despite the lack of general rules, some trends in nanocarrier uptake have been observed. For example, soft nanoparticles that can be easily deformed have been shown to have prolonged circulation lifetime. They have also shown reduced accumulation in the spleen, which is, in addition to the liver and kidneys, one of the organs that plays an important role in nanoparticle degradation and elimination. An increase in the size of nanocarriers has been observed to lead to a higher clearance rate, although there is no agreement on the optimal size of the nanoparticles to be used for the drug delivery as this will largely depend on the type of target cell.

Some of the issues with nanoparticle delivery could be overcome by the introduction of a more systematic nanomaterial classification, and uniform and shared protocols for nanoparticle assessment. Some researchers even suggest the design of a 'periodic table' of nanomaterials, which would serve as a reference for researchers working on the design of structures for biomedical applications.

9.3   Tracking Nanomaterials in Biological Systems

The choice of the imaging strategy to study the interaction of therapeutic nanomaterials with cells, in particular concerning their uptake and drug release, depends on the type of biological system explored. When simple 2D or 3D cell cultures are used, fluorescence microscopy is a suitable method of choice. However, the penetration of visible light is limited to several millimetres, so that the thickness of the sample needs to be taken into account. As we move from cell cultures into whole organs and the body, we need to be able to image nanomaterials within the micro- and macroscale environment. Medical imaging strategies such as **magnetic resonance imaging (MRI)** or **positron emission tomography (PET)** can be adapted to explore interactions of nanostructures within the body (Figure 9.6 and Back to Basics 9.6).

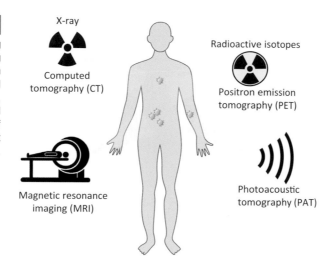

Figure 9.6

Medical imaging strategies for tracking nanomaterials. Each method is characterised by specific resolution, which can be enhanced by the use of nanostructured contrast agents.

Back to Basics 9.6 Medical Imaging Techniques

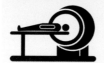

Magnetic resonance imaging (MRI) uses a very powerful magnet (1.5–3 T) to align the magnetic moments of protons in the sample, producing an equilibrium magnetisation along the longitudinal axis. A radio frequency (RF) pulse at the resonant frequency (5–100 MHz) transfers energy to protons, which can then rotate their magnetic moments away from the longitudinal axis to an angle called the flip angle. When radiation is removed, the magnetic moments of the protons relax to equilibrium over a time known as the relaxation time, which depends on the chemical and physical nature of the tissues (Grover et al., 2015). MRI contrast in soft tissue (brain, muscle, tumours, connective tissue) stems from the local differences in the proton density due to the variations of water concentration.

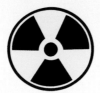

Positron emission tomography (PET) is based on the detection of radioactivity emitted after a radioactive probe is injected into the blood. The radioactive probe emits a positron (anti-electron), which collides with an electron in the tissue, and the subsequent annihilation generates gamma rays that are recorded by photomultiplier–scintillator detectors. Commonly used radioactive probes are radioisotopes oxygen-15, fluorine-18, carbon-11 and nitrogen-13, which have half-lives of about several minutes, but heavier elements such as copper, zirconium or indium are also employed. PET scans are usually completed within 10 to 40 minutes and have been used to track neurotransmitters, blood components such as glucose, and for the detection of cancer.

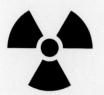

Computed tomography (CT) uses X-rays to record a pattern of densities within a particular tissue. An X-ray generator/detector rotates around the object within the scanner, and the internal structure of the object can then be reconstructed from the large number of images obtained. X-rays are attenuated differently by different tissues, and in such a way the contrast can be achieved. For example, bones and calcified tissues attenuate X-rays very well, and appear very bright in the CT image, whereas air and water appear black. Contrast agents are often used to increase the contrast between normal and pathologic tissue. For example, iodinated contrast agents can be added to visualise vascular structures.

Photoacoustic tomography (PAT) is a technique based on the acoustic detection of optical absorption from biological chromophores or added contrast agents. PAT generates high-resolution images due to the lower scattering of the acoustic waves when compared to the optical waves. Although PAT is based on absorption, it can penetrate deeper than fluorescence imaging, while sustaining high spatial resolution. The penetration depth can reach up to 10 cm and higher. PAT also uses non-ionising laser illumination and it is faster and less expensive than MRI imaging. PAT is based on a photoacoustic effect, in which an object absorbs light, which is then converted into heat. This causes a temperature rise and thermoelastic expansion of the tissue, which results in the emission of acoustic (ultrasonic) waves. Natural PAT probes are haemoglobin and melanin, whereas contrast agents might be composed of various chromophores.

At the same time, the sensitivity of these techniques can be improved by the use of nanoprobes as contrast agents. The first family of inorganic nanoparticles approved for clinical use was iron oxide nanoparticles, used as contrast agents for MRI of soft tissues. Magnetic resonance imaging is based on measurements of local differences in the proton density due to the variation of water concentration in soft tissues such as the brain, muscle, connective tissue and various tumours. To achieve diagnostically relevant contrasts, MRI requires an increase in the applied magnetic field or use of effective contrast agents such as small paramagnetic complexes, metalloporphyrins, polymeric and macromolecular carriers of paramagnetic complexes, or paramagnetic and superparamagnetic nanoparticles (Estelrich et al., 2015).

The efficiency of MRI is improved if the contrast agents are not rapidly cleared from the body and if they can target a particular tissue, which makes functionalised magnetic nanoparticles particularly well-suited for MRI-based cancer detection (Research Report 9.3).

Research Report 9.3 | Magnetic Nanoparticles As Contrast Agents for MRI of Cancer Tissue

Particularly interesting MRI contrast agents are monocrystalline engineered iron oxide (MEIO) nanoparticles such as those based on MFe_2O_4 spinel structure (M can be Mn, Fe, Co or Ni). Such NPs show different magnetisation ability based on the size (12 nm $MnFe_2O_4$ NP, MnMEIO, have higher magnetisation than 5 nm nanoparticles), and the presence of different ions (Mn-containing NPs have higher magnetisation than Ni-containing NPs). Lee and coworkers (2007) explored MnMEIO NPs for cancer imaging. The surface of MnMEIO was modified with Herceptin, an antibody that binds to HER2/neu marker expressed in a large number of cancer cells. When MnMEIO-Herceptin conjugate was used to detect breast cancer cells (MCF-7 and MDA-MB), it showed high magnetisation and targeting ability. As a result, higher MRI contrast and more efficient detection of cancer cells were achieved compared to negative control (without HER2 receptor) or pancreatic cells (BxPC-3), which contain a single Herceptin receptor. NIH3T non-cancerous cell line rich in HER2 receptors was used as a positive control.

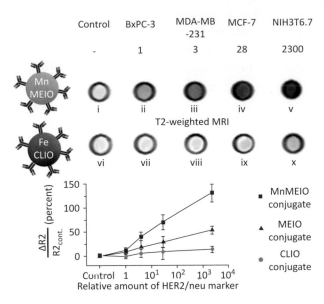

Source: Reprinted by permission from Springer Nature: Lee et al. (2007).

MnMEIOs were much more efficient than traditional cross-linked iron oxide (CLIO) nanoparticles which showed little difference across explored cancer cell lines (Lee et al., 2007).

The main limitation of MRI diagnostics and other medical imaging techniques is the lack of specific targeting. A library of specific targets could help us not only to improve the sensitivity of imaging techniques to improve early diagnostics but also to design more efficient drugs and drug delivery systems. This brings us to the next important application of nanomaterials and this is their use for the design of **theranostic probes**.

9.4   Theranostic Nanomaterials

Theranostics is a multimodal approach to disease treatment, which couples therapy and diagnostics. **Theranostic nanomaterials** combine the therapeutic activity of the nanoparticles with their ability to act as contrast agents or imaging probes. Such nanoparticle systems can be imaged by traditional imaging techniques, and they are usually activated by application of an external stimulus such as magnetic field, light or radio waves. The therapeutic activity can be achieved either by the triggered release of a drug (stimuli-induced drug release, Figure 9.7a) or by the intrinsic response of an excited nanoparticle which can lead to the production of reactive oxygen species or an increase in local temperature (stimuli-induced damage, Figure 9.7b).

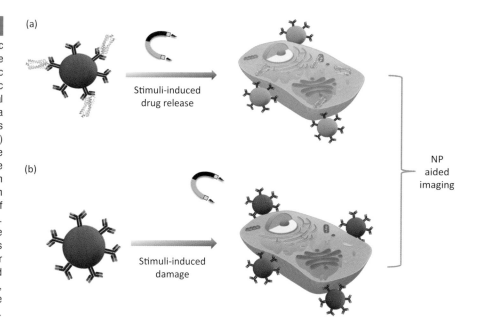

Figure 9.7

Magnetic theranostic nanomaterials can be used both as diagnostic probes and therapeutic agents. An external stimulus such as a magnetic field is employed to either (a) induce the release of the drug or (b) cause damage to the cell directly through an increase in temperature or level of reactive oxygen species. Intrinsic properties of the theranostic nanoparticles can also be used for nanoparticle aided imaging, for example, with magnetic resonance imaging.

An example of therapeutic activity is the increase in temperature (usually several °C) known as **hyperthermia** in the vicinity of certain nanoparticles, which can cause the death of temperature-sensitive cancer cells. Due to their fast metabolism and growth, cancer cells are less robust and more sensitive to temperature increase than healthy cells, which makes hyperthermia-inducing nanoparticles such as magnetic iron oxide or plasmonic noble metal nanoparticles particularly well-suited for removal of cancer cells (Back to Basics 9.7, Huang and El-Sayed, 2010).

Back to Basics 9.7   Light-Induced Hyperthermia

Temperature increase at the cellular level causes changes in blood flow rate, tissue elasticity, protein synthesis, and can lead to dissociation and inactivity of cells. Controlled and localised heat generation is a principle of thermal therapy.

Hyperthermia (overheating) requires the local temperature to increase from 37 °C, which is a normal physiological temperature, to 41–48 °C. At this temperature denaturation and aggregation of proteins occurs, and the rates of biochemical reactions change, which results in cell inactivation and death. Such overheating is particularly effective for the removal of cancer cells, which are more sensitive to temperature changes than healthy cells.

Light-induced hyperthermia exploits laser energy to generate heat by triggering photothermal conversion agents.

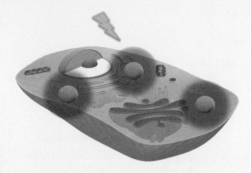

Near-infrared (NIR) light with wavelengths of 600 to 1000 nm can penetrate through the tissue and be converted into heat with the help of nanomaterials such as gold, silver and palladium nanoparticles, and some carbon nanostructures. Due to minimal light scattering, the penetration depth of light in the NIR region can be 1 to 10 cm depending on the type of tissue.

Upon irradiation, the oscillating electromagnetic field of light triggers the polarisation of the conduction band electrons on the surface of the nanostructures. Polarised electrons go through collective coherent oscillation with respect to the positive ions in the metallic lattice. This process is known as surface plasmon oscillation or surface plasmon resonance (SPR) since the frequency of the incident light is equal to the oscillation frequency (they are in resonance).

The relaxation of the excited electrons occurs either through SPR scattering (light emission of the same energy as incident light) or the transfer of absorbed energy to the metallic lattice in the form of thermal energy. This thermal energy is subsequently transferred to the surrounding medium, resulting in a local temperature increase.

Both the relaxation and scattering can happen during the relaxation process and are affected by the shape and size of nanoparticles. For gold nanorods (Au NR), which have both longitudinal and transverse SPR peaks, the scattering component increases and the absorption component decreases with the increase of aspect ratio (length divided by width). As a consequence, large Au NR that have high scattering efficiency are preferred in imaging, whereas smaller Au NR that have high absorption efficiency are preferred for photothermal therapy.

Any nanosystem which can be used with traditional medical imaging platforms capable of delivering or acting as therapeutic cargo might be considered a theranostic system. The limitations encountered in the design of nano-based drug delivery systems, such as identification and attachment of targeting molecules, cell/tissue targeting, circulation time, toxicity profiling, all apply to the design of theranostic probes.

In the next few decades, improved understanding of nanomaterial–cell interactions, and the biology of diseases will lead to the design of new diagnostic and therapeutic materials and devices, and ultimately the development of intelligent drugs and personalised medicine. Significant advances in understanding the interactions between the cells and engineered materials on both the nano- and macroscale have been made in the field of tissue engineering, in which the nanocomposites and biofunctionalised nanomaterials have led to the design of novel implants and responsive hybrid materials.

9.5   Nanomaterials in Tissue Engineering

Tissue engineering is a field that aims to design three-dimensional scaffolds that contain suitable biomolecular cues to enable **cell differentiation** (change of one type of cell into another) and **proliferation** (an increase of the number of cells). Such engineered tissue can be used to regrow or replace tissue after injury or disease, and to study biological processes, which could eventually eliminate the need for the use of animal models.

Tissues are built of cells and an extracellular matrix (ECM) composed of various nanoscale elements and biomolecules (see Chapter 3 and Back to Basics 9.8). Due to their size and properties, nanomaterials are suitable building blocks for the design of 3D scaffolds. They can improve mechanical stability, minimise the detrimental immune response, provide antimicrobial activity and be used to monitor the health of the implanted tissue.

Each tissue has a unique structure and function, and this has to be reflected in the engineered tissue as well. For example, bone requires precisely engineered scaffolds that provide unique mechanical properties, while softer porous scaffolds that can embed different types of cells are needed for liver engineering.

Engineered tissue is composed of three main components: (a) a **3D scaffold** that provides a suitable environment for the growth of the cells, (b) **tissue-specific cells** and (c) **growth factors and regulatory signals** that enable cell adhesion, migration and proliferation (Figure 9.8).

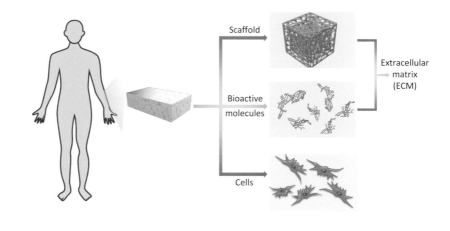

Figure 9.8

Main components of engineered tissue. The scaffold provides structural integrity and mechanical stability enabling attachment, migration and growth of the cells in the presence of growth factors and signalling biomolecules. Scaffold and biomolecular elements are known as the extracellular matrix. Biomolecular elements shown in the figure are bone morphogenic proteins BMP-1 (Griffith et al., 1996) and BMP-9 (Mi et al., 2015).

The 3D scaffold and the regulatory biomolecules are known as the extracellular matrix, which provides structural and biochemical support to tissue cells. Its complex and dynamic nature makes it difficult to mimic and as a result, the design of the extracellular matrix has been one of the key challenges in tissue engineering, which benefitted significantly from the introduction of nanostructured materials.

9.5.1   The Extracellular Matrix

The **extracellular matrix (ECM)** is a structural matrix that regulates the growth, metabolism and health of tissues through cell adhesion, cell migration and transfer of biochemical cues (Back to Basics 9.8).

Back to Basics 9.8	Composition of the Extracellular Matrix

The extracellular matrix is a heterogeneous structure unique to each tissue, it contains many physical, biochemical and biomechanical components that create a healthy environment for cell proliferation and communication.

The main components of the ECM are **fibrous proteins** such as collagen, elastin, fibronectin and laminin, **enzymes** such as metalloproteinases, **regulating proteins** such as growth factors and cytokines, and **proteoglycans**, proteins with covalently linked carbohydrate chains.

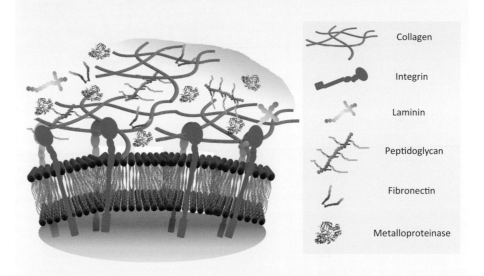

Fibrous proteins are mainly responsible for the mechanical structure and properties of the ECM, although fibronectin is also involved in the control of cell adhesion and migration.

Various enzymes directly contribute to the dynamic nature of the matrix through the continuous remodelling of its structural elements. The main class of remodelling enzyme is **matrix metalloproteinases (MMPs)** responsible for collagen degradation. Degradation of ECM proteins is the tightly regulated process responsible for the control of tissue development. Indeed, MMPs are known to play an important role in processes such as bone growth, wound healing and tissue regeneration. MMPs are also involved in the control of cell adhesion through interaction with numerous adhesion molecules on the cell surface. Currently, there are 24 known MMPs identified in vertebrates including 23 in humans. Shown here is MMP-10 with 3 calcium (Ca^{2+} in green) and 2 zinc (Zn^{2+} in orange) ions involved in the regulation of enzymatic activity of MMPs (Batra et al., 2012).

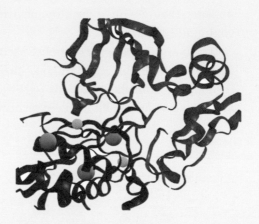

Signalling and other regulatory processes within the ECM are controlled by **growth factors** and **cytokines**. This large and heterogeneous group of proteins influences expression and turnover of specific ECM molecules, impacts the proliferation of cells by binding to cell membrane receptors such as **integrins**, and have also been shown to interact widely with proteoglycans in a highly cooperative fashion.

Proteoglycans, composed of protein and sugar units, play different roles depending on their structure and position. They can be involved in the control of collagen orientation and cell adhesion, and in the regulation of hydration and tissue swelling properties (Iozzo and Schaaefer, 2015). For example, the chains of aggrecan, a principal load-bearing proteoglycan of cartilage, aggregate (and hence the name) into large supramolecular structures (larger than 200 MDa) (Nap and Szleifer, 2008).

The ECM is a dynamic and heterogeneous structure composed of water, polysaccharides, fibrous proteins such as collagen, elastin (discussed in Chapter 3) and the glycoprotein fibronectin. Collagen and elastin are mainly responsible for mechanical properties, whereas fibronectin is involved in cell attachment and the regulation of cell function.

The extracellular matrix is continuously remodelled through non-enzymatic and enzymatic processes, for example through the action of metalloproteinases. Such remodelling affects mechanical and biochemical properties and it is reflected in each tissue having different elasticity, tensile strength and the ability to retain water. These properties even vary across the individual tissue itself, all due to the heterogeneity of the matrix. Cancer tissue is often characterised by a large degree of heterogeneity, and by stiffness not observed in the surrounding tissue. This is a result of the extracellular matrix deposition and extensive remodelling through cross-linking of structural proteins, which generates larger and more rigid fibrils. Such mechanical changes affect the function of growth factors and impacts cell behaviour, ultimately leading to abnormal growth or inflammation-like states within the tissue, which characterises cancer.

Balance within ECM is important for tissue health, and ECM models and mimics are not only valuable tools for tissue engineering but also for studying behaviour and interaction of cells in a 3D environment. However, the design of ECM is difficult because of molecular components and structures within the matrix spanning different size scales. For example, with a diameter between 35 and 600 nm collagen fibrils dominate the nanometre scale, but also extend well into the micrometre range.

Another factor to consider is that the nanosized regulatory proteins and micrometre-sized cells need to be able to diffuse and migrate over larger distances, and designed extracellular matrices need to provide mechanical integrity and stability over micrometre-scale while remaining dynamic enough to accommodate nanoscale elements, which are continuously replaced or regenerated.

Significant advances in ECM engineering were made by the introduction of various nanomaterials and small-scale technologies such as electrospinning and 3D printing, which will not be discussed here but more information can be found in papers suggested for further reading. Instead of exploring the technology behind macroscale design using nanoscale elements, here we focus more on the basic aspects and advantages of nanomaterials in tissue engineering.

9.5.2   Nanomaterials for Tissue Scaffold Engineering

Nanotechnology is changing tissue engineering through the design of extracellular matrices with nanofeatures, either through the production of **nanofibres**, design of **nanopatterns** or the use of various **nanoparticles** (Figure 9.9). These materials enable assembly of interfaces suitable for attachment and differentiation of stem cells (Research Report 9.4), carry growth factors and signalling peptides, but also often provide mechanical stability needed for cell proliferation and tissue regrowth.

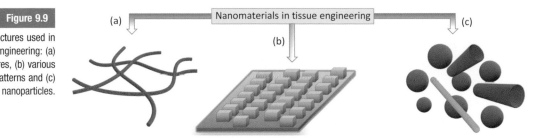

Figure 9.9

Nanostructures used in tissue engineering: (a) nanofibres, (b) various nanopatterns and (c) nanoparticles.

Research Report 9.4	Nanopatterns Influence the Differentiation of Stem Cells

Stem cells are unspecialised cells, which can turn into tissue-specific cells under certain physiological and experimental conditions. In some organs, such as bone marrow, stem cells regularly divide to replace damaged or old cells, whereas in other organs this process is rare or much slower. There are three main types of stem cells: adult stem cells, embryonic (or pluripotent) and induced pluripotent stem cells, which are reprogrammed adult cells first prepared in 2006.

Stem cells have been very important for the development of regenerative medicine, and in particular for tissue engineering. Stem cell differentiation is a complex and tightly controlled process, which is still not well understood. Among other things, studies have shown that the presence of various interfaces can impact differentiation pathways. For example, when human mesenchymal stem cells hMSC (derived from mesenchymal embryo tissue) are differentiated in the presence of surfaces that contain linear nanopatterns, the differentiation into neurocytes (nervous system building blocks) depends on the spacing within the pattern (Kim et al., 2013).

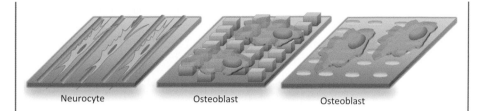

Neurocyte   Osteoblast   Osteoblast

hMSC can respond both to the type (post vs pits) and density of the nanopatterns as shown here in the case of osteoblast growth (Ahm et al., 2014). Osteoblasts are large cells responsible for mineralisation of the bones, and nanopatterning has been extensively explored as a way to induce the differentiation into bone cells during bone tissue engineering.

Nanofibres are often obtained using the process of electrospinning, which uses the electric field to shoot the liquid polymer out of a needle. In such a way polymer fibres can be produced that can range in scale from a few tens of nanometres to micrometres. Synthetic polymers such as polyglycolic (PGA) and poly L-lactic acid (PLLA) (PGA and polylactic acid are shown in Research Report 2.4) are commonly used for electrospinning, but for tissue engineering biocompatible polymers such as collagen, gelatin, silk and chitosan are preferred. However, protein-based polymers such as collagen and silk can be damaged during the fibre-preparation processes which often require increased temperature or use of electric fields. One of the solutions to overcome this challenge is to use the hybrids of synthetic and biopolymers, which can additionally be enhanced with nanoparticles.

Nanoparticles are used in tissue engineering to enhance the mechanical properties of the scaffold, impact the proliferation or differentiation of cells, or be used as carriers of regulatory components both for the cells or extracellular matrix (Figure 9.10). **Metallic nanoparticles** such as gold and silver are mainly explored as scaffold enhancers and therapeutic agents. The hyperthermia effect (Back to Basics 9.7), during which pulsed laser light can be used to generate heat in the presence of gold nanoparticles, can be used to **modulate muscle movement** (Gentemann et al., 2017) and nerve cells communication, while the **antibacterial activity** of nanoparticles is often employed in wound-healing applications. Chronic and burnt wounds can easily get infected, and a high incidence of antibiotic-resistant microorganisms requires the use of new strategies to deal with severe post-graft infections. This can be achieved by the design of wound-healing tissue, which contains embedded nanoparticles such as silver that can act as a nano-based antibiotic (Research Report 9.1) or semiconducting nanoparticles, which can produce cell-damaging reactive oxygen species (see Research Report 2.1). Nanoparticles that can be affected by external stimuli such as magnetic nanoparticles can be used to direct the growth of the cell or control the release and delivery of particular growth factors (Yuan et al., 2018).

Figure 9.10

Nanoparticles in tissue engineering. (a) Surface modified nanoparticles can be used to improve mechanical properties and act as cell anchors. Nanoparticles can also be used (b) to direct the differentiation of stem cells or (c) to deliver cell or tissue altering biomolecules to cell-seeded scaffolds.

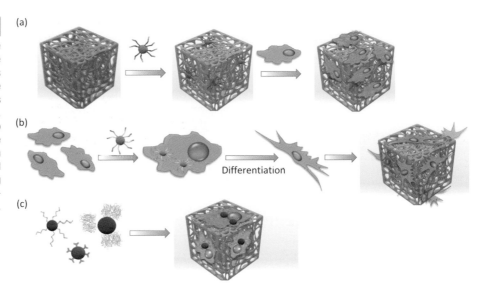

In terms of tissue engineering, the biggest advances have been made in the engineering of bone (Back to Basics 9.9) and dental tissue, partially due to the application of nanoparticle composites such as porous bioactive glass nanoceramics (see Chapter 2). The main components of bioactive glass nanoparticles are silicon dioxide (SiO_2), calcium oxide (CaO) and phosphorus pentoxide (P_2O_5), all of which are found within the native bone tissue, and therefore well-tolerated by the body once they are implanted.

Back to Basics 9.9   Bone Engineering

Bone tissue is a complex hard tissue composed of two distinct parts, a compact shell called cortical bone and a porous core spongiosa. Both are made of **osteon units** that contain **osteocytes** (*osteo* is Greek for 'bone' and osteocytes are bone cells), **collagen fibres** and **calcium phosphate (hydroxyapatite) crystals**.

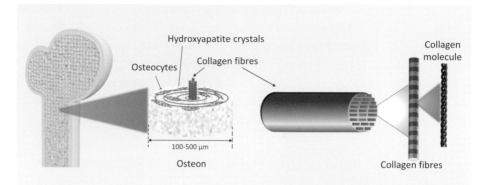

The collagen fibrils are characterised by 67 nm periodicity and 40 nm gaps between collagen molecules filled by hydroxyapatite crystals, which increase bone rigidity. The extracellular matrix of the bone is organised hierarchically and spans several orders of magnitude ranging from nanometre to centimetre.

The engineering of the bone tissue requires mechanically stable scaffold material which can support the growth of blood vessels and differentiation of cells. Osteogenic stem cells are seeded within the scaffold and require particular physical and biochemical factors to afford mature osteocytes. Depending on the type of bone replacement strategy, the scaffold material can be either injectable or rigid. It is usually made of biopolymers (collagen, silk, chitosan) mechanically enhanced with bioactive glass or carbon nanomaterials, and it can either be assembled or patterned in such a way to provide both the nanoscale and microscale features necessary for bone growth. Growth factors such as bone morphogenetic proteins (BMPs) are incorporated within the scaffold together with vascularisation factors to enable the formation of blood vessels to supply the tissue with nutrients.

One of the major issues in tissue engineering is the **regrowth of blood vessels** or **vascularisation** to ensure a continuous supply of nutrients. Such a process requires a cocktail of growth factors which need to be delivered in particular concentrations and at specific sites. Nanoparticles, such as polymeric nanoparticles, which can be prepared in such a way to enable a continuous release of molecules over time, are particularly well-suited for delivery of the growth factors and other regulatory proteins. But one of the most widely applied classes in tissue engineering is the family of **carbon nanomaterials**. Graphene, carbon nanotubes and even carbon nanodiamonds have been used both in the design of scaffolds and for delivery of bioactive molecules. The advantages of carbon nanomaterials lie in their thermal and electrical conductivity, mechanical strength and low toxicity, which has proved useful for engineering of muscle, nerve and bone tissue. Carbon nanotubes are similar to branched extensions of neurons and due to their electrochemical properties, have been used for neuroregeneration, regrowth and repair of nerve tissue (see Research Report 2.2). The versatility of nanoparticle classes has prompted the development of nanocomposite hydrogels, porous and water-loving materials that can act both as scaffolds and drug delivery platforms.

9.5.3 Nanocomposite Hydrogels in Tissue Engineering

Hydrogels are three-dimensional polymer networks with high water-binding capacity and porous structures that can accommodate cells, which are excellent scaffolds for tissue engineering (see Back to Basics 2.5). They can be made from biopolymers such as peptides (Back to Basics 9.10), DNA (see Research Report 6.2) and protein-based polymers (collagen, gelatin), man-made polymers, or combinations. The three-dimensional network is achieved by physical cross-linking such as ion chelating, or strong covalent cross-linking of smaller elements known as **hydrogelators**. The number and the strength of interactions between hydrogelators determine the mechanical properties, and hydrogels can be designed in such a way to be controlled by external stimuli such as pH, temperature or light.

Back to Basics 9.10   Peptide Hydrogels

Different classes of peptides have been used to design **peptide hydrogels** for applications in engineering of tissues such as bone, cartilage and the central nervous system. One of the biggest advantages of peptide hydrogelators is the sheer number of functional groups and moieties that can easily be added to the core peptide structures through chemical modification. In addition, many peptide structures can be tuned to respond to external stimuli. For example, one of the first dipeptide hydrogels, which was made of leucine and aspartate, was shown to be **thermoreversible**. This meant that it could cycle between the liquid and soft solid state using a change in temperature. Thermoreversible hydrogels are particularly suitable for loading for small molecules, which can be added in a liquid phase and then solidified into a gel state on demand. Formation of dipeptide hydrogels usually proceeds in several stages; smaller structures are formed first, followed by self-assembly into amyloid fibres, which ultimately gel at higher concentration in aqueous solutions.

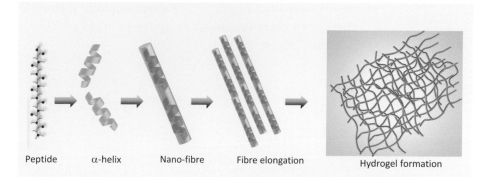

Peptide   α-helix   Nano-fibre   Fibre elongation   Hydrogel formation

The control over hydrogel properties can be achieved by the careful design of hydrogelators, which can be assembled or disassembled using various external stimuli. This is particularly useful for the preparation of on-demand drug delivery systems or adaptable biological implants. Besides temperature and pH-sensitive hydrogels, peptides can be used to make hydrogels sensitive to chemical actuators such as small molecules or metal ions, light and enzymes that cleave or add functional groups to the hydro-gelator backbone.

Light actuation of hydrogel properties has been achieved by either binding or cleavage of functional groups under irradiation, but such processes are not reversible, and once formed, hydrogels cannot cycle between liquid and solid states. This can be overcome by the use of molecules such as azobenzene, which undergo a conformational change and can cycle between cis–trans isomers under irradiation. Such a change in conformation induces a change in the relative position of benzene rings, which affects the π–π stacking between the azobenzene and peptide backbone resulting in a less solid gel containing cis- and more solid gel trans-azobenzene (Huang et al., 2011).

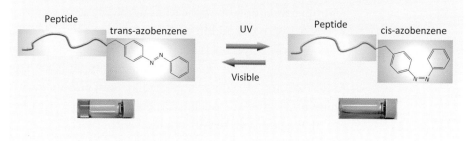

Peptide   trans-azobenzene   UV   Peptide   cis-azobenzene
                                           Visible

Due to the large water content, hydrogels are brittle and weak when dehydrated, so that their handling and application in medicine is limited. Most hydrogels lack mechanical strength and electrical conductivity, which can be overcome by the use of **nanocomposite hydrogels** prepared either by physical or chemical cross-linking (or both) of organic polymers with nano-materials (Figure 9.11).

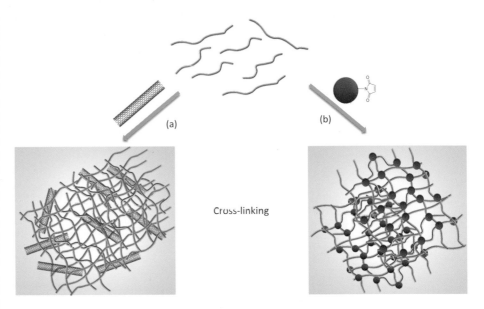

Nanocomposite hydrogels. Hybrid hydrogels can be made by cross-linking of nanomaterials with polymers. Cross-linking is achieved either by (a) physical cross-linking by employing weak interactions (electrostatic, hydrogen bonding, π–π stacking) or (b) chemical cross-linking by the formation of strong bonds through a range of chemical reactions (shown is maleimide nanoparticle, which can interact with thiol-containing polymers).

The resulting hydrogels combine the properties of polymers (elasticity, hydrophilicity and porous structure) and nanomaterials (mechanical stability, large surface area, conductivity, light sensitivity), and can be used to obtain smart materials which can self-heal and be attenuated by external stimuli.

Stimuli-responsive hydrogels are particularly useful for tissue engineering and wound healing because they undergo changes that can be induced by heating, irradiation or application of magnetic or electric force, or in the case of DNA hydrogels addition of a particular DNA strand. Thermoresponsive nanocomposite hydrogels are often made in such a way that they can undergo reversible changes in properties. For example, they can transition from a liquid (sol) to gel state at a particular temperature such as the physiological temperature of 37 °C. Such hydrogels can be used for the design of injectable gels that solidify when in contact with the body, or for drug release by temperature-induced expansion. Magnetoresponsive hydrogels with embedded magnetic nanoparticles are particularly interesting as they respond to the external magnetic field, and in this way can be used in the design of structures that exhibit controlled motility, which is the property of soft robots (Research Report 9.5).

Research Report 9.5	Magnetically Responsive Hydrogels for Tissue Engineering and Soft Robot Design

Biological tissue is characterised by a high level of heterogeneity and exhibits different physiochemical properties across the range of scales (such materials are referred to as anisotropic). One of the biggest challenges in tissue engineering is to develop strategies that can introduce this heterogeneity into designed materials. Different strategies have been demonstrated based on printing different layers of hydrogels, or the use of photolithography and light-triggered cross-linking to obtained areas that differ in mechanical properties. But one of the most interesting routes is to employ an external magnetic field and use magnetic nanoparticles to create patterns within the gels.

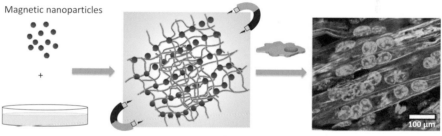

Magnetic nanoparticles

+

Methacryloyl gelatin

100 μm

Source: Tognato et al. (2018), by permission of John Wiley and Sons.

In one such example, researchers from AO Research Institute in Davos designed anisotropic hydrogel using methacryloyl gelatin, which is a widely used hydrogelator and results in thermoresponsive and biocompatible hydrogels. In a first step 45–60 nm spherical iron oxide nanoparticles were prepared and mixed with the liquid hydrogelator. The nanocomposite liquid was then exposed to the magnetic field to align nanoparticles into filaments after which the gel was cross-linked using UV light. The size and length of the magnetic filaments were controlled by the application of a magnetic field to obtain patterns suitable for the growth and differentiation of stem cells. This was demonstrated by the use of human mesenchymal stem cells (hMSC) which were seeded onto gels and shown to orient themselves in the direction of the filaments.

In addition to being useful for tissue engineering, the magnetically responsive hydrogel was also employed to design a soft robotic system in the shape of a starfish, whose motility could be controlled by the application of the external magnetic field (Tognato et al., 2018).

Natural polymers such as collagen, gelatin and chitosan have all been used in combination with physically or chemically cross-linked nanoparticles to make stimuli-responsive nanocomposites with enhanced mechanical stability and increased resistance to enzymatic degradation. The latter can be useful for the design of materials with a long shelf life, or those that need to persist in the body over long periods.

One of the biggest challenges in tissue engineering is mimicking the heterogeneous structure of the natural extracellular matrix, which is characterised by physical and chemical gradients. This challenge can be addressed by the use of stimuli-guided gelation of nanocomposites, for example, induced by light, to enable temporal and spatial control over the strength and position of strong and weak cross-links.

Another challenge is the printing of the hydrogel material in three-dimensional geometries, which not only requires the design of stable materials, but also a combination of techniques. Besides, high-resolution imaging is needed to provide a detailed structure of the tissue, and the advanced spectroscopic techniques to obtain data on molecular components. Once this information is known, deep learning algorithms can be employed to provide the best protocol for 3D assembly of nanocomposite scaffolds suitable for cell seeding and growth.

However, all of these strategies for making the most suitable scaffolds cannot be used for the design of clinically relevant engineered tissues without having a clear picture of toxicological effects of embedded nanomaterials and their interactions with cells, and overall impact of tissue health. Such studies are important aspects of **nanotoxicology**, a field that has steadily grown over the last three decades, and has been important for shaping the policies related to the regulation of manufacturing and applications of engineered nanomaterials.

9.6   Nanotoxicity and Environmental Impact of Nanomaterials

Engineered nanomaterials are increasingly being used not only in medicine but also in various consumer goods such as TV screens, cars and clothing items, to name a few. In 2014, around 2000 nanotechnology-based consumer goods were commercially available in over 20 countries (Vance et al., 2015) and this number continues to grow. As they become increasingly important for the design of biomedical devices and the formulation of new drugs and used in everyday consumer products, it is important to asses and regulate the risk associated with their manufacturing and use. There are several agencies around the world, most notably the European Chemicals Agency (ECHA) in the EU and the US Food and Drug Administration, that have taken the lead both in terms of classification and regulation of known and emerging nanomaterials. That said, there is still plenty of work to be done, as preparation and characterisation protocols used are as diverse as the nanomaterials made, which makes the field of nanotechnology difficult to regulate. Both the FDA and ECHA have been working to identify the sources of nanomaterials, classify the products that use them and estimate their environmental impact.

Although there is no single template available, there are two main stages in the assessment of the risk associated with engineered nanomaterials. First, the hazards associated with a particular material need to be identified and second, the risks associated with that hazard need to be analysed. The most challenging step is the identification of potential risks, and this is the main role of nanotoxicology, a field closely linked to nanomedicine.

When we discussed the use of nanomaterials in drug delivery, we mentioned that we still do not know how to rationally design nanomaterials in such a way to control their cell uptake. But we know that there are several aspects of nanomaterials that have to be taken into account when designing materials suitable for biomedical use, such as size and shape, surface charge and composition, mechanical properties and affinity to the formation of aggregates (Figure 9.12).

Figure 9.12

Properties that need to be taken into account during the toxicological profiling of nanomaterials.

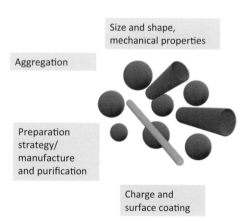

Size and shape, mechanical properties

Aggregation

Preparation strategy/ manufacture and purification

Charge and surface coating

Besides, the information on the manufacturing protocol and purification steps is important to obtain a complete toxicological profile. For example, toxic chemicals used during the synthesis of nanomaterials might end up in the final product. Some studies have shown that the observed toxicity of carbon nanotubes stems from the trace metal catalyst that remains embedded within the structure after the synthesis (see Chapter 2 for more on carbon nanotube synthesis).

In general, risk assessments help us not only to understand the potential hazards associated with the materials but can also guide the choice of recycling and disposal strategies. Some preliminary toxicological predictions can be based on physiochemical properties alone. For example, nanomaterials that produce oxidising species in aqueous solutions such as copper nanoparticles will be more toxic to certain cells or organisms than inert gold nanoparticles. However, the risk assessment is not complete without the data on the physicochemical properties of the nanomaterials and their interaction with biological systems, which are obtained from in vitro studies using 2D or 3D cell cultures followed by animal studies (Figure 9.13). Most common nanotoxicity studies are done by exploring the dose–response in in vitro models after the assessment of physicochemical properties and stability (Research Report 9.6).

Figure 9.13

Workflow for assessment of nanomaterial toxicity. Physiochemical properties of nanomaterials are first characterised and then followed by in vitro and in vivo studies using animal models. Efforts are made to design organ-on-chip to obtain biologically relevant data and eradicate, or at least minimise, the use of animal models. Organ-on-chip image courtesy of Dr Roisin Owens, University of Cambridge.

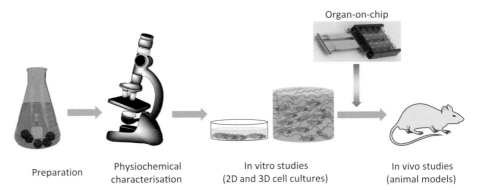

Organ-on-chip

Preparation | Physiochemical characterisation | In vitro studies (2D and 3D cell cultures) | In vivo studies (animal models)

Research Report 9.6   Exploration of the Cellular Toxicity of Nanomaterials

After they reach the cell, nanoparticles can induce oxidative stress or organelle injury and enhance immunological response by stimulating secretion of cytokines that activate immune system cells.

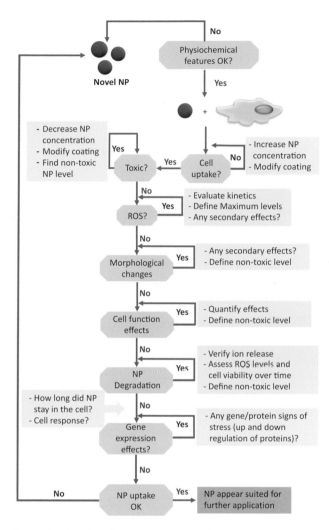

Source: Reprinted from Soenen et al. (2011), with permission from Elsevier.

The most commonly used protocol for assessment of nanomaterial toxicity is the viability study of cells exposed to different doses of nanomaterial in cell cultures. However, cell death is the ultimate effect of many disrupted pathways, and physical and chemical damages introduced by the presence of nanomaterials within or on the surface of the cell. To understand the nanomaterial toxicology, it is important to assess those changes by careful design of in vitro studies.

Proper in vitro evaluation needs to include relevant **tissue types**, and preferably an unmodified cell line, take into account the possible

interference of nanoparticles with the commercial cell assays and include the evaluation of physiologically **relevant amounts** (Krug, 2014). It should also include studies in the presence of serum proteins, which mimic biological fluids.

Soenen and colleagues (2011) proposed the in vitro workflow to ease the cell toxicity studies of novel nanomaterials, which introduces a more systematic approach that could provide useful information over a range of nanoparticles. This workflow takes into account not only the cell viability (death of the cell) but also the production of reactive oxygen species (ROS), morphological changes within cells, effects of nanoparticle degradation and changes in gene expression, which impact the protein levels (Soenen et al., 2011).

However, toxicity data obtained using 2D cultures often do not translate in vivo. This can be overcome by the use of more complex 3D models such as organoids and organ-on-chip devices. Besides studying their uptake into cells and impact on the overall health of a particular tissue, the effects of long-term accumulation need to be taken into account and these require the design of complex studies that allow monitoring over time.

The biggest obstacle to assessing nanomaterial toxicology is the **lack of standardised protocols**. Often a particular type of nanomaterial is explored using one cell line and looking at the limited number of parameters leading to an incomplete picture of toxicological profile. Another persistent issue is the use of concentration values that do not always reflect the nature of nanomaterials and their active surface area which might differ significantly between different nanomaterial classes, despite them having the same mass/volume concentration. Researchers from the Swiss Federal Institute for Materials Science and Technology proposed **data quality management for engineered nanomaterials** to be implemented after some toxicological data are obtained (Figure 9.14).

They distinguish between an approximate risk assessment when few or contrasting toxicological data are available, and comprehensive risk assessment when enough data have been gathered to make a decision (Som et al., 2013). Such a decision-making process can significantly ease the early development of nanomaterials, and identify those that either have a detrimental effect on the environment or require some investment to minimise such an effect in the early phase of development, for example, through modification of the preparation strategies.

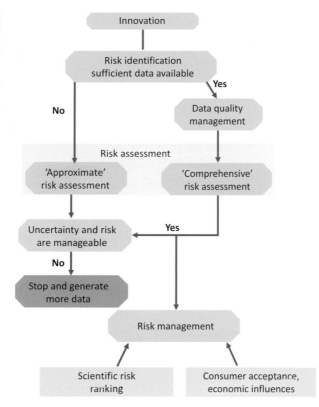

Figure 9.14

Data quality management workflow for engineered materials. Adapted with permission from Som et al. (2013). © 2013 American Chemical Society.

Key Concepts

Biological barrier: a physical barrier that can effectively sort out circulating molecular species, particles or whole cells into those to be eliminated and those to be used. Such are blood vessels, epithelial layers in intestines, blood–brain barrier and cell membranes.

Cell culture: a process by which cells of interest are grown under controlled conditions and in an artificial environment. Two- and three-dimensional cancer cell cultures are particularly useful to study different therapeutic nanomaterials and drug formulations.

Endocytosis: trafficking mechanism across the cell membrane which involves the formation of membrane buds or vacuoles inside the cells.

EPR effect: enhance permeation and retention effect characterised by physiological changes which result in enhanced permeability of blood vessels in infected or cancerous tissue.

Extracellular matrix: a heterogeneous structure unique to each tissue, which contains several physical, biochemical and biomechanical components that create a healthy environment for cell proliferation and communication.

Ligand-mediated cell targeting: active targeting of cells, which involves the design of ligands that bind or interact with cell-specific biomolecules.

Nanocarriers: nanosized structures with either embedded or immobilised therapeutic cargo, which aid its delivery to the target cells.

Nanocomposite hydrogels: hydrogels that contain a polymer component and engineered nanomaterials which enhance the mechanical stability, provide anchoring points for cell attachment or carry biomolecules needed for cell growth and proliferation. The ultimate goal is to use nanomaterials that can respond to external or internal cues and act as stimuli-responsive and self-healing materials similar to those found in biological systems.

Nanotoxicology: research field concerned with the study of the toxicity of nanomaterials and the design of proper protocols and risk assessments for engineered nanomaterials.

Protein corona: a layer of proteins such as serum albumin formed around a nanoparticle in blood.

Theranostic nanomaterials: nanosized materials that couple diagnostics and therapy. They can be used both as probes that detect the presence of a target cell and also as therapeutic agents, which either deliver a drug cargo or cause induced damage due to their intrinsic properties. Such is hyperthermia induced by nanoparticles that can be activated by light, acoustic waves or magnetic field.

Tissue engineering: design of tissue scaffolds seeded with cells and various biomolecular components to be used for replacement or regrowth of damaged or diseased tissue.

Problems

9.1   How can nanocarriers aid the uptake of drugs into the body?

9.2   What are the strategies to improve the stealth of nanocarriers and make them invisible to the immune system?

9.3   Name two strategies to load a nanocarrier with a drug cargo.

9.4   Chemotherapeutic drug doxorubicin was encapsulated within liposomes to improve the treatment of breast cancer.
   (a) How many 10 nm liposomes would it take to deliver the medicine contained in a single pill of a drug? The density of a typical drug is $1250 \ kg \, m^{-3}$.

(b) Doxorubicin is not soluble in water. Where would you expect most of the doxorubicin to be found within the liposome and why?

(c) Discuss the potential routes by which the drug could be released once it reaches the cell.

9.5 Describe how gold nanoparticles and gold nanorods can be used for the design of theranostic materials. Which other materials can be used for theranostics?

9.6 What is the most likely cell uptake mechanism for positively charged, 80 nm spheric silica nanoparticles?

9.7 Hydrogels are excellent materials for tissue engineering. What are their advantages compared to other materials? Name at least three strategies that can be used to embed silver nanoparticles within the chitosan-based hydrogel, and name functional groups (if any) that need to be introduced to the hydrogel backbone.

9.8 Folate receptor (FR) is a cysteine-rich glycoprotein with a specific binding pocket for folic acid (scheme below), and it is often used as a cancer biomarker. In one application, silver-coated magnetic nanoparticles (Ag@MNPs, 30 nm) with attached folic acid are used for the detection and removal of lung cancer cells.

(a) Describe one covalent and one non-covalent method, and draw appropriate structures, for the attachment of the folic acid to the surface of the Ag@MNP surface. The structure of folic acid with the marked protein-binding region is shown below.

Protein-binding region

(b) Describe two analytical methods which can be used to prove that nanoparticles bind to lung cancer cells, clearly stating the instrumental requirements and advantages and disadvantages of each method.

(c) Name two ligands other than folic acid which could be coated onto magnetic nanoparticle to ensure the specific binding to the folate receptor. State briefly which strategy you could use to attach them onto the nanoparticle surface.

(d) Which control experiments are needed to ensure that folic acid binds specifically to lung cancer cells?

9.9 Iron oxide nanoparticles coated with cancer-targeting ligands can act as theranostic systems. Explain the principle of magnetic nanoparticle theranostics clearly describing the experimental set-up required for theranostic treatment of patients. What happens to the nanoparticles once the treatment is completed?

9.10 One of the biggest threats to public health is the emergence of antibiotic-resistant bacteria such as methicillin-resistant *S. aureus* (MRSA) strain in hospitals. Detection of such bacteria is usually done by colony growth and cell counting, or genome sequencing, both of which take days to complete.

(a) Describe how you would remove antibiotic-resistant MRSA from the surface of the surgery tables using a nanomaterial-based strategy.

(b) Discuss the classes of nanomaterials which can be used, modifications (if any) which are required as well as the advantages and disadvantages of nanomaterial-based antibiotics.

9.11 Mesoporous silica nanoparticles (mSiO$_2$ NPs) can be used to deliver chemotherapeutic drug Taxol selectively to pancreatic cancer cells.

(a) How can loaded and coated NPs be protected from the removal by macrophages on their route to cancer tissue?

(b) Which analytical method(s) can be used to study internalisation of mSiO$_2$ and drug release?

(c) Name at least one route for clinical administration of mSiO$_2$ NPs to cancer patients. Discuss the advantages and disadvantages of the proposed route clearly stating the biological barriers that need to be overcome to reach cancer tissue.

9.12 Design a simple workflow for the quick assessment of the toxicity of a new type of carbon nanotube.

Further Reading

Drug Delivery and Nanotherapeutics

Behzadi, S., Serpooshan, V., Tao, W., et al. (2017). Cellular uptake of nanoparticles; journey inside the cell. *Chemical Society Reviews*, **46**(14), 4218–4244.

Gao, W., Thamphiwatana, S., Angsantikul, P. and Zhang, L. (2014). Nanoparticle approaches against bacterial infections. *Wiley Interdisciplinary Reviews in Nanomedicine and Nanobiotechnology*, **6**(6), 532–547.

Golombek, S. K., May, J-N, Theek, B., et al. (2018). Tumour targeting via EPR: strategies to enhance patient responses. *Advanced Drug Delivery Review*, **130**, 17–38.

Jain, A., Singh, S. K., Arya, S. K., Kundu, S. C. and Kapoor, S. (2018). Protein nanoparticles; promising platforms for drug delivery applications. *ACS Biomaterials Science and Engineering*, **4**(12), 3939–3916.

Mendes, L. P., Pan, J. and Torchilin, V. P. (2017). Dendrimers as nanocarriers for nucleic acids and drug delivery in cancer therapy. *Molecules*, **22**, 1401–1422.

Paranjpe, M. and Müller-Goymann, C. C. (2014). Nanoparticle-mediated pulmonary drug delivery: a review. *International Journal of Molecular Sciences*, **15**, 5852–5873.

Ventola, C. L. (2017). Progress in nanomedicine: approved and investigational nanodrugs. *Pharmacy and Therapeutics*, **42**(12), 741–755.

Tissue Engineering

Motealleh, A. and Kehr, N. S. (2016). Nanocomposite hydrogels and their applications in tissue engineering. *Advanced Healthcare Materials*, **6**, 1600938.

Shi, Q., Liu, H., Tang, D., et al. (2019). Bioactuators based on stimulus-responsive hydrogels and their emerging biomedical applications. *NPG Asia Materials*, **11**, 64.

Tan, H-L., Teow, S-Y. and Pushpamalar, J. (2019). Application of metal nanoparticle-hydrogel composites in tissue regeneration. *Bioengineering*, **6**(1), 17.

Nanotoxicology

Francis, A. P. and Devasena, T. (2018). Toxicity of carbon nanotubes: a review. *Toxicology and Industrial Health*, **34**(3), 200–210.

Nel, A. E., Xia, T., Meng, H., et al. (2013). Nanomaterial toxicity testing in 21st century: use of a predictive toxicological approach and high through-put screening. *Account of Chemical Research*, **46**, 607–721.

Nowack, B., Müller, N., Krug, H. F. and Wick, P. (2014). How to consider engineered nanomaterials in major accident regulations? *Environmental Science Europe*, **26**, 2.

Yildirimer, L., Thanh, N. T. K., Loizidou, M. and Seifalian, A. M. (2011). Toxicological considerations of clinically applicable nanoparticles. *Nano Today*, **6**, 585–607.

References

Ahm, E. H., Kim, Y., Kshitiz, et al. (2014). Spatial control of adult stem cell fate using nanotopographic cues. *Biomaterials*, **35**, 2401–2410.

Bartesaghi, A., Merk, A., Borgnia, M. J., Milne, J. L. S. and Subramaniam, S. (2013). Pre-fusion structure of trimeric HIV-1 envelope glycoprotein deter-mined by cryo-electron microscopy. *Nature Structural Molecular Biology*, **20**, 1352–1357.

Batra, J., Robinson, J., Soares, A. S., et al. (2012). Matrix metalloproteinase-10 (MMP-10) interaction with tissue inhibitors of metalloproteinases TIMP-1 and TIMP-2: binding studies and crystal structure. *Journal of Biological Chemistry*, **287**, 15935–15946.

Bertrand, N., Wu, J., Xu, X., Kamaly, N. and Farokhzad, O. C. (2014). Cancer nanotechnology: the impact of passive and active targeting in the era of modern cancer biology. *Advanced Drug Delivery Reviews*, **66**, 2–25.

Blanco, E., Shen, H. and Ferrari, M. (2012). Principles of nanoparticle design for overcoming biological barriers to drug delivery. *Nature Biotechnology*, **33**(9), 941–951.

Chang, B-M., Pan, L., Lin, H-H. and Chang, H-C. (2019). Nanodiamond-supported silver nanoparticles as potent and safe antibacterial agents. *Scientific Reports*, **9**, 13164.

Drost, J. and Clevers, H. (2018). Organoids in cancer research. *Nature Reviews Cancer*, **18**, 407–418.

Estelrich, J., Sanchez-Martin, M. J. and Busquets, M. A. (2015). Nanoparti-cles in magnetic resonance imaging: from simple to dual contrast agents. *International Journal of Nanomedicine*, **10**, 1727–1741.

Gaenger, S. and Schindowski, K. (2018). Tailoring formulations for intrana-sal nose-to-brain delivery: a review on architecture, physiochemical charac-teristics and mucociliary clearance of the nasal olfactory mucosa. *Pharmaceutics*, **10**(3), 116.

Gentemann, L., Kalies, S., Coffee, M., et al. (2017). Modulation of cardio-myocytes using pulsed laser irradiated gold nanoparticles. *Biomedical Optics Express*, **8**, 177–192.

Griffith, D. L., Keck, P. C., Sampath, T. K., Rueger, D. C. and Carlson, W. D. (1996). Three-dimensional structure of recombinant human osteo-genic protein 1: a structural paradigm for the transforming growth factor-beta superfamily. *Proceedings of the National Academy of Sciences of the USA*, **93**, 878–883.

Grover, V. P., Tognarelli, J. M., Crossey, M. M., et al. (2015). Magnetic resonance imaging: principles and techniques: lessons for clinicians. *Journal of Clinical and Experimental Hepatology*, **5**, 246–255.

Huang, X. and El-Sayed, M. A. (2010). Gold nanoparticles: optical properties and implementations in cancer diagnosis and photothermal therapy. *Journal of Advanced Research*, **1**, 13–28.

Huang, Y., Qiu, Z., Xu, Y., et al. (2011). Supramolecular hydrogels based on short peptides linked with a conformational switch. *Organic and Biomolecular Chemistry*, **9**, 2149–2155.

Iozzo, R. V. and Schaaefer, L. (2015). Proteoglycan form and function: a comprehensive nomenclature of proteoglycans. *Matrix Biology*, **42**, 11–55.

Junghanns, J-U. A. H. and Müller, R. H. (2008). Nanocrystal technology, drug delivery, and clinical applications. *International Journal of Nanomedicine*, **3**(3), 295–310.

Kapalczynska, M., Kolenda, T., Przybyla, W., et al. (2018). 2D and 3D cell cultures: a comparison of different types of cancer cell cultures. *Archives of Medical Science*, **14**(4), 910–919.

Kim, J., Kim, H. N., Lim, K-T., et al. (2013). Designing nanotopographical density of extracellular matrix for controlled morphology and function of human mesenchymal stem cells. *Scientific Reports*, **3**, 3552.

Krug, H. F. (2014). Nanosafety research: are we on the right track? *Angewandte Chemie International Edition*, **53**, 12304–12319.

Lee, J-H., Huh, Y-M., Jun, Y-W., et al. (2007). Artificially engineered magnetic nanoparticles for ultra-sensitive molecular imaging. *Nature Medicine*, **13**, 95–99.

Lonhienne, T. G. A., Sagulenko, E., Webb, R. I., et al. (2010). Endocytosis-like protein uptake in the bacterium *Gemmata obscuriglobus*. *Proceedings of the National Academy of Sciences of the USA*, **107**(29), 12883–12888.

Matsumura, Y. and Maeda, H. A. (1986). A new concept for macromolecular therapeutics in cancer chemotherapy: mechanism of tumour tropic accumulation of proteins and the antitumour agent smancs. *Cancer Research*, **46**, 6387–6392.

Mi, L. Z., Brown, C. T, Gao, Y., et al. (2015). Structure of bone morphogenetic protein 9 pro complex. *Proceedings of the National Academy of Sciences of the USA*, **112**, 3710–3715.

Nap, R. J. and Szleifer, I. (2008). Structure and interactions of aggrecans: statistical thermodynamic approach. *Biophysics Journal*, **95**(10), 4570–4583.

Oh, J. Y., Kim, H. S., Palanikumar, L., et al. (2018). Cloaking nanoparticles with protein corona shield for targeted drug delivery. *Nature Communications*, **9**, 4548.

Peer, D., Karp, J. M., Hong, S., et al. (2007). Nanocarriers as an emerging platform for cancer therapy. *Nature Nanotechnology*, **2**, 751–760.

Soenen, S. J., Rivera-Gil, P., Montenegro, J-M., et al. (2011). Cellular toxicity of inorganic nanoparticles: common aspects and guidelines for improved nanotoxicity evaluation. *Nano Today*, **6**, 446–465.

Som, C., Nowack, B. Krug, H. F. and Wick, P. (2013). Toward the development of decision supporting tools that can be used for safe production and use of nanomaterials. *Accounts of Chemical Research*, **46**, 863–872.

Tognato, R., Armiento, A. R., Bonfrate, V., et al. (2018). A stimuli-responsive nanocomposite for 3D anisotropic cell-guidance and magnetic soft robotics. *Advanced Functional Materials*, **29**(9), 1804647.

Vance, M. E., Kuiken, T., Vejerano, E. P., et al. (2015). Nanotechnology in the real world: redeveloping the nanomaterial consumer products inventory. *Beilstein Journal of Nanotechnology*, **6**, 1769–1780.

Wong, A. D., Ye, M., Levy, A. F., et al. (2013). The blood–brain barrier: an engineering perspective. *Frontiers in Neuroengineering*, **6**, 7.

Yuan, M., Wang, Y. and Qin, Y.-X. (2018). Promoting neuroregeneration by applying dynamic magnetic fields to a novel nanomedicine: superparamagnetic iron oxide (SPIO)-gold nanoparticles bounded with nerve growth factor. *Nanomedicine*, **14**, 1337–1347.

Appendix

Three-Dimensional Lattice Types

CUBIC

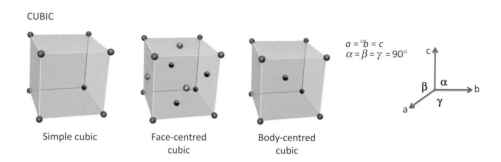

| Simple cubic | Face-centred cubic | Body-centred cubic |

$a = {}^\circ b = c$
$\alpha = \beta = \gamma = 90^\circ$

TETRAGONAL

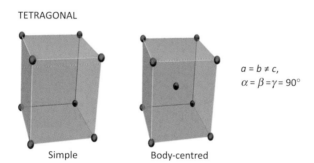

Simple   Body-centred

$a = b \neq c,$
$\alpha = \beta = \gamma = 90^\circ$

ORTHOROMBIC

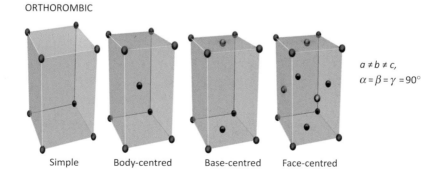

Simple   Body-centred   Base-centred   Face-centred

$a \neq b \neq c,$
$\alpha = \beta = \gamma = 90^\circ$

RHOMBOHEDRAL

HEXAGONAL

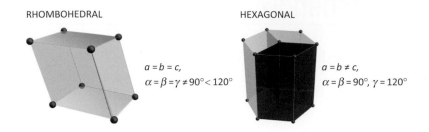

$a = b = c,$
$\alpha = \beta = \gamma \neq 90° < 120°$

$a = b \neq c,$
$\alpha = \beta = 90°, \gamma = 120°$

MONOCLINIC

TRICLINIC

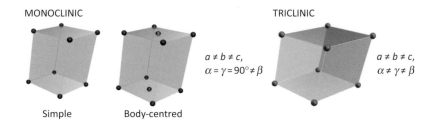

$a \neq b \neq c,$
$\alpha = \gamma = 90° \neq \beta$

$a \neq b \neq c,$
$\alpha \neq \gamma \neq \beta$

Simple   Body-centred

Index

Locators in *italic* refer to figures; those in **bold** to tables